CARDIAC ATHLETES
Real Superheroes
Beating Heart Disease

By

Lars Andrews

Foreword
by

Dr Andre La Gerche

CARDIAC ATHLETES

DEDICATION

This book is dedicated to the memory of the late John Gilmore Hopkins (RIP 1984 aged 47) who indirectly inspired me to start my cardiology career as a trainee cardiac technician all those years ago after hearing of his tragic death caused by a faulty artificial heart valve. John was one of many thousands around the world who had their lives prematurely and cruelly cut short because profit was put before people.

I am a 'people's person' and I am 47 as I type this ...

ACKNOWLEDGEMENTS

I would firstly like to thank a very special person. My career in cardiology and the eventual creation of Cardiac Athletes, the huge growing global support network and the monies being raised to help combat heart disease and even this book would not have happened if I had not had a chance meeting with a certain Sheila Hopkins all those years ago and if Sheila had not shown me her late husband's death certificate. I will always be indebted to Sheila for sowing the seeds of interest in cardiology in my then young mind, for giving me a direction and purpose in life, for all the love and encouragement over the years and for all the wonderful meals and cups of tea whilst I studied for and passed yet another exam. It has not been a waste 'She'. You have helped save others' lives too.

Secondly I would personally like to thank all the loyal members of the Cardiac Athletes forum who got behind the idea for writing a book about their varied cardiac and sporting experiences and to the 17 who were first in sending me their very personal and moving stories. As far as I am aware this is the first book of its kind and somehow I think it won't be the last. I wanted to bring awareness to the general public what great people you all are and to give you another medium in which to reach out and inspire others out there like you, perhaps at a key low turning point in their lives. Together as a team I think we have accomplished this.

I would like to thank Russ Bestley once again for helping me create the CA logo design way back in 1998 and working with me on the early Newsletters.

Finally I would like to personally thank world leading Sports Cardiologist Dr Andre La Gerche for agreeing to write the Foreword to this book and for being interested in Cardiac Athletes. I look forward to reading the scientific advancements made by Dr La Gerche in the coming years.

Thank you all.

CONTENTS

FOREWORD

Exercise represents one of our most powerful therapies in cardiology and yet it is frequently overlooked. There are very few cardiac conditions where exercise restriction is required and, in the overwhelming majority of patients, there is no limit to what can be achieved. For athletes, the diagnosis of a heart condition is unexpected and presents many questions specific to their sports passion: *what exercise can I do? How quickly can I get back into my normal exercise patterns? Is there any restriction on what I can do?* Etc, etc. Perhaps surprisingly for many athletes, they find their health practitioner looking back at them with blank looks: *you were running how far? Why? Are you mad?*

Athletes represent the perfect patient. They are often super-motivated, interested in their health and have an ability to accept their health issues as their own challenge to face. Sometimes the medical profession fail them. The athlete's specific demands for information stretch many health professionals' knowledge leading to frustration of both parties. There is a specific knowledge gap which needs to be filled.

Lars Andrews has had the inspiration to realise this. In 2001 he created the website www.cardiacathletes.com for athletes with cardiac conditions to share experiences and advice. In the modern interconnected age, this provides a forum for athletes from around the world to find others with similar heart conditions, experiences and goals. Thus, cardiacathletes.com represents a "support forum" which empowers people to both seek and provide advice whilst also allowing the freedom to make informed decisions about how appropriate any advice may be. Lars Andrews wisely chose to provide a relatively unfiltered format for open discussion rather than a didactic site with professional advice. He provided the ingredients for people to inspire and now his book documents this result.

I remember reading a book by "The Man" Dave Scott, multi-winner of the Hawaii Ironman in the 80's, who said: "don't be afraid to set ambitious goals, but always remember to celebrate every small step along the way". Nothing could be more apt for the athlete who develops a cardiac condition. On the road back from treatment it may seem difficult to know what you can expect and what may be possible. Although there are a few exceptions, exercise is a mainstay therapy of rehabilitation from most cardiac illnesses (heart attacks, cardiac surgery, even heart failure) and the athlete should be encouraged to set ambitious goals. However, the path to achieving those goals may present unique obstacles and challenges.

Exercise regimes may need to be specifically tailored to the constraints of the cardiac condition, medications or devices and goals may need to be repeatedly adjusted. This does not diminish the elation gained from exceeding expectations. For all but the very best athletes, sports participation is all about proving something to yourself. This is no different for cardiac athletes. In addition, cardiac athletes have the ability to inspire others, cardiac patients and the general community alike, who can instantly recognise the additional dedication and discipline required to push on when so many would sit down and switch on the TV. There are now numerous heart transplant recipients who have competed in marathons and triathlons proving that a new lease of life can be used as an opportunity to inspire others.

One of the great challenges for athletes can be to find the professional medical advice to manage the unique hurdles presented by their cardiac condition as they pursue their athletic passion. My experience is that there are relatively few cardiologists with a specific interest in the assessment and management of athletes. There are few exercise rehabilitation programs which cater for athletes with cardiac conditions and the unfortunate athlete who has suffered a heart attack, for example, can receive varied advice on when and how to re-start a structured exercise program.

www.cardiacathletes.com represents a really positive response to this health provision gap. If there are insufficient services to meet the athlete's specific needs then athletes will have the motivation to seek the necessary advice. I strongly support this initiative but would also encourage athletes to point out their failed expectations in health provisions so that we doctors and allied health professionals can try and do something about it.

My personal experience is that there are few things more rewarding than helping someone get back across the finish line.

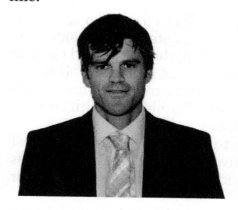

Dr. André La Gerche MBBS, PhD, FRACP, FCSANZ, FESC
Clinical Cardiologist - St Vincent's Hospital Melbourne, Australia
Cardiac Investigation Unit | 41 Victoria Parade, Fitzroy 3065 | www.svhm.org.au
T: +613 9288 4423   F: +613 9288 4422   andre.lagerche@svhm.org.au

Hamilton Fairley Research Scholar – University of Melbourne, Australia
St Vincent's Department of Medicine | 29 Regent Street, Fitzroy 3065 |
www.unimelb.edu.au

Visiting Professor - University of Leuven, Belgium
UZ Leuven | campus Gasthuisberg | Herestraat 49 | B - 3000 Leuven | www.uzleuven.be

PREFACE

Why has this book been created ?

This book has many potential audiences. It is for anyone recently diagnosed with a heart condition. It is for the person who has just gone through a cardiac procedure or surgery. It is for the doctors, nurses and allied health staff treating such people. It is for everyone and anyone interested in maintaining a good level of health and fitness. It is for anyone seeking inspiration. It is for anyone with a heart.

In this book I will not simply tell you a story or serve you a plate full of facts. I will ask you to stop and consider key points. I will ask you questions along the way. I and Cardiac Athletes need your help. There is a lot still to do. If whilst reading something within these pages you think to yourself "I know the answer to that ! " or " I could help with that ! ", then please get in contact with me.

The 17 case stories set out in this book offer the widest insight into the various relatively common heart conditions and how they impact an individual's life and the lives of their nearest and dearest.

Their stories are extremely important to hear and digest. There has to be a mass attitudinal change towards people who have recorded medical conditions be they cardiac or some other part of the body especially if that person is taking part in sports that you yourself would be unable to complete with your ' normal, healthy, average fitness '. Why should this person be discriminated against, labelled, stigmatized and infringed in other areas of their lives ? Does a medical condition define someone ? What if this person with a recorded cardiac condition finishes full Ironman Competitions and within a respectable finishing time ? Do you focus on the negative (the heart condition) or do you focus on the positive thing about that person (their true grit and mental will) ? As we all live longer more and more of us will have one medical condition or another.

There is a revolution happening now. It started many years ago but no-one was keeping record and no-one was particularly interested, but I am. We are seeing more and more people with missing limbs, with replacement prostheses taking part in competitive sports.

The 2012 Paralympics were a huge success because now these individuals are respected as true competitive athletes in their own right rather than being seen as the ... and yes I am going to use the words I heard not that many years ago ... in the early days the Paralympics were watched by many who thought it was just a ' freak show ' ... but now able bodied people tune in to watch the Paralympics seeking motivation and inspiration to lift themselves out of their own malaise and depression. Such athletes as these are guiding lights for the masses. These athletes can have the most noticeable 'handicaps ' and yet once you see them get going ... there is no handicap ... the human mind can overcome more than we realise. One ' disabled ' athlete if televised can be the role model who suddenly ignites a flame of inspiration in many more ' abled ' and ' disabled ' wannabies around the globe who just happen to be watching the event.

I applaud the IOC for taking Paralympians seriously. Also by allowing these incredible individuals to display their prowess at overcoming their physical ' challenges ' we all gain new insights into the science of athletics and sports training and competing.

When we learn the psychology of an athlete who has a 'handicap ' and yet they still bring home the medals ... we can all learn a lot from that individual.

Who am I ?

I don't want to say too much about myself because this book is about the achievements of others but I realise a Preface is where I am supposed to establish my credibility. Briefly then, so that you understand how a set of circumstances can lead to the creation of **Cardiac Athletes**, my story goes like this. Stick with it, it is relevant and is not me stroking my ego but me showing how quirky things in life can link together to create something new. Much of this can be viewed and listened to as a YouTube video on the main CA website **Video Gallery** page here:

http://cardiacathletes.com/1/videos/

My appreciation for anyone trying to overcome a disability began way back in 1980/81 when I broke my own neck whilst playing rugby. I knew nothing of correct diet or recovery and I was over-training. All the warning signs were there in terms of loss of muscle mass, general tiredness, and a growing number of lesser injuries but I ignored them. Luckily I had only temporary paralysis but needed surgery to re-attach my head and neck to my shoulders. A Mr Brian Elliott, Consultant Orthopaedic Surgeon performed the Cloward procedure (surgery pioneered by a Dr Ralph Cloward after the Japanese attack on Pearl Harbour) and fused my C6/C7 cervical vertebrae. This brought an end to my rugby days.

I started reading books on exercise and physical therapy and rehabilitating myself in the coming weeks, months and years. I was not an academic before the injury but had to become one now that sports were out, for a while anyway. At first, my choice of college subjects was selfish. I chose topics such as human biology, psychology and physical education purely to help myself get back to some level of health, fitness and confidence. I thought at first that I would become a sports coach and so started a BA (Hons) Degree in Sports Studies/Science, but later realised I wanted to help others to help themselves more. An NDE or Near Death Experience I had at the time of breaking my neck had altered my world view and left me with some social integration problems. I saw many around me now as being superficial and selfish so I chose to work as a sports activities instructor, with adults who had learning difficulties such as Down's Syndrome, Autism, Cerebral Palsy, etc.

I completed a course with the American College of Sports Medicine and became a Certified Health and Fitness Instructor in Preventive and Rehabilitative Exercise Programming working in a Sports Centre doing fitness testing and 1:1 and 1:10 gym training.

Then I discovered by chance the work of Cardiac Technicians as they were then called within the NHS (National Health Service within the UK). I was kindly offered a place as a trainee at Conquest Hospital, Hastings, England.

Whilst at Conquest I started my training in cardiac theatre monitoring, pacemaker implantation and follow up testing, heart scanning, exercise stress ECG recording, Advanced Life Support and a whole host of other relevant skills, qualifications and experiences.

I was then invited to help with Conquest's excellent Cardiac Rehabilitation programme.

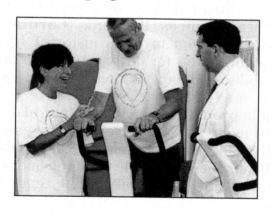

I gave talks to 20–30 heart patients twice per month on "Safe & Effective Exercise". Much of this was then adopted into the British Heart Foundations standard Cardiac Rehab Programme.

My final year Dissertation looked at the effectiveness of Conquest's own Cardiac Rehabilitation programme and uncovered significant ECG changes occurring in patients who are not normally or routinely monitored during these cardiac rehabilitation exercise sessions.

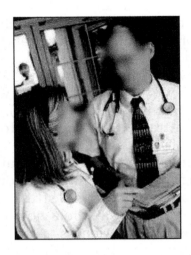

Whilst a Senior Cardiac Technician one day I happened to pass by two junior doctors in a corridor discussing a patient and I heard them use the words **"Cardiac Cripple"**.

As you can see from my own history I had a greater respect and appreciation for anyone trying to overcome an illness or disability and didn't share these doctors belief that some people are just hopeless cases. I have seen improvement in people with the worst physical disabilities so was (and yes using an ' expletive ') *bloody* annoyed with them using this label because once you have a label attached to you then that is the way people treat you and worse still ... how eventually an individual might end up seeing themselves.

Having read many books on psychology and NLP particularly I understood the power hidden in words and how we can use words to either build or destroy a person. So just for the fun of it I started to ask myself ... *" what would be the exact polar-opposite of a 'Cardiac Cripple' ?"* ... and then after a short while bouncing ideas around in my head it hit me. Wouldn't it be a ... **"CARDIAC ATHLETE"?**

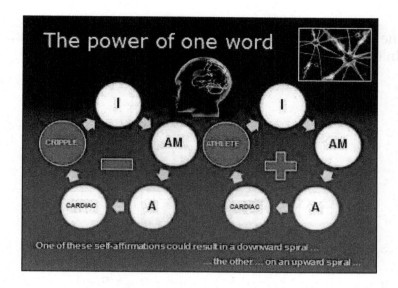

The Evolution of Cardiac Athletes

You see whilst I was giving my talks to groups of cardiac rehabilitation patients I would usually get one or two individuals in the group of say twenty who were frustrated that they were now in the midst of people who were never athletic and were never going to be athletic. These few were usually of very active sporting backgrounds who through no fault of their own had eaten and exercised correctly for years, avoided smoking, saturated fats, etc, but due to one unpredicted genetic chromosomal abnormality had experienced one of the many heart diseases.

These individuals were usually angry, frustrated, impatient, wanted answers now and wanted to get back to their favourite sports asap and to forget this major cardiac event had ever happened to them.

At first I decided to put together a basic ' Newsletter ' with the hope of pulling these like-minded people together.

I realised I had a unique set of personal experiences, education, training and qualifications. I recognised their frustration and hunger for answers just as I had to search alone myself many years earlier after breaking my neck. I didn't want them to have to search as hard as I had to.

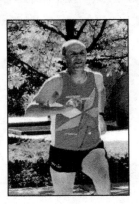

It was around 2000 that I met a Russ Bestley a lecturer and graphic designer with a pacemaker himself and yet who was out there breaking all kinds of endurance records and yet these achievements were going unrecorded and unrecognised by the general population. I knew there were many more thousands if not millions like Russ out there. I asked Russ if he could put my design ideas together for a group logo and the present one you see is Russ's final draft which was trademarked in 2001.

Together with Russ I decided to produce a more formal newsletter and called it ' The Association of Cardiac Athletes Newsletter ' to try and bring this special group of people together. this was sponsored for a while by heart pacemaker company Medtronic who generously covered the cost of printing.

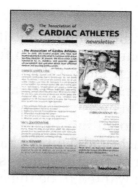

It proved popular but as the internet was developing I realised that this would offer access to a wider audience and so started to make enquiries into how a Cardiac Athletes website could be created.

On 19 September 2001 **www.cardiacathletes.org.uk** domain was first registered and on 21 September 2001 the Cardiac Athletes website went 'live' for the first time.

I started to receive emails from people all over the world and realised I needed to create a Forum so that people could talk to each other directly. I looked at a number of Forum packages from various companies and decided to go with what I considered to be the best at that time. On 2 February 2006 the Cardiac Athletes Forum was launched. The rest ... as they say ... is history ...

In 2010 I was kindly invited to fly to Pennsylvania, America to attend a large gathering of **Cardiac Athletes** who had decided to meet up each year and run as individuals and relay teams in marathons.

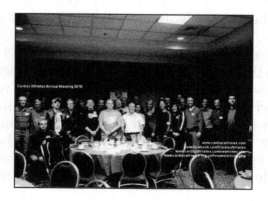

Harrisburg was the venue and it was a wonderful experience to meet many of my forum friends and heroes. I felt obliged to add even more value to this great gathering and say my own personal thanks by way of a presentation on Sports Cardiology. This was well received and resulted in a stunned and hushed room in which I could hear brain cells mulling over all the facts and figures I had just presented and also the faint squelch of creative juices starting to flow. The precise reaction I had wanted to be the catalyst for. We even managed to raise enough money to buy our first defib and I proudly presented this to both the Mayor of Harrisburg and also the Fire Chief for use the very next day in the Harrisburg Marathon.

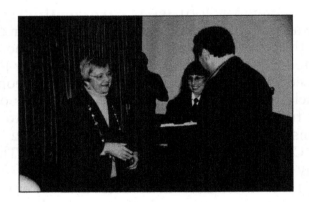

It remains one of my main goals for Cardiac Athletes to buy and donate more AED defibs back into the sporting communities around the world, effectively ' closing the circle of life ' ... heart survivors saving the lives of other heart victims.

Before I move on to the next sub-heading I would just like to make this personal statement to all Americans ...

When I was trying to get Cardiac Athletes working and growing I wrote to all the big heart and cardiac societies around the world. Guess what ? It was only you Americans who literally ' ran with ' the idea. America, the American pioneering spirit, it's deep appreciation for trying new things, challenging new frontiers, ... you gave me a chance where others turned up their noses. You Americans embraced this new idea and got excited about it and spread the word. So I would just like to say this to you all ... " God bless America and all Americans ... and thank you ! "

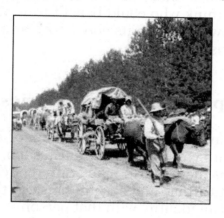

Image reproduced from:
http://www.scientificamerican.com/article/why-pioneers-breed-like-rabbits/ ;)

So why this book ?

I could see such a book as this in print way back in 1998 when I was giving talks to cardiac rehab patients but it has taken me a 'little longer' than anticipated to actually getting it done. I could see value in people's stories. They are incredibly uplifting and take us out of ourselves and we learn from each other how to view life's hardships in a different way and to bounce back despite them. A book you can pop in your luggage bag and read on a flight or at a bus stop. A book you can pass on to another person.

A book such as this could potentially uplift and inspire many hundreds or even thousands if handed forward often enough, perhaps starting a new ' mini revolution ' who knows, and that is the spirit of this book I hope you the reader will enter into with us.

Once you have enjoyed this book, and I know from my own personal experience reading it through in preparing it for publishing, you really need to read it through 2 or 3 times in order to hear every hidden message and nuance, don't let it collect dust on a shelf, pass it forward to someone you might know or think who could benefit from reading it. Tell them to also download it in its ebook format if a soft back or hard back copy isn't available.

Why a compilation of short stories ?

As a boy I always loved receiving a book of different short stories. I am sure you had your favourites too. The beauty of this book is that there are so many different characters each with a different cardiac and sporting history that it is hoped you the reader can identify with that person.

Maybe your characters are similar in the way that you see the world and think, reflected in the words and expressions and pace of speech and humour which causes you to connect to that person and so then that person becomes your mentor and motivator. I have deliberately left spellings and expressions as spoken by the Cardiac Athletes in their own 'mother tongues'. A compilation of short stories is easier to digest and you can dip in and out when you have the time or inclination.

Although not a heavy lofty academic tome there are many important issues raised within these pages and which occasionally reappear and repeat within different members stories. See if you can identify them. See if you can come up with answers to them too. If you do then write and tell us about them.

I must warn you of something else though. You will find yourself laughing out loud at key points in this book and crying when you read other pages. So if you are worried about strangers or even friends seeing you all emotional then maybe it would be best to read this book when alone and unobserved.

Why bother ?

So much of my work as a Chief Cardiac Physiologist and recently as a Cardiac Technologist / Echocardiographer in Australia, has been all doom and gloom, seeing one very infirm elderly patient after another, which can drag down the spirits of even the most resilient medical professional so I felt compelled to develop this group and community and immerse myself in it each day and the characters there would unknowingly uplift my spirits. I offer you their 'special medicine' now.

Through my eyes everyone is equally important. If we fail to listen closely to one person's story we will likely miss some key learning points for our own lives and everyone has an extremely valuable and important story to tell others. Until now these human achievements have gone little detected, little known by the wider world. There has been a steady drip of people achieving sporting successes at the astonishment of their cardiologists but none of it has been recorded. I am helping to change that.

That ' special characteristic '

Some people when dealt a bad hand in life, when suffering injury, disfigurement, loss, etc., ... become victim to their circumstance and no amount of counselling or friendly advice will help that person recover their lost spirit. And then there are those people who despite every adversity thrown at them, despite their pain and suffering, they bounce back, often stronger and happier than they were before.

I like this second sub-class of people. Is it just their inner stubbornness ? How is it they never lose their spirit and love of life and in some ways relish the challenges life throws at them. There is something very special about the human mind when it gets it right. An injury or disfigurement is absorbed, assimilated into that persons personality. It becomes 'no big deal' and with time appears to have vanished in its importance and that person may need reminding that a year or two ago yes they did have their chest cracked open and an artificial valve was truly inserted. Really ?

Some psychologists refer to these people as " rebound personality " types and this is the stuff champions are made of.

A book such as this fits neatly in between other books on psychology, maybe the psychology of achievement, but as any of the Cardiac Athletes would remind you ... lose your mind-body connection ... and you do so at your own peril.

During many of these stories see if you can identify where each person experiences their own very personal epiphany. That defining moment they let go of fear and truly start their ' new ' lives.

I remember mine, there were more than one actually. The first day I took off my neck brace and just sprinted so hard and fast it was great to feel the wind in my face again. That marked my start of experimenting.

Then another marked the end of my experimenting. The day I was doing neck-springs off a gymnastics box on my physical education teachers course and the demo with others got out of sequence and I had to miss the box altogether to avoid a mid-air collision with others and was hurtling head first at the floor but had the presence of mind to get into a tuck position as I had been taught and land and roll on the back of my neck and shoulders and end up standing to an ovation, shaken AND stirred.

That day I decided no more unnecessary risks. I had my confidence back. I drew a bench mark and told myself no-one was ever going to push me into risking my health ever again. PE instructors included. I was in control of me again.

See if you can spot those moments in the coming stories. They are critical. As are the low points, the turning points. It often starts by changing just one thought, one word in the internal conversation in the mind.

I want to hear from you

I would be delighted to hear from readers of the book who feel the book has impacted their lives in a positive way. Please feel free to email me at lars@cardiacathletes.com with any interesting stories from your own past or current cardiac history, and to share your experiences with us. You never know, your experiences may make it into ' Cardiac Athletes Book II ' along with an acknowledgement !

Where does the money go ?

Proceeds from the sale of this book go into the ' **Cardiac Athletes Trust Fund** ' which in turn goes towards combating and beating heart disease. We (Cardiac Athletes) buy AED Defibs for sports centres and clubs to protect young athletes from SCD – Sudden Cardiac Death.

Donate here:
http://www.cardiacathletes.com/cardiac-athletes-trust-fund.php

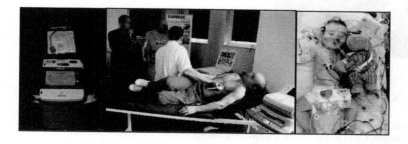

It is hoped that some of the money will be able to go towards Pre-Competitive Sports Participation Cardiac Screening Days, towards research into preventing babies being born with Congenital (Genetic) Heart Disease, and towards many other areas of cardiac prevention, surgery, and rehabilitation.

You might like to get more involved than just simply buying this book and you can do so if you so wish by going to the Web Forum and joining ' **Team Cardiac Athletes** ' as one of the various levels of supporter. Again your donation at registration will go towards our many worthy cardiac causes.

Join and **Register** here:
http://www.cardiacathletes.org.uk/forums/register.php

Thank you for buying and reading this book, I hope you enjoy it and learn lots from the Cardiac Athletes, ...

Happy exercising and ... look after that heart ...

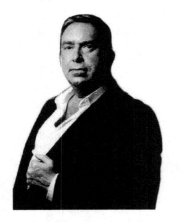

Lars Andrews MSc, AIR, ASAR, PiCSA, CSANZ.
Founder, CEO & Editor of Cardiac Athletes

Formally Chief Cardiac Physiologist -- Portsmouth NHS Trust, England, UK.
Presently Cardiac Technologist – Box Hill Hospital, Victoria, Australia.

Cardiology Department | Nelson Road, Box Hill, VIC 3128 |
https://www.easternhealth.org.au/

T: +61 3 9895 3333   M: +61 0432 0591 23   lars@cardiacathletes.com

INTRODUCTION

Know your enemy

Imagine for a moment if you will that you are looking down at our planet Earth from space. Maybe you don't have to imagine because you are a NASA astronaut or Russian Cosmonaut or International Space Station Scientist reading this book ? (There's wishful thinking). You look out your port hole window and down on this pretty blue planet and everything appears calm and serene ... but it isn't. There is a war going on down there. An enemy who respects no country boundaries. A global war that is resulting in millions of deaths and many millions more casualties needing lifesaving surgery, medical devices and life-long health-care. Who is the enemy causing all this human suffering and tragedy ? The enemy is **Heart Disease**.

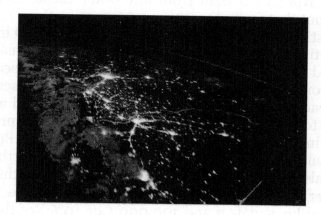

NASA photo reproduced from:
http://smallwarsjournal.com/jrnl/art/escalating-from-terrorism-to-nuclear-war-on-the-asian-subcontinent

How big is the battle ? The truthful answer is we just don't know precisely. Why don't we know ? Well because the stats, the figures are wrong ...

1) there is no standardized post mortem assessment procedure around the world,

2) classifications differ around the world,

3) not everyone who dies has an examination of their heart to determine its condition at the time of death,

4) stats quoted are projections based on best evidence,

... and there are many more flaws in the systems other than these four I just quoted.

What we do know is that it is **<u>MASSIVE</u>**.

Much of the following data comes from the World Health Organisation [1]. CardioVascular Disease (CVD) is the number one cause of death globally: More people die annually from CVD than from any other cause. Stop and think about that for a moment ...

An estimated 17.3 million people died from CVD in 2008, representing 30% of all global deaths. Of these deaths, an estimated 7.3 million were due to coronary heart disease and 6.2 million were due to stroke. By 2020, heart disease will be the leading cause of death throughout the world and will increase to reach 23.3 million by 2030. CVDs are projected to remain the single leading cause of death. Presently congenital heart defects are every country's #1 birth defect and are also the #1 cause of birth defect related deaths. Each year over 1,000,000 babies are born worldwide with a congenital heart defect and 100,000 (or 10%) of them will not live to see their first birthday and thousands more die before they reach adulthood. Bloody depressing !

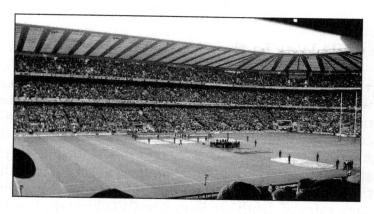

A horrible image but picture in your mind's eye for a very brief moment a 'blue baby' on EVERY spectators seat within a major sports, soccer or athletics stadium as they usually seat around 80 to 100 thousand spectators. Then think of that many baby deaths happening every year ! Not good. Think of all the potential talents lost to the world. All the good that could come from a child knowing they were saved by others because they are valued and worthy and loved. Such a waste. An unnecessary waste. We can do something about this heart disease enemy. Help Cardiac Athletes to eliminate it.

War zones

Let's zoom in with our space telescope on a few countries to get an idea of the size of the battle going on down there and see who is winning, whether it is the humans or whether it is Heart Disease. As a mark of respect let us pay homage to the countries of the contributors to this book. Let us look at the battles being waged in the USA, in the UK, in India and in Australia. I won't bore you with too many facts and figures. I will present you with just enough so that you get a feeling for the scale of this battle front. The following numbers have been plucked directly off the pages of recent and up-to-date and reliable reference sources at the time of this manuscript being sent to the publishers.

The CVD War in the USA

Heart disease is the number one cause of death for both men and women in the United States, claiming approximately 1 million lives annually. Every 33 seconds someone in the United States dies from cardiovascular disease which is roughly the equivalent of a September 11th-like tragedy repeating itself every 24 hours, 365 days a year. More die of heart disease than of AIDS and all cancers combined. Although rates of death attributed to CVD have declined, the burden of this disease remains high. Cardiovascular disease (CVD) is the term used for heart, stroke and blood vessel diseases.

This year more than 920,000 Americans will have a heart attack [2-3] ; nearly half of them will occur without prior symptoms or warning signs. 250,000 Americans die annually of Sudden Cardiac Death. That's 680 every day of the year. One-half of the victims of Sudden Cardiac Death are under the age of 65. An estimated 80 million Americans have one or more types of heart disease. About 8.9 million Americans have chest pain (angina). Currently about 7.9 million Americans are alive who have had a heart attack.

In 2008, the total cost of cardiovascular disease (coronary heart disease, hypertensive disease, heart failure and stroke) in the U.S. was estimated at $448.5 billion. (This includes direct costs such as costs of doctors, hospital services, medications, etc., and indirect costs such as lost productivity.) In comparison, the estimated economic cost of cancer in 2007 was $219 billion. Less than half that for Heart Disease.

By 2030, 40.5% of the US population is projected to have some form of CVD. Between 2010 and 2030, medical costs of CVD are projected to triple, from $273 billion to $818 billion. Knock-on costs due to lost productivity, etc, for all CVD are estimated to increase from $172 billion in 2010 to $276 billion in 2030, an increase of 61%. Effective prevention strategies are needed if we are to limit the growing burden of CVD.

Please help Cardiac Athletes fight Heart Disease in America.

Donate here:
http://www.cardiacathletes.com/cardiac-athletes-trust-fund.php

The CVD War in the UK

In 2010 CVD was and still remains the biggest killer in the UK [4] , resulting in more than 45,000 deaths amongst individuals less than 75 years of age. Almost 180,000 people died from CVD around 80,000 of these deaths being from coronary heart disease (CHD) and around 49,000 from strokes. It caused around 46,000 premature deaths, the majority 68% of these were men. There are around 150,000 incidents of stroke every year. Over 87,000 percutaneous coronary interventions (PCIs) are now carried out every year, more than three times as many as a decade ago. In 2009, CVD cost the UK health care system £8.7 billion and the UK economy £19 billion in total. The cost per capita for CVD in the UK is €156, which is lower than average for the European Union.

Please help Cardiac Athletes fight Heart Disease in the UK.

Donate here:
http://www.cardiacathletes.com/cardiac-athletes-trust-fund.php

The CVD War in India

WHO (World Health Organization) statistics show that India has 200 million affected, out of which nearly 1 million die every year, that's an amazing 3,000 per day or 2 deaths per minute. Asian Indians develop heart attacks 6-10 years earlier than other populations. There has been a significant increase in the prevalence of coronary artery disease (CAD) in young men (20-40 years) and women (20-50 years) in India. In India, an alarming 40% of first heart attacks occur in people <45 years of age and two-thirds in people younger than 55 years. In sharp contrast only 3% of all heart attacks (10,000 women and 30,000 men) occur among Americans <40 years of age. An alarming 50% of CAD deaths occur in people <50 years of age. For comparison, only 1% of all CAD deaths among US whites occur in people younger than 45 years of age and 87% of CAD deaths occur in those >65 years of age. The WHO has also estimated that India lost $9 billion (USD) in national income from premature deaths due to heart disease, stroke, and diabetes in the year 2005.

It is estimated that by 2020 cardiovascular disease will be the largest cause of death and disability in India with over 3 million deaths every year and accounting for 40 per cent of all deaths [5] . It has also been forecasted that more than 2.6 Million people will die from coronary heart disease, which constitutes 54% of all cardiovascular disease deaths. Approximately half of these deaths will occur in young and middle aged individuals, making the impact to society and the economy even more significant. India is set to be the 'heart disease capital of the world' in just a few years time. Not good reader. Not good at all.

Please help Cardiac Athletes fight Heart Disease in India.

Donate here:
http://www.cardiacathletes.com/cardiac-athletes-trust-fund.php

The CVD War in Australia

Data for 2010 and 2011 from the Australian Heart Foundation [6] reveals the following. CVD is the leading cause of death in Australia, accounting for 31.7% of all deaths. Heart Disease now affects 1 in every 6 Australians and 2 out of 3 families. In total it affects 3.7 million (3,700,000) Australians. One Australian dies from Heart

Disease every 12 minutes. Australian women are 4 times more likely to die from heart disease than breast cancer ! Each year around 55,000 Australians suffer a heart attack. This equates to one heart attack every 10 minutes and in 2011 heart attacks claimed 9,811 lives or on average 27 people died of a heart attack each and every day.

Please help Cardiac Athletes fight Heart Disease in Australia.

Donate here:
http://www.cardiacathletes.com/cardiac-athletes-trust-fund.php

Who is winning this war ?

Again I am not going to bore you by quoting lots of numbers at you but the forward projections for Heart Disease are upward. This data is readily available from many sources across the internet libraries of the world and all showing the same. Pacemaker and stent companies publish their future sales figures for their shareholders and both show handsome upward trends. The same for heart valve replacements too. Cardiac drug sales will continue to rise also. Heart transplant and heart failure figures have slowed as medical professionals become quicker and better equipped for dealing with acute cardiac emergencies and stop them from becoming chronic conditions. As more people live longer and longer obviously the likelihood that they will each get a cardiac condition increases. Atrial fibrillation is a common ailment of the ageing heart for instance.

So why am I mentioning these trends ? Well in time there will be more and more people around you who will have treated and managed cardiac conditions. More and more of these people with heart conditions will want to continue with active athletic lifestyles until one day the majority of those running the Boston Marathon for instance will have heart conditions and the minority will not yet have a diagnosed heart condition. There will then have been a switch. Those at most risk will be those who have not had a medical heart screening. Those at least risk will be the heart patients who have had all the cardiology tests and scans and who know their individual exercise heart rate ranges and how hard they can push themselves. They will have become the new safe exercise ambassadors to others.

Cardiac Rehabilitation ... any good ?

Answer ? Yes and no. Yes they have been scientifically proven to reduce all risk factors, second heart attacks and extend life. You can expect a 17% reduction of having a second heart attack a year later and the chance of you dying two years later will be reduced by 47% [7]. There are many more benefits too. We have come a long way from the 1960's six week enforced bed rest.

It's a bit like steering a ship. If you adjust the direction of your heading or course by just a tiny degree, over time that will take you miles from the person you once were with all those heart risky bad habits. So yes they are good for you if you can get on a CR course. No because there are far too few of these programs around. Your nearest one may be a two hour journey away. You are not going to do that. There is sporadic funding and still a lack of respect for it. Some conditions are excluded from cardiac rehab programmes because they have been deemed as being high risk such as having an implanted ICD and yet I know ICD patients completing Half ('Tinman') and Full 'Ironman' Triathlons and in good times too. Can you ?

There is uneven and unequal cover. Many patients don't attend although they were visited on the wards and offered it so they are left to find out information on their own and online. There are fewer female and ethnic patients attending too. Trained supervisors differ in their knowledge and expertise. It all seems so ' hit and miss ' and that is a real shame. Because there are far too few cardiac rehab programmes many people find themselves too far from organized community based phase 5 cardiac rehab so an online group such as **Cardiac Athletes** helps a great deal.

If you are reading this as a potential cardiac rehab patient then you would do yourself and your heart a great deal of good by doing the following 5 key things right now, today, without delay and change the direction of your life and extend your life by at least 10 years, very possibly much more. Ten additional years for one hours work ? That's proper use of time !:

1) join **Cardiac Athletes** without delay and chat with people similar to you:

http://www.cardiacathletes.org.uk/forums/forum.php

2) read all the answers to the **FAQ's** on this Cardiac Athletes web page:

http://www.cardiacathletes.com/faqs.php

3) buy yourself a **Heart Rate Monitor** and make friends with your heart again:

http://www.garmin.com/en-US/explore/intosports/

4) join a free **HRM community website** like this one and find training buddies:

http://connect.garmin.com/en-US/

5) use the more accurate **Karvonen formula (%HRR)** heart rate calculator here:

http://www.cardiacathletes.com/heart-rate-calculators.php

Trends in online communities

More and more people are creating their own online heart communities and groups and this is happening at an accelerated rate as ideas bounce around the internet and are copied. This is a good thing. The same way planets form from space dust and rock debris the internet is helping these separate online communities discover each other, clustering together to share common knowledge and experiences which then benefits everyone. Fewer people are left feeling alone and isolated and over-burdened with what they once thought was a unique medical problem only they had. Comfort comes in knowing others also have an identical medical condition and these are the ways they are dealing with it in a more effective way. In the animal kingdom there is not only safety in numbers but also comfort in numbers for us social ape-humans.

It's not all electronic now either. Humans are social creatures and love to meet other people similar in character and views. Online internet groups are now enabling people to commute and actually meet up face to face with others who are similar but just across the border. To meet up, chat, share experiences and tips and maybe run in a relay team in a collective celebration of a second chance at life feels great. Humans like to gravitate to others similar to themselves, and gain much from belonging to a self and mutually supporting group.

What the reader is going to read

You are not about to read heavy, stuffy academic case studies but actual ' real-life ' (and death) personal accounts revisited and relived in written words.

What the book covers

In this CA Book 1 the stories come from male and female members of Cardiac Athletes, from the USA, from India and from Australia. They include people born with Congenital Heart Defects but who didn't know it until later in their lives. It includes those predisposed to developing Coronary Heart Disease and who had a surprise heart attack. It includes those who got heart disease as a result of a viral or bacterial infection. Oh yes it could happen to you too. A scary thought isn't it !? This book includes those who were competitive athletes and sports stars before contracting heart disease and it also includes people who were not competitive athletes but who have, since their heart condition, turned their lives and fitness around so that they too are now enjoying the heart healthy benefits of regular progressive exercise training and competitive sports events.

Overall ' theme ' of book

The overall theme of this book is a rather one-sided, upbeat, light-hearted look at a very serious subject, that of heart disease. Only successes are reported here and no apology is offered for compiling such a book as this. The goal is to uplift, inspire and turn lives around with the words on these pages.

Repeating themes

Certain ' themes ' keep re-emerging from the CA Forum and are again echoed in this book. They are worth mentioning and thinking about. As you read the following Cardiac Athlete's stories be aware of the following ten themes ...

Theme 1:

We need to relearn our sixth sense

From the stories you are about to read you will see how the human brain is far too powerful for the human body and athletes exemplify this dis-ability, this dis-association. They are able to tolerate higher levels of physical discomfort for longer and repeat it more often. They can if not careful switch off from the tiny sensory ' danger warning signals ' their bodies are sending their brains. They lose that all-important mind-body connection which other creatures in the animal kingdom remain highly attuned to and do not over-exert themselves, unless pushed by a human that is ! In self-denial they suffer repeated bouts of overtraining until one day they get an autoimmune condition whether osteo-arthritis or a cardiomyopathy or a heart conduction defect or even a lung disorder.

There is a physiological safe zone to train and compete within and a threshold which when exceeded will result in cardiac cell trauma and increased fibrosis. We are only just beginning to realise this and trying to unravel all its mysteries. Technology in the form of the many myriad biofeedback gadgets will help us to not over exert ourselves and to train more ' scientifically ' and safely and logically.

See if you can identify in the following stories the exact moment each of the following Cardiac Athletes actually get back in touch with their own bodies. Some state it clearly in print. They are relearning their own mind-body connection and listening harder for the weak 'background' (body) signals that mean they are starting to over exert or over train. Cardiac Athletes have to become ' grand masters ' at listening to their bodies. Cardiac Athletes have renewed respect for their bodies.

Theme 2:

Cardiac Athletes are pioneers

Where there is a lack of cardiologists with a deeper appreciation of the cardiac ' patient ' who is also an athlete, these individuals are left to their own devices (literally) and ' experimenting ' with their own medications and doses and treatment protocols. Sporting patients are left to experiment on themselves. This is tantamount to playing Russian Roulette for some and humans being humans some will do it if they cannot get good advice.

There have been many pioneers within the field of cardiology over the years, from the first angiogram, first bypass graft, first balloon angioplasty and stent, the first valve replacement, the first heart transplant, and so on ... until now we have created a situation where many of these people are now living longer and fitter lives than previous survivors of heart disease. These survivors are (to borrow from a favourite TV series) ' going where no cardiac patients have been before ' ... they are now pioneers of their own lives and challenging conventional medical wisdom which is always stubbornly slow and resistant to change.

I recognised very early on that there was a small sub-section within my cardiac rehab talk groups who reminded me of myself. They were the more sporty and active ones. The ones who had, always been involved in competitive sports and athletics but who had found themselves in a group of less active, elderly and historically sedentary individuals and they were desperate to have their questions answered on how and when they could quickly resume their competitive sporting lifestyles ... although mine was a spinal injury and theirs a cardiac injury ... we were the same and I had already trodden the path they were about to ... I knew they would become pioneers of their own lives just as I had to experience many years earlier ... when no-one has the answers you have to tentatively experiment with your own physical barriers each and every day ... a scary and unsettling situation for an adult to find themselves in again ... to start over again ... to have lost that feeling of invincibility ... I recognised this ' type ' of person and recognised them as a 'friend' and felt compelled to do all I could for them ... because I found myself in a moment in time with just the right experiences, insights and qualifications ... I felt it was my duty to do all I could to help this special group of people to regain their athletic lifestyles which I have always admired. I just love ' rebound personalities ' ... the people who refuse to give up no matter what the odds ... the people who you watch on the sports field and you see them get closed down by big burly defenders and there is no way out for them and then suddenly they break free and they are away sprinting faster than they have ever sprinted before and the opponents can't catch them and they score ... they did the ' impossible ' ! Wow !!! Doesn't that feel great ? Doesn't that just lift your spirits ? Doesn't that make you wonder about the human ability ? The human spirit ?

In creating the Cardiac Athletes website and Forum I hoped to pull in more of these characters so that we could all learn from each other and uplift our collective spirits in the same way and as more and more members joined this gravitational pull would accelerate tornado-like ... Cardiac Athletes may not have Super Human bodies but they do have Super Human spirits ... have no doubts about that ...

Theme 3:

We need more Sports Cardiologists

These stories reveal cardiac patients searching, often blindly, for ' the best ' sports sympathetic heart doctors and yet it is still a bit of a lottery because how do you as the patient really know ? Cardiac patients are still getting treated badly out there and often having to ' shop around ' for an understanding Cardiologist who gives good sound advice and has more sympathy for the more athletic heart patients. There is no official register of cardiologists with a special interest in the subject and no way of knowing to what depth their knowledge goes to in this specialist field of Sports Cardiology which is still in its relative infancy anyway.

Theme 4:

We need Sports Cardiology Centres

There is also a lack of technical staff out there who would know how for instance to optimize a particular patient pacemaker so that the patient could perform at their very best in an endurance event such as a marathon, triathlon or even Ironman Triathlon.

Many pacemakers are still being left in ' factory settings ' and not being adequately tailored to the person's typical daily activities which may include long swims, cycle rides or runs during every week. What is happening still is that this patient-athlete goes back to the pacing clinic with stories of " hitting the wall " far too early and yet they are being fobbed off by non-sporty and not very fit technicians that it is their underlying deconditioned fitness level until one day that pacemaker patient sees a different clinician who is more willing to make a pacing parameter adjustment. This first adjustment might make the athletic performance situation worse because few clinicians have a full appreciation of how one or two adjustments to pacemaker timing parameters might affect an individual's athletic performance. Getting the timing of pacemaker firing out by a few milliseconds can adversely affect how the four heart chambers fill with blood and then contract.

Often ECG monitoring during the actual sporting activity after these pacemaker adjustments are made is necessary but rarely done and so it more usually takes a second or third visit back to the pacing clinic until the device is optimized. Now this is time consuming and costly and very ' hit-and-miss '.

Cardiac Athlete 'Chooka' who you will read about in a moment, has recently had an upgraded pacemaker implanted which has dual sensors on-board, an

15

accelerometer and also a minute ventilation sensor which work in harmony to try to mimic the natural physiological heart rate changes with increasing and decreasing exercise intensity. So far, as I type this, poor Chooka has had this top of the range pacemaker implanted now for about a month and yet it is still not tailored to her so that she can get a decent exercising heart rate. She is still stuck at a heart rate under 100 ppm and has booked a third follow-up appointment with company pacemaker specialist to be present this time so that it can be setup correctly.

There really needs to be special Sports Cardiology Clinics where knowledgeable and specialist Cardiologists, Registrars and Technical staff follow-up the sporting heart patients as I am describing. I know that there are moves to set such centres as these up in a few cities around the world but it is still very early days and very sparse coverage sadly.

By pulling Cardiac Athletes together into one centre new avenues of discovery will open up. To illustrate this let me take two of the athletes you are about to read about. I won't tell you their names but let you see if you can spot the similarities in their post op experiences. Both had similar heart valve repairs and both noticed a reduction in their sports performances. Now this was due to a paradox of repairing that particular heart valve. You get rid of the everyday, day to day symptoms but can decrease sports performance as a consequence. The repair can actually make the effective orifice area or opening smaller and so the heart has to work harder ... a 'mechanical' or post-operative stenosis.

There also seems to be an increasing number of ultra-distance athletes having strokes. This includes long-distance runners and high kilometre cyclists. Why is this happening ? Is it because they are becoming dehydrated and then their blood becomes viscous and sticky making them susceptible to forming blood clots in the blood vessels supplying their brains and resulting in these strokes ?

Common occurrences like these would become more evident in a medical centre dedicated to athletic heart patients and solutions could then be sought to rectify them.

Theme 5:

Are we starting to see a post athletic epidemic ?

An increasing volume of scientific research is highlighting an increasing number of life-long serious competitive athletes now developing heart related problems. If this is due to repeated over training and over-exhaustion this shows just how powerful the human mind is at overcoming physical discomfort and certainly brings into question the old physical cultural adage " No pain, no gain ". Dr Andre La Gerche who has been very kind in writing the Foreword to this book is researching this phenomenon and has written many well respected and peer reviewed scientific papers on the growing number of veteran athletes developing heart conditions and what physiological and biochemical changes may be behind it [8-12]. Perhaps " the wall " that sports commentators refer to an endurance athlete hitting is there for good reason ?

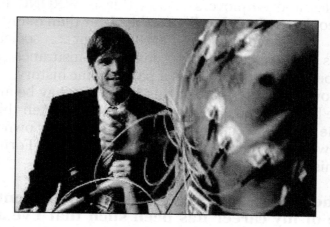

Are we really beginning to see the start of what may become an epidemic of retiring elite athletes with various cardiac and respiratory illnesses ? Just as there is a lower limit of exercise in order to maintain a fit and healthy heart and body, there also appears to be an upper limit threshold of exercise which if exceeded daily over a number of years can result in a dilated and scarred poorly contracting right ventricle which is more prone to life-threatening heart arrhythmias. Dr La Gerche is trying to determine what the safe upper training threshold is. Stay tuned folks !

Theme 6:

We must get rid of ' Cardiac Discrimination '

It is interesting for me as a hospital worker to read how the patient sees and experiences the hospital setting. It is sad that some of the stories you will read in a few moments still show an attitudinal stance from some medical professionals which is now outdated and outmoded ... advise these patients not to exercise at your own peril !

Some of the members have decided not to include their names for personal fears and for good reason because they do not want to be discriminated against by insurance companies and employers ... and this is WRONG because these people are fit and well, possibly fitter than many people not yet diagnosed with a heart ailment ... society and attitudes and policies have to change ... insurance policies cannot be weighted because of a past cardiac history.

I know if you are reading this Mr X you may be annoyed with me because you asked me to edit and shorten this but I think the message is clearer and stronger in your own words. Here is what one member of the Cardiac Athletes Forum says about this issue:

" The issue for me is related to employment. The nature of my career has been such that I've always been in precarious employment situations. Well compensated when things are going well, subject to abrupt dismissal when they are not. Being a 'heart patient' isn't helpful for being assigned important organizational roles or finding a new job. Companies want a guy who isn't going to create a big

problem by suddenly dropping dead. It's also a hindrance to finding a new job after getting sacked. In the US, employers provide health insurance for their employees. Cost is commensurate with the population they cover. Old guys (and particularly old sick guys) will significantly drive up health insurance costs if you allow too many of them onto the payroll. I am particularly sensitized at the moment. I had always been able to avoid the sack until last November, when we got a new managing director, who shot a bunch of us so he could replace w/ his own peeps. I am now approaching 60 and looking for employment. I am well educated, have a good resume, but am past my sell-by date. Not physically attractive or very charming. Really struggling at the moment, I can't afford to have one more reason for someone not to consider me for employment. Google search is both wonderful and dangerous, and EVERYBODY now uses it to check out prospective employees. If I was some French guy who couldn't get promoted or sacked, and had guaranteed health coverage, then I would just sit back with my cigarette and stinky cheese and not give a damn about exposing my identity.

So that's the gory explanation -- and you certainly don't want to put all of that crap in a preface, but I hope that gives you an appreciation for why some of us want to keep a low profile. I think the preface could say something generic like 'Due to their personal circumstances, some of our members require anonymity in sharing their stories' and leave it at that. Aside from the book, I expect that you will continue to find many Americans who don't want their identities exposed on the CA site (or elsewhere) in order to keep their heart disease under cover."

People who overcome a physical or psychological trauma, surgery, whatever .. should be applauded. That would be the person I would employ if I was an employer. It is those who don't even try and leach the social welfare system who should be " booed " and ostracized.

If it was me I would not employ you until you have had a full cardiology screening AND finished a recent half or full marathon within a decent time ! How about that ? Anyway how many bosses and managers and health insurance salespeople are out there who have pristine coronaries and finish marathons, triathlons, half and full ironman races ? I don't know any. Do you ?

In time and as people live longer CEO's of big companies will have various heart problems and corrective surgeries so maybe that is when there will be attitudinal change ?

Theme 7:

Are we really becoming ' trans-humans ' ?

It is becoming more and more acceptable to have your own body melded with that of technology. It does not change the essence of us being ' human '. For a while it looked like we might be able to talk about ourselves as being 90% carbon life form, 5% titanium screws, 3% plastics and 2% silicone but now with bio-engineering even this analogy becomes blurred. Where does being ' human ' begin and end is another question these Cardiac Athletes are challenging. Are they 'transhuman' , enhanced humans or just plain human ?

There is and has been an increasing ripple of human transformation happening. Humans are being fused with more and more bio-technological advancements. In some corners of the internet these people are referred to as 'transhumans' ... but I find that term insulting too, just like I did the term ' cardiac cripple ' because humans have always had the spirit to overcome hardships and adapt. We are at the threshold of engineering 'better than human' physiologies. We had 'patch and repair' ... then metal screws and plates ... then bone grafts ... on the internet you can now watch stems cells being dripped onto a collagen fibre ghost heart model until it starts twitching in an organised and recognisable fashion. Who knows what else is going on in the research labs around the world ? What when we can replace a person's faulty heart valve with an exact copy grown in a test tube and replaced via key hole surgery ? Will this person be labelled a " heart patient " ? After all their replacement valve will be a pristine new one. So will their insurance premiums drop ?

There is presently another revolution going on but it is a steady one so not many people are seeing its influences on our day to day lives. The silent creeping medical revolution is stem cells. More and more and every day it seems I am hearing how stem cell therapies are curing this and that illness or disease. Soon cardiology may have stem cells for all its diseases. I can see a time when the cardiologist may be able to inject some new natural pacemaker cells inside the heart and directly into the zone where defective SA nodal or AV nodal cells are. Metal implantable pacemakers will become a thing of the past, resigned to the dusty shelves of museums and personal collections.

Scar tissue caused by heart attacks may be removed by scavenger cells and a different syringe of myocardial stem cells may be injected directly into the injury site. Diseased heart valves may be removed by robots controlling intravascular lasers and a new valve may be inserted after being made by 3D collagen scaffold printing in a solution bath of native stem cells. Fantasy, fiction or factual reality ?

Theme 8:

Would preschool screening be a bad move ?

There is a real and present fear of cardiac screening of all preschool sports participating youngsters. Although Italy leads the world in this and has dramatically reduced sudden cardiac deaths in young sports participants by a massive 89%

between 1979 and 2004 [13] will even the smallest, most insignificant murmur then result in that child being discriminated against for the rest of their lives as portrayed in movies like 'Gattaca', hence labelled a ' heart patient ' and discouraged from taking part in certain sports and activities and later hit with higher insurance premiums and be less attractive for employers ? After all here we have the Cardiac Athletes breaking sporting records so why should you curtail that individuals sports participation if they have had the fault 'fixed' ?

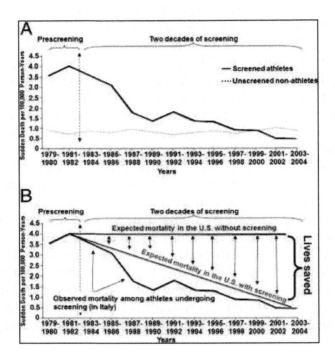

Chart reproduced from:

Corrado, D.; Basso, C.; Pavei, A.; Michieli, P.; Schiavon, M.; Thieman, T. J., Trends in Sudden Cardiovascular Death in Young Competitive Athletes After Implementation of a Preparticipation Screening Program. Journal of the American Medical Association 2006, 296 (13), 1593-1601

It wasn't until after I was a cardiac technician and I did an echo on myself that I discovered I had a mild mitral valve leak too. I have possibly had this heart valve regurgitation all my life but if I had been put through an Italian model heart screening I would possibly have been discouraged from taking part in competitive sports and would certainly not have enjoyed all that I have in my rugby, skiing, athletics, karate, etc. My life would have been far poorer. Especially when many of life's lessons and resilience are learned on the sports field and in the athletic arena. This need not be a compulsory screening and yes there are some brilliant voluntary screenings going on in America, for instance **Holly Morrell's 'Heartfelt Cardiac Projects'** screening days ...

http://heartfeltcardiacprojects.org/

... and also **CRY**'s screening days in the UK which I used to enjoy very much being part of ...

http://www.c-r-y.org.uk/

... but this is too sparse and there really needs to be many more of these initiatives. I am not aware of this kind of thing going on in India or Australia but maybe someone out there reading this could enlighten me by way of an email ? Let's create a register of these screening projects.

Theme 9:

We need more CPR and AED Defibrillators

You will read how important it was to their survival that an AED (Automated External Defibrillator) was nearby and that prompt and effective CPR was administered. If you haven't done a CPR course yourself I urge you to do so without delay. You may need those skills for one of your family, loved ones or friends TOMORROW ... or in the coming hours, days, weeks, months, ... Maybe you would consider making a kind donation to the **Cardiac Athletes Trust Fund** so that we can purchase and place defibs in more sports centres to help save the lives of future sports participants ?

Donate here:
http://www.cardiacathletes.com/cardiac-athletes-trust-fund.php

Theme 10:

Can Cardiac Athletes really destroy all Heart Disease ?

Although a nice ' BHAG ' (Big Hairy Audacious Goal) for Cardiac Athletes ... will we ever eliminate the planet of Heart Disease ? Maybe it would be possible through genetic screening and engineering but there will always be people with ' cardiac surgeries ' resulting from trauma accidents for instance and ' cardiac histories ' caused by viral and bacterial diseases.

If we all joined forces and worked together we could I believe significantly reduce the death and suffering caused by heart disease around the world, reduce it to no more than a low background noise ... With the knock-on benefit of billions if not trillions of capital expenditure saved.

Wouldn't you like there to be more swimming pools, sports arenas, more heart survivor athletes to share training sessions with and to laugh at life together with ? I know I would be healthier and happier surrounding myself with that kind of environment. More Cardiac Athletes celebrating life through sports.

Cardiac Athletes need you

If having read this book you feel you fit the profile of a 'Cardiac Athlete' and also feel you have a great story to share with others, then please join us and get typing because I am already putting together a second CA Book and I should be able to put it together much quicker now that I know how to do it. Send your story to: lars@cardiacathletes.com and be sure to include one or two photos and a link back to your own website or Facebook page if you have one.

About the Glossary

Please note, I have compiled the Glossary at the rear of this book myself using as much plain English as I could manage (and you could put up with) so the terms will not be described by way of a concise literary definition and no apologies are offered for this by the editor (me again). It is the same with both my spelling and grammar. I apologise now if you spot a mistake but I have done this all on my own and on a budget.

The goal is for the Cardiac Athlete stories to flow. If you make it to the end of this book having read every word and understood every glossary entry you will already have become quite an authority on heart disease and its cure. You will have joined the ranks of us other ' heart geeks ' and have a deeper understanding and appreciation of what it is like to be a Cardiac Athlete and you will be better prepared if and when you have to join our ranks.

I hope you enjoy the following stories.

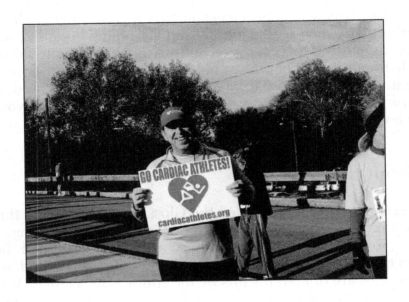

CHAPTER 1

Brian ' Echoguy ' :

" I had tears in my eyes as I crossed my first post op finish line."

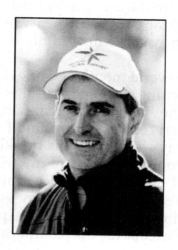

CARDIAC ATHLETE 1

First name: Brian
Forum name: " Echoguy "
Country: USA
Diagnosis: Aortic stenosis
Treatment: Aortic valve replacement, Ascending Aorta graft
Other facts: Medtronic Global Hero

My wife was the runner in the family. She got up early in the morning and ran around the neighbourhood while I tried to get back to sleep. She worried that I was putting on weight and not getting enough exercise. I tried to convince myself that I was getting enough physical activity from golf, but I knew differently. Finally, I decided to jog a bit with her so that I would no longer need to pretend that golf would help get me into shape.

On July 4th 1998, I reserved a tee time at one of the nicest public golf courses in town. The problem was that I could not find three friends to join me. One of my golfing friends mentioned that he was running in a 5k race and invited me to join him. I had been running for several months at that point and decided to cancel the tee time and see if I could beat him in the race. I had no idea of pacing, but by the end of the race I had learned that I could push myself pretty hard for 22 minutes. I was rewarded with a cap as an age group award winner in my very first race. I was hooked.

Over the next several months I worked on increasing the distance of my morning runs and was able to tackle a 10k by Thanksgiving. The inaugural Flying Pig Marathon was coming to Cincinnati the next spring and I made the mistake of mentioning to my wife that I was thinking about trying a marathon. She promptly told all of my friends my plans. I was committed. I closely followed a training plan for the race and was successful in meeting my goal finish time. I checked marathon off my life list and expected to move to the next challenge except for one complication; a friend had qualified for Boston.

Soon I was training with a group of friends, all with the intention of increasing speed to achieve that Boston qualifying time. After several attempts, I qualified in my eighth marathon. By that time running had become an important part of both my health and my social life. I was able to increase both distances and speed with significant improvement nearly every race. We started a small running club on our side of town and we became regulars at all of the local races.

By Labor Day of 2003, at the age of 43, I was ready to see how far I could push my limits in a flat 10k race. I went out faster than ever before and tried to run faster when the pain started to get to me. I was counting on a "puke in the chute" experience. What I had not counted on was heat stroke and passing out just short of the finish line. After they cooled me down and rehydrated me in the emergency department, the doctor noticed that I had a significant heart murmur. The cardiologist ordered an echocardiogram that showed a bad heart valve known as aortic stenosis. He advised that I should not run or exercise significantly again until after I had the valve replaced. In one day I went from one of the better master's runners in town to a "cardiac cripple" ...

Part of the work up of my heart condition included a cardiac catheterization that was done about two weeks after my heat stroke. During the cath they could directly measure the pressure gradient across my diseased aortic valve and found it to be normal. When I woke up after the procedure, the cardiologist told me that while my valve was not normal, I should be able to run again with very little restriction. The valve would need to be followed regularly by echocardiograms, and would be expected to worsen over time, but I could go back to enjoying the sport that I had come to love.

I started back slowly and over time built confidence in myself that I could recognize when I was getting overheated or dehydrated and back off the pace a bit. Over the next five years I joined friends in lots of wonderful running adventures. We participated in running events ranging in distance from 5k to 100 miles in fun and interesting places all over the country. In 2008 a friend and I completed all of the certified marathons in the State of Ohio, a total of 12, in one calendar year. I noticed that my times were slowing a little over the years, but nothing significantly more than expected for a 48 year old. My semi-annual checkups with the cardiologist also showed that my valve was slowly worsening, but nothing of particular worry.

One frosty morning in January 2009, I was jogging to the park to meet my friends when I noticed that I felt a little lightheaded. We were scheduled to run a tempo run that morning as the first hard running day of our Boston Marathon training cycle. I decided the anticipation of running hard had caused me to start out too fast and was pleased when my head cleared when I slowed the pace a little. By the time I was with my friends running our warm up mile, I had forgotten all about any earlier abnormal feelings.

Initially the faster pace of the tempo mile felt good, like usual in a challenging run. But after just a quarter mile or so I noticed that my hands and feet felt very odd and cold. Soon I felt lightheaded again and decided that I needed to slow down and warm up better before I pushed. After climbing a small uphill knob, I felt very dizzy and decided I better walk a little. The next thing I remember was one of my friends shining a flashlight in my face looking at my cuts. I had hit my face on a mailbox trying to catch myself as I blacked out and fell to the ground.

Symptoms are what turns a medical aortic valve problem into a surgical aortic valve problem. Passing out and hitting my face on a mailbox sure sounded like a symptom to everyone around me, but I was in denial. I looked for every other possible explanation for the events of that morning. But, it was obvious that I would need surgery; it was just a question of how soon.

We spent the next year researching our options of valve types, surgical procedures and timing of surgery. I met with two different cardiologists and four different cardiothoracic surgeons to discuss my options. I was also able to find on-line help about cardiac valves and valve surgery from several different sources, particularly a forum for athletes returning to sport after cardiac surgery at:

www.cardiacathletes.com

It was at this site that I first learned that open heart surgery did not necessarily mean an end to all athletic endeavors. Several members posted results from marathons, ultra-marathons and triathlons. This made facing surgery much more palatable.

My pre-surgical workup included a cardiac catheterization which, like the one five years before, showed normal pressures across the valve. I was advised that I could begin to exercise carefully again. I ran slowly through the summer and fall and decided by October that I was back in good enough shape to tackle a half marathon. I decided to run the half marathon associated with the nearby Columbus Marathon. This race would not have any significant hills and several running friends would be participating. I started easy and carried my camera with me and stopped at the governor's mansion long enough to have my photo snapped with the governor and his wife. I felt great until about mile 10 when I had to stop and walk a few times due to light-headedness. A small uphill near the finish was the final blow. I could not find room to slow enough to walk and I passed out before I made it to the finish.

This time I hit the back of my head, so no more facial scarring. But, now with two strikes, it became obvious that the surgery would need to be sooner rather than later. After I recovered from my injuries, I found that I could no longer run at all without getting lightheaded. Walking up hill also seemed to bring out symptoms. It was time.

Now that it was time for surgery, we needed to finalize which type of valve and which surgeon would operate. After much hand ringing, we decided on a "tissue" valve so that I would most likely not need to take major anti-coagulating medications. The price for that luxury is the need for replacement of that valve in a decade or so. As for a surgeon, we picked Dr. Eric Roselli at the Cleveland Clinic, located less than a day's drive from Cincinnati.

In the months between my symptoms and my surgery, I learned a lot about myself and my time on earth. I learned that I really liked running and that I liked to talk about running even when I could not run. I learned that running had afforded me the luxury of eating volumes of food that I would not be able to continue to consume if I changed to a sedentary lifestyle. I learned that I loved the camaraderie of an easy run talking with friends. I learned that even though I thought I was being cautious, that running had the potential to do more harm than good for me if I took it too far. I learned that I was not too terribly afraid to die.

I think that the most important thing I learned during

this period was that I needed to be less critical of how other people spend their time on earth. I am aware that people look at my running as a waste of my time. I know different. Nobody likes to be judged, and I need to do my best to not be judgmental toward others in any aspect of life.

As the day of surgery approached I considered less rigorous activities I could pursue after my recovery. Gardening. No. Woodworking. No. Back to golf. No. Maybe hiking. If I could just do some fast packing.... OK. That is actually nearly running. So if that is what I am going to do, I might as well go back to running. I was encouraged by the results that I saw in the Cardiac Athletes and held out hope that one day I would be able to run again.

Finally in early March of 2010, the day of surgery arrived, about 6.5 years after I was first diagnosed with aortic stenosis and a little over one year since I developed some symptoms related to the valve. My small support team included my wife, 22 year old son, and sister in law. My wife's support team included my uncle and aunt who had been through the same procedure, in the same place, several years ago. As we walked to the surgical staging area, I realized how much I liked my role in the procedure more than my wife's. I was getting a new valve and hoped to be fixed. She had nothing much to gain and lots to lose if things did not go well. I did find myself worried a bit about loss of mental function that is sometimes seen after open heart surgery, a.k.a. "pump head", but in general felt pretty much at peace with our decisions and with whatever might happen.

Our pre-op education the few days prior to surgery prepared us very well for what to expect before and after surgery. With very few minor delays my procedure went according to plan. I ended up with a bovine pericardial valve and a new ascending aorta. I was in and out of surgery in the expected time and woke up in the intensive care unit as expected.

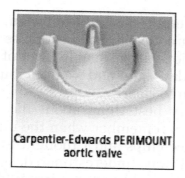

Carpentier-Edwards PERIMOUNT
aortic valve

Image reproduced from:
http://www.yourheartvalve.com/productinformation/pages/aorticvalvepericardial.aspx

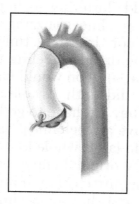

Illustration reproduced from:
http://www.ucaorta.org/ascending-aortic-aneurysms.html

In the intensive care unit, I found myself with two primary challenges. First was trying to relax my chest muscles enough to allow the ventilator to do the work for me when I awoke from anaesthesia. I was relieved that I did not have to spend much time in that situation and while the tube coming out was uncomfortable, it was wonderful to be able to breathe independently again.

The second challenge was dealing with the intensity of the chest pain that I was experiencing. I thought of myself as an athlete and tolerant of significant pain, but I found that even dosing my narcotic pain medication as fast as allowable, I could never achieve a reasonable level of pain control. It was not until two days later and we tried ibuprofen that I was able to get the pain to clear.

By far the very best thing about the ICU was the ice chips. I will always remember when the nurse asked me if I would like some ice chips and I thought to myself, yes, that would be nice. I way underestimated. After nothing by mouth for hours, then a tube in my irritated throat, those ice chips helped hit ecstasy areas in my brain that I had no idea even existed. For the rest of my life I will never turn down an offer for ice chips.

On my second post op night, I woke up in the middle of the night with an odd fluttering feeling in my chest. Not pain, but a very strange, almost buzzing sensation. I was in a cardiac telemetry floor by that time, so I was being monitored. I had the dreaded feeling that the surgery was going bad and that the surgeon would have to go back in and re-operate like they did with Arnold Schwarzenegger. I decided then that if they did have to go back in the next day, I would choose to have a mechanical valve the second time and hope that it would last a whole lot longer. That decision made me question my original choice of my tissue valve. I was relieved when the nurse came in and said that my heart rhythm looked great and she saw nothing of concern on the monitor. I got to keep the cow valve.

My biggest obstacle to getting discharged on time was to get my gastrointestinal system working again. I had dosed myself with all of the narcotic pain medication available the first day and a half and it had a profound constipating effect on me. Now that my pain was easily managed with ibuprofen and acetaminophen, I was paying the price of those narcotics two days later. Because constipation is almost never a problem in my normal life, I did not have much of a strategy to deal with it, other than to be frustrated. Finally, with a bit of an assist from Milk of Magnesia, things started to move again and I was able to get back to normal.

On the day before my discharge from the hospital I

experienced an emotion that I don't think I had ever experienced before or have since, significant melancholy. I was aware that many cardiac patients experience periods of depression, but this seemed to be very early for that. I was not interested in eating food, watching tournament basketball, or taking a shower. All of these things had brought me great pleasure in the past. When I mentioned it to my wife, she said she could not see any difference in my outward affect compared to the previous day. But I clearly felt significantly different. Those feelings slowly diminished over the next several days after I got home.

I was discharged from the hospital on the fourth post-operative day and my wife drove me home across the State of Ohio the next day. It was nice to be able to spend time in the car together to give us a chance to gather some perspective before we got home. My pain was well controlled with ibuprofen and acetaminophen unless I sneezed. I did have a pillow to hold to my chest when I coughed or sneezed, and it did great for coughs but not so hot for sneezes. Luckily, I only sneezed three times in the five days after surgery.

Soon after we got home, it became obvious that it would be helpful for me to track my exercise tolerance progress like I had for my training in the past. I took out my running log book and started recording how many walks and how many times I went up and down the stairs during the day. By post op day #8 I was walking over ¼ mile per trip and taking three or four walks per day. A little over two weeks I was able to walk for a mile at a time. I decided that I would be interested in the local cardiac rehab program and asked my cardiologist about the details.

Because the majority of cardiac rehab patients are not particularly athletic, the standard beginner program would probably not be challenging enough, so I was started on phase III cardiac rehab. I started the program one month after surgery and appreciated being watched on a monitor while I worked out on the bike and the elliptical machine. By that time I was walking between four and eight miles per day. At my third session, five weeks after my surgery, the rehab nurse said the words I longed to hear. In order to get my heart rate where she wanted it, I was going to have to start running.

The first running steps did not feel as good as I had hoped. It had been a long time since I had both feet off the ground jogging so I should not have expected it to feel comfortable. Also, I was carrying ten extra pounds since I had stopped running several months ago. But, I was running again, slowly, and there was some hope that I would be able to run with my wife and my friends again someday.

After three weeks of working with the cardiac rehab nurse, she turned me loose to begin training on my own. I had not shown any rhythm problems or blood pressure problems while monitored and I could now work on my own as long as I used my heart rate monitor.

Progress seemed very slow over the next few months, but I was greatly encouraged by the friends I had made on the Cardiac Athletes on line forum. It was reassuring that I was not alone in the world trying to come back to an active lifestyle after open heart surgery. I was able to share ideas and get feedback nearly every day with folks in a very similar situation from all over the world.

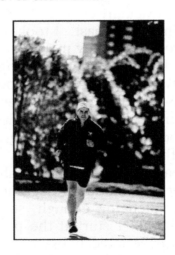

About the time I started running again, I noticed that the Cardiac Athletes had scheduled a reunion event at the Harrisburg Marathon in mid-November. Athletes would be coming from several states as well as England and Australia to enjoy a banquet together and participate in the marathon or relay. I started thinking that finishing a marathon eight months after surgery might be possible and started a slow progression of build-up to that distance.

My first goal in the build up toward Harrisburg was to gain confidence in my new valve by participating in shorter distance races. At ten weeks post op, I found myself standing on the starting line of a local 5k race for the first race of my new running life. When the gun went off, I was tempted to push the pace to see just how fast I could go. But, the goal that day was to run with confidence at a moderately challenging pace and finish strong. I needed to prove to myself that I could control the effort. I was one of the slower ones from our running club that day, but several of our club members came back to the finish area to see that I had tears in my eyes as I crossed my first post op finish line.

Through the summer I was able to slowly increase distances and I was strangely satisfied when some of my old overuse injuries started to show themselves again. How nice it was to be able to overuse those leg muscles, tendons and bones! I told myself that my heart surgery made me a more mature and appreciative runner. I tried to appreciate every day that I could join my wife and friends on a run around the neighborhood. Most of all I looked forward to participating in events, but realized that every run is a gift and should not be taken for granted.

Finally the weekend of Harrisburg arrived. My training had included three half marathons and several long runs indicating that I was ready to go the distance. I was able to whittle my weight down to closer to my former racing weight. This would be marathon #58, but it sure felt like #1.

At the Cardiac Athletes banquet the night before the race, I was encouraged by hearing the stories of those who had now been racing for many years post op and continue to do well.

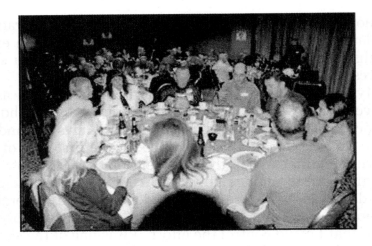

Standing on the starting line with my new found friends I again got choked up considering my good fortune over the past year. It was such a joy to be able to participate again. When I looked down at my watch I realized that it was not showing my heart rate. I had forgotten to put on my chest strap to monitor my heart rate and it was now too late to get back to the hotel. I considered stepping off the course and taking it as a sign that I should not run, but decided instead that I had ten years of experience in monitoring my effort and I should be able to keep myself below the danger zone. So it ended up that my first unmonitored run after surgery was a marathon.

I did start fairly slowly and got into a comfortable rhythm for the first several miles. At around the halfway point, I met a fellow runner who said she was hoping to qualify for Boston with a time that was close to what I had planned to run. We ended up running most of the rest of the race together and we were able to cross the line in a time fast enough to qualify her for Boston. Crossing the line was a sweet return to marathon running, made even sweeter by sharing a victory with someone else.

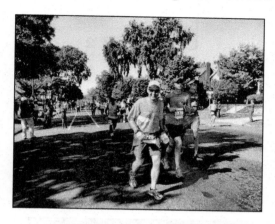

I learned long ago in marathon running to avoid the post marathon blues by planning the next race even before crossing the finish line. By the time I finished Harrisburg, plans were in the works for the Myrtle Beach Marathon three months later and several more races in the spring. I am confident that I will be healthy enough to do those events, but now have the perspective that I cannot take any race or any run for granted. I need to appreciate every healthy day and live it to the fullest. And who knows, maybe that long ago planned trip to South Africa for the Comrades (ultra) Marathon may someday actually happen.

CHAPTER 2

Rick ' 2ndchance ' :

" My death was painless "

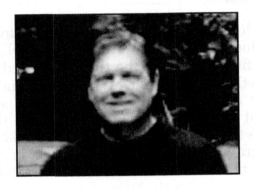

CARDIAC ATHLETE 2

First name: Rick
Forum name: "2ndchance"
Country: USA
Diagnosis: Coronary Artery Disease
Treatment: Six Bypass Grafts

I was telling my USTA doubles tennis partner that I needed an extra minute during the changeover because I had felt faint and winded in the middle of the game we had just finished mid-set.

The next thing I was aware of was four or five firemen looking down at me as I lay on the hard floor of the indoor courts. I sincerely asked, " what happened ? " One of the faces responded sharply, " Your heart stopped." Next, my daughter who had witnessed my resuscitation after what my emergency medical report termed ' Sudden Cardiac Death with spontaneous return of circulation ', was bending over me. I said, " Sorry, Steph." She explained to me that one of the other figures in the periphery of my vision had saved me with immediate CPR. Miraculously, on the evening when fate determined that I would suffer a cardiac arrest, a cardiologist just happened to be playing for the other team. A paediatric intensivist was also in the house enjoying a drink after his team had finished a match. These two heroes performed world class CPR for at least twelve minutes until the fire department rescue squad arrived to shock me back to life with the AED.

The squad transported me to the nearest hospital where the cardiologist who saved my life and brain had privileges and called ahead. After a rapid assessment in ER, I was carted up to the cath lab, where my saviour performed an angiogram which disclosed a complete blockage of my left coronary artery and other narrowed sections on the left. Soon, I was talking with the surgeon who performed an emergency six vessel bypass that started at midnight.

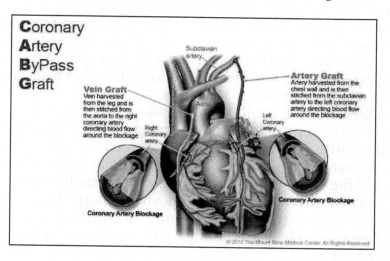

Illustration reproduced from:
http://www.mountsinai.org/patient-care/service-areas/heart/areas-of-care/heart-attack-coronary-artery-disease/treatment

My wife, mother and other close family members had rushed to the hospital and held vigil during the several hour procedure. When I came to in recovery, I still had the breathing tube and recall a feeling of choking while I gestured in some way that led to immediate relief as the tube was pulled.

My family was allowed in after I had been wheeled to cardiac intensive care. I recall much of the conversation. My wife reminds me that the first thing I said was, " Don't even think about cancelling the shower." My daughter's wedding was a little more than a month away and a long-planned shower was scheduled for the following weekend.

I sometimes tell people that I proved the adage that the first symptom of heart disease is death. But that's not quite true in my case. I had always maintained some kind of workout regimen. Until knee surgery at the age of fifty, I had been a runner. I always fancied myself a bike rider but rode for fun more than training. After the knee surgery, I followed medical advice and stopped running except for tennis. I had always lifted weights. In the couple of years before my " event," I had participated in a twice a week spinning classes designed for serious riders and triathletes. Then, a couple of months before the arrest, I signed up for a VO2 max test – the first in a couple of decades. I was very disappointed with my result. It should have been a warning shot. That was April.

When I began some longer outdoor rides in May, I was perplexed that I would become winded on hills that I had no problem with in prior years. I entertained the fantasy that I was suffering from exercise induced asthma. I even bought an over the counter inhaler. I knew that a cardiac issue was a concern. Even though I had devoted a large block of my career as a trial attorney to defending the medical profession and had relatively deep training in the science of cardiology, I exercised a degree of denial that nearly cost me my life but for the miracle of arresting a few feet from a cardiologist. When he learned that I had often defended cardiology cases, he asserted that karma was in play.

He is still my cardiologist, and I was very pleased the day he showed me a blow-up of the picture of my holding my infant granddaughter in a frame on a table in his office.

My recovery from surgery was not as rapid as I expected. Even though I was playing tennis three months later, my aerobic capacity seemed to be lagging. I was determined to come back better than before and made slow progress on the treadmill. I rejoined the advanced spinning class and gradually gained confidence and strength over the winter.

A year after the surgery, I was running and biking at a level where I contemplated entering road races and duathlons. I envisioned myself a finisher rather than a competitor. Then, I was slapped down when a follow-up nuclear stress test and angiogram disclosed that two of my grafts were closed, no doubt from the time of the surgery. I now had an explanation for why my recovery had been slower than I hoped. But I also learned that my training had led to development of pretty good collateral flow in the affected portions of my heart. I was initially depressed but got over it as continued training led to my ability to finish some road races.

In the past year, (I am now three years out), I have run 10k races and completed three sprint duathlons. One of these days, I will get serious about improving my swim so I can do triathlons. Of course, I still play a lot of tennis. My training also includes weights and yoga.

Within weeks after the arrest, I found Dr. Caldwell Esselstyn's book, Reverse and Cure Heart disease. I was so impressed by the results of his program and studies, that I immediately adopted his recommendation of a plant-based diet. I expect to continue this path the rest of my life with the hope that I will enjoy the result that his compliant study subjects experienced – no cardiac events.

At the age of sixty-four, I am not upset at not being in the front half of the pack at the races. But I feel grateful every day for the sunrise, the company of my family, and the miracle of being able to progress on the bike and run. I hope

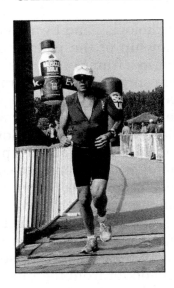

to continue my present occupation of law professor into my seventies.   Along with my wife, I am one of the primary babysitters for my granddaughter a couple of times a week (I volunteer to teach some of the night classes to free some earlier hours) and during those hours, I often think of how close I came to missing the blessing of being a grandpa.   The " event " taught me an obvious but elusive lesson – don't take a new day for granted.   I also wonder about the lore of coincidence.   Both I and the hero cardiologist were last-minute subs for our teams. If my arrest had occurred almost anywhere else, ...

CHAPTER 3

John :

" If I was not in as good of shape as I was, I may not be here "

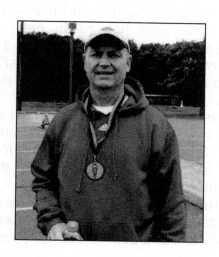

CARDIAC ATHLETE 3

First name: John
Country: USA
Diagnosis: Coronary Disease; Heart Failure; Heart Attack
Treatment: Angioplasty and Stent x 1

My name is John Jones and I am currently 55 years old. I live in The United States, Wapwallopen Pennsylvania. I worked in manufacturing management and was a Plant manager for a national Semi trailer manufacturer. I worked long hours and had a good deal of stress. I thought that I did not have much time for exercise and eating right.

By the time I reached 40 years old I was very much out of shape and 80lbs over weight. After attending a company sponsored seminar that gave us a questionnaire on our health, I realized I was in poor physical condition. I took this as a wakeup call and decided to start by losing weight.

At 41 years old I started a daily walking program and lifted weights. I looked over my diet and started changing it by first eliminating soda which I drank morning, noon and night. I went to drinking mostly water and started to lose weight. After I lost some weight I started to try and run. I had small goals in the beginning and just wanted to be able to run from one telephone pole to the next. It took a few months and I increased myself to 3 miles. I loved running and it began to consume me, I ran my first 5K a few months after starting to run and I was hooked. I ran 5K's almost every week end.

I began to run longer races and then set a goal to run a marathon. I ran my first marathon about a year after starting to run. I did not know how to train for this and with the long hours on my job the training beat me up, 2 weeks before the marathon I could hardly walk. I did run the marathon and finish but was in pain for several weeks. I said " that is it, no more marathons " but after the pain went away I was ready to set a goal to run a marathon again but this time I would find out the proper way to train. I ran another marathon and did much better, felt much better and realized maybe I could qualify for the Boston Marathon.

Now my goal was to qualify for the Boston Marathon. The Boston Marathon is one of the few or maybe the only marathon that the only way in besides running for a charity is to run a qualifying time at another marathon. I trained harder and ran more miles, I tried 4 times to qualify and either missed it by a few minutes or injured myself with stress fractures.

In 2007 I was having heart palpitations and was referred to a cardiologist. I was about to run another marathon so the cardiologist wanted to make sure all was ok. He had an echo cardiogram and a CT scan with dye of my heart done. The results showed at that time I had just a spec of plaque in one artery and normal heart function except for some heart enlargement which he attributed to athletes heart. As far as my heart health everything was good.

In 2008 I was 51 years old, I was running another marathon and it was my 5th attempt to qualify for Boston. I was not feeling good the morning of the marathon and told my wife I may not even run, she said you did all this training just go out and run and enjoy yourself don't worry about the time. I decided to run and took the goal of qualifying off the table, I don't know if it was because I took the pressure off myself or what it was but when I seen my wife at mile 25 I was over 10 minutes ahead of the qualifying time I needed. I ended up qualifying with time to spare !

In 2009 I ran the Boston Marathon and at mile 9 something happened and I could hardly bear weight on my right leg. It took 5 marathons, multiple injuries and a lot of pain to get to the Boston Marathon so I was not going home without the finishers medal. I walked with a limp from mile 9 to 26.2 to finish and received my finisher's medal, it turns out I had a stress fracture between my hip and femur. Before I was satisfied that once I made it to Boston I would not be pressuring myself to qualify again. But this changed everything now I felt I had to go back and be able to run the whole 26.2 miles and enjoy myself.

It took a long time to heal and get myself back up to running the miles I needed to train for a marathon. In the fall of 2010 I felt I was ready to start marathon training again and set a goal of running a spring 2011 marathon. At the same time the Boston Marathon was changing the qualifying standards, which made it a little more difficult to qualify.

I ran a Marathon in March of 2011 and qualified for the Boston Marathon with 8 minutes to spare but now with the new standards that may not get me in. To try and make sure I would get in I ran another Marathon in May 2011 and qualified with 11 minutes to spare but stress fractured my tibia. In the September Boston registration I found out I made it in for the 2012 Boston Marathon. I was healed from my stress fracture and started to increase my miles.

I started my marathon training in January 2012 and felt

that I was in very good condition. Training was going very well and I was cross training doing cycling classes at the YMCA twice a week.   In January 2012 I did an indoor triathlon and placed in my age group.   I was continuing my marathon training and on Jan 28th 2012 I ran 13 miles with a group of friends and felt good.

On Jan 30th 2012 I went to my 8 am cycling class at the Y and for that class we were going to race each other on computerized bikes with screens that we normally did not use.   There were not enough bikes for the entire class so we went in two groups.   After we finished we were to go back to our normal cycling bikes which were in another room.   I finished and as I was walking down the hall I felt dizzy, I went into the room, climbed onto my bike and was trying to lock in my shoes and that is the last thing I remember ...

From what I have been told after getting on the bike I fell forward hitting my head on the console of the bike and not moving.   The person on the bike next to me thought I had slipped and asked if I was alright, I did not respond.   She yelled down the hall to the cycling instructor while she was trying to hold me from falling off the bike.   Other members of the class helped her get me to the floor.   Another member of the class ran down the hall pulled an emergency alarm and told people to call 911.   He came back to the room and said I was gasping for air and then had no pulse; he started CPR and yelled for someone to get the AED.

Staff from the Y came and assisted with CPR; additional staff from the Y brought the AED and used it.   From what I been told the ambulance arrived quickly, they shocked me with their defibrillator and determined that I should not be taken to the local hospital but should be life flight to the trauma hospital.   I was told I was shocked one more time while in flight to the hospital.   I had an 80% blockage of the left anterior descending artery which was stented.

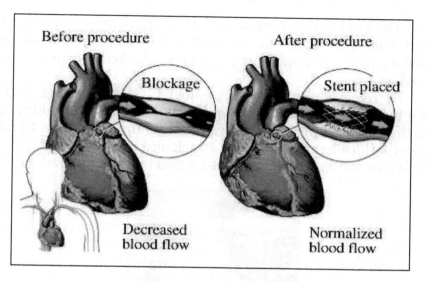

Illustration reproduced from:
http://kentuckianahealthwellness.com/understanding-
stents-and-treatment-of-coronary-artery-blockages

The quick action of my cycling class, the Y staff and the fact they had an AED saved my life !   I don't remember anything that happened on Jan 30th after getting back on the exercise bike but doctors and nurses at the hospital said that all I kept asking them was will I be able to run the Boston marathon.   I was not allowed to run even a portion of the Boston marathon which was in April but I did go to the Boston marathon and unofficially walk the first 3 miles.

I was in the hospital 3 days and left the hospital with a life vest which is an external defibrillator. I had to wear the life vest 24 hours a day for 30 days until they scheduled me for a stress test. I started a 12 week Cardiac Rehabilitation program the week after I came home from the hospital.   I had to wear the life vest for the first 3 weeks of rehab.

In the end of Feb 2012 I was given an echo cardiogram and stress test.   I did well on the stress test but the echo cardiogram showed some wall motion abnormality with my heart. I was then given a cardiac MRI.   After the stress test and eco cardiogram I was able to stop wearing the life vest and the electrophysiologist said that his opinion was that I had a 80% blockage of the LAD and a piece of plaque or blood clot came along and completely blocked it causing the cardiac arrest.

He released me to the cardiologist. After looking at all the tests my current cardiologist opinion is that in addition to the blockage problem I have heart failure. He feels I had heart failure before the heart attack and cardiac arrest. He feels that the cardiac arrest was caused by the heart failure.

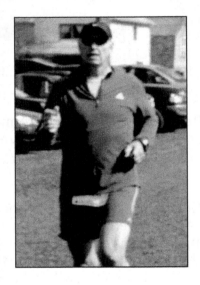

I finished cardiac rehab; I wish it lasted longer because I felt more secure while being monitored. I was more confident to push myself while I was being monitored. I really feel that I did not have any warning signs before my cardiac arrest but maybe if I was paying closer attention to my body I may have had signs. I am much more aware of what my body is feeling now and ended up twice in the emergency room because I thought I was having chest pains. Both times the pain was not heart related.

Since my cardiac arrest I have had fear and anxiety of another cardiac arrest. It was very bad the first few months after my event.

While I was in the hospital my wife brought me my IPAD

and I spent a great deal of time researching what happened to me. I also was searching for help with running after a heart attack when I came across the Cardiac Athletes page. I could not believe it, there were other people out there with similar situations. I had people around me think I was nuts because I wanted to run again. But here at CA I found people that felt the same way I do, I spent a lot of time reading the stories and following the forums. Then I began to participate in some of the discussions, it made me feel there was hope to once again be active. I found the members very welcoming and always positive. I hope to participate in the 2012 get together in Baltimore MD.

If there was any advice I could give it would be to pay close attention to your body and when something does not feel right get it checked ! When you look at my situation it is hard to see why I had this cardiac event. I have no family history of cardiac issues. I had acceptable cholesterol limits, I have never smoked and rarely used alcohol. For the last 11 years I have exercised regularly and probably for last 9 years have been in the best shape of my life.

Some people will say to me look you spent all that time getting yourself in great shape and see what happened. I say and my doctors will agree that if I was not in as good of shape as I was I may not be here and I would not be recovering as fast as I am !

CHAPTER 4

Kathryn ' Chooka ' :

" Seeing 'someone like me' achieve such a lofty goal, was too confronting for them "

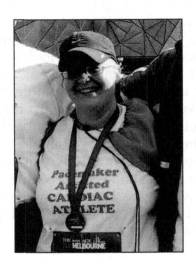

CARDIAC ATHLETE 4

First name: Kathryn
Forum name: " Bionic Chook "
Country: Australia
Diagnosis: Paroxysmal Tachyarrhythmias
Treatment: SA and AV Node ablations; dual sensor pacemaker

My name is Kathryn but everyone calls me "Chooka" which is slang for chicken. I am 46 years old and live in Melbourne Australia. I got the name ' Chooka ' because I was born 6 weeks premature and was kept in a heated cot until I could be bought home from the hospital a few months later. My GP said at the time that I was like a hatchling and I've been called ' Chooka ' ever since.

In November 2006 I completed my third New York City Marathon. I am not a runner, nor do I have a background in athletics, but I have a dream.

My friends call me Chooka but my cardiologist calls me 'non-physiologic' because I am totally dependent on a cardiac pacemaker and rely on it for every single heartbeat. My heart cannot generate any heartbeats of its own. Just think about that for a minute; no pacemaker ... no heartbeat ! And I've been like this for a smidge under 30 years.

My pacemaker is fitted with breathing and motion sensors which analyse how active I am and generate my heartbeats accordingly. How fast my heart beats, how slow, the when and the how is all completely computer controlled. Technically that makes me more of a battery hen than a chook.

I can't remember when I first started to experience palpitations. It's probably more accurate to say I can't remember NOT experiencing them. Even before I started kindergarten it was noticed that exercise often caused my heart rate to go up (as it should), but sometimes it would stay up for a couple of hours, and sometimes for days. Of course, exercise wasn't the only trigger and my heart would often go berserk for no good reason at all, even while I slept.

Until the age of 11 or 12, I thought everyone's heart did that, I thought everyone experienced chest pains if they ran around too much. I never had the stamina other kids seemed to have, and as exercise often triggered the rapid heart rates, I was usually the mascot or scorer on school sports days. Growing up, I dreaded sports days because I often had to watch my friends having fun from the sidelines.

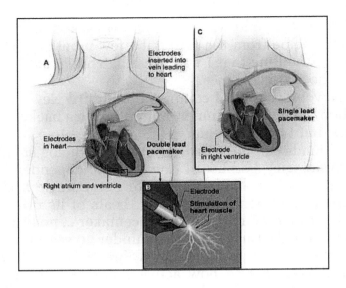

Illustration reproduced from:
http://www.nhlbi.nih.gov/health//dci/Diseases/pace/pace howdoes.html

I was implanted with my first pacemaker when I was 17 years old after undergoing surgery to try and correct the rapid heart rates. By then, the episodes of palpitations were so severe that I would faint several times a week and tests showed that my heart rate was as high as 250 ... in my sleep.

Part of the main nerve pathway in my heart was destroyed and a pacemaker was needed to bypass the damaged area and keep my heart beating in a regular rhythm. The surgery cured the rapid heart rates but turned me into a complete invalid instead, unable to do the most basic everyday things. There were days when I couldn't stand up long enough to take a shower, or walk the length of my drive-way to collect the mail. I had to leave school when I could no longer walk from one classroom to the next. On a good day I could slowly go about my daily business but there was always a feeling of tightness or pressure in my chest, intense squeezing in my neck and it was difficult to breath. On my worst days I wouldn't be able to feed myself. Stairs were excruciating no matter what kind of day I was having.

After about 15 months doctors discovered that the reason I was an invalid was because my heart was beating in an unsynchronized manner. The top half of my heart was still beating erratically, but the bottom pumping chambers (the chambers that were being regulated by the pacemaker) were beating at a much slower and steadier rate. In short, the top half of my heart was beating up to four times faster than the bottom half.

I was incredibly fortunate at the time in that there was ground-breaking research going on at a hospital in Sydney. Research into surgical cures for heart rhythm disorders.

Doctors there came up with a radical solution. As a result of the first surgery, I was dependent on my pacemaker to bypass the damaged areas of my heart's electrical system. There was no getting around that. The rapid rates in the upper heart chambers were caused by my own heart generating abnormal heartbeats, so the solution? If all the tissue that generates a natural heartbeat was surgically removed and the pacemaker was left to make all my heartbeat decisions, then my heart would beat and in regular steady rhythm. New pacemakers with motion sensors were also just being newly developed and it was thought that if my current pacemaker was replaced with one of these, then the pacemaker would more closely mimic a normal heart rhythm when I exercised. The biggest obstacle was that if the surgery was performed, it could not be reversed, I would be totally and completely dependent on my pacemaker for every single heartbeat for the rest of my life.

It sounds like a difficult decision to make, to render my own heart incapable of ever producing a natural heartbeat again, especially at the age of 18, but it wasn't. There was my own gut instinct that said ' go for it, the rationale behind it made sense ' and there was my GP who said I had the heart of a 70 year-old and was running out of options. But the biggest push to go ahead with the surgery came from a cardiologist who I saw for a second opinion. He said I shouldn't have the surgery at all ...... because I wouldn't survive it ..... but then conceded that if I did nothing, then I would most likely be dead in less than a year. Of that, I had absolutely no doubt.   So it was a trip interstate from Melbourne to Sydney for the surgery.

The doctors in Sydney were a little more optimistic. They laughed and joked and said I wouldn't be running any marathons in the future, but on a more serious note, they said I probably wouldn't be able to do anything more strenuous than walking afterwards. But after the surgery my life just took off.   I was able to go back to school and on to university to study medical science.   I was even able to join a gym and do beginner classes, and no-one knew I was battery operated unless I told them.   Each year was better than the last and I thought things would just keep on getting better.   I was wrong......

Around 12 years ago I came to the realization that my health had not only stopped improving, but was in fact, deteriorating.   Over time, gym workouts no longer left me feeling good, they left me feeling sick and exhausted, so I stopped going.   It took two hours for me to get out of bed every morning.   I found myself unable to go out socially after work, and if I went out on the weekend, I often had to pull a sick day on the following Monday (and I don't drink !).   I was struggling to work a 40-hour week and was considering cutting my hours to part-time (when I have the world's most sedentary job !).

I can't tell you how long I lived like this only that it had become my ' norm '.   The change was so slow and insidious that I barely noticed.   For a long time I was in denial and blamed a stressful job and getting older (at the age of 34) for my predicament.   I didn't even think to mention any of these symptoms to my cardiologist.   In retrospect, I didn't think any of what I was experiencing to be heart related because I wasn't in any physical pain or short of breath like I had been as a teenager.   It wasn't until I got the results of a routine heart test that I began to think differently.

The tests showed that I had three enlarged heart chambers, three leaking heart valves, and a diseased right ventricle (the chamber that pumps blood to the lungs). These changes were to be expected, explained my cardiologist, and quite normal for ' someone like me ', a legacy of the initial disease process that caused my heart problems in the first place, 2 operations and almost twenty years of having my heart artificially driven by a pacemaker. In fact, my heart was in better condition than he expected it to be. I was in great shape, he said ...... considering.

He was right of course. Given everything I had been through, I couldn't expect my ' normal ' to be like everyone else's. And while it was the kind of normal my cardiologist was expecting, it wasn't the kind of normal I was expecting. I began to question, that if this is what my life is like at 34, what was it going to be like at 44, or 54, or even 64 ? I had been deluding myself for years that everything was fine, but the test results forced me to take a good hard look at how I was living. I wanted better.

Since the first surgery as a 17 year-old, my goal was always to be fit and healthy, but just wanting to be fit and healthy is such a vague goal, no wonder I was only moderately successful in achieving it. I needed a goal with a more definite outcome, something more specific, something BIG.

What I desperately wanted was endurance just so I could get through a normal day without struggling. Endurance was something I'd never had before, so I began to look specifically at endurance training. Imagine being fit enough to run a marathon when, at the time, I couldn't even run for a bus. I thought that if I were fit enough for a marathon I'd be fit enough to do ANYTHING, so the goal became a marathon .... but which one ?

I spent months surfing the Internet. It had to be a marathon that was held in a cool climate. Exercising in the heat puts extra stress on the heart, and my pacemaker doesn't know what the temperature is. It had to be a marathon that had extensive medical backup, one that had a generous time allowance, one that I could gain entry into without a qualifying time, but most importantly, one that was big enough, grand enough, and spectacular enough to keep me motivated and focused. I had no fitness whatsoever, and so to even begin a training program was going to be tough. Training for a marathon was going to be, by far, the hardest thing I had ever done, so it had to be one hellava race to keep me committed to it.

Then I stumbled upon the NEW YORK CITY MARATHON: 37,000 competitors running through the city streets of New York, in the coolness of late autumn, with 2 million spectators to cheer you on, a medical station at every mile, 2000 medical personnel on the course, an 8.5 hour time limit, and I could " buy " a place as an international entrant. It doesn't get any more perfect than that. I initially set my sights for 2007 (the year I would be turning 40) as I thought it would take me more than 4 or 5 years to train for something that big, and I thought I had all the time in the world. Again, I was wrong.....

So by June/July 2002 I had pretty much decided to run in New York in 2007, that is, until my mum became ill. A simple ear infection left her bedridden for over 6 weeks. She lost all sense of balance and couldn't do a single thing for herself. I had to rely on friends, neighbours, and relatives to come in to help me wash her, feed her, take her to the bathroom, and to keep an eye on her while I was at work. I felt incredibly guilty when I had to call in help when I should have been able to do much of the work myself. She had looked after me when I was a teenager, but I wasn't able to do the same for her. And this was just an ear infection, what if it had been something more serious or more-long term ? I was forced to ask the question - ' how could I possibly look after my mother when I couldn't even look after myself ? ' So my plans had to change.

I went out and spent most of my savings on a treadmill and decided that I was going to be ready for New York 3 years earlier than originally planned. I set my sights for 2004. I was sick of waiting for things to get better when it was becoming glaringly obvious that " better " just wasn't going to happen without some hard work on my part. I was determined to never find myself in a position like that again. It's bad enough not being able to do the things you WANT to do, but it's demoralizing when you can't do the things you NEED to do.

Even after my mum was up and moving again, it was still

quite some time before she even started to resemble her old self again. It was a good six months before she was confident enough to leave the house and venture out on her own. The marathon training had to take a back seat for a while longer, but while my mother recuperated, I had my treadmill and I tried walking a little bit every week which was hard. Then I discovered I had a knee problem, and realized that even if I got the walking down pat, I still wouldn't be able to run.

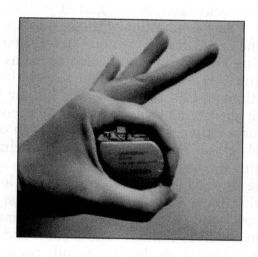

I thought I had injured my knee back in the days when I was able to go to the gym, but it's now thought to stem from having a very inactive childhood. The knee didn't worry me too much over the years, but I wasn't training for a marathon back then, and I had never really attempted to run before. I persevered with it for a while longer, but the knee wasn't improving and was holding me back, which meant that I wasn't able to work on my fitness either. My knee, which was just a minor nuisance in the past, suddenly became a significant obstacle. I had to get my knee right, so that I could work on my fitness, which I hoped would result in a stronger heart, which would give me the endurance I wanted.

I went to my GP who prescribed various anti-inflammatories, but they were of limited benefit. I needed more expert advice, so I made an appointment to see a physio my GP highly recommended. Three weeks before my first appointment I injured my other knee. Getting two knees fixed for the price of one sounded like a pretty good deal.

Enter sports physiotherapist Steve Sandor: Steve quickly worked out what the problems with my knees were and showed me how to tape my kneecaps into proper alignment. He also gave me exercises that I had to do every day to strengthen the muscles which keep the kneecap in place. A few weeks later he suggested jogging on a mini-trampoline. I was unfamiliar with the motion of running and using the mini-tramp would strengthen my knees without hurting them and would also serve as a bit of an intro to jogging. When I started out I could only do a few minutes at a time and I thought it would kill me ! But Steve set tiny weekly goals, and each week saw an accomplishment in one form or another. Baby steps, but each one bringing me that much closer to New York. Steve challenged me without pushing me beyond my limitations.

For a long time I feared that I might have left it too late to start training for a marathon and that I just didn't have enough to work with. I had no background in athletics, no foundation on which to build a fitness base, and a heart that wasn't like everyone else's, but thankfully Steve persevered. A brave move on his part. In the past, it was always difficult to find a personal trainer or anything remotely similar. As soon as I mentioned " heart condition ", they would literally run a mile. If I did happen to find a gym instructor to help me with any type of exercise program, they would either push me so hard that I wouldn't be able to keep up, or they would be fearful of the condition and not push me hard enough. Either way, the results just didn't eventuate and I would give up.

One gym instructor said I was a " waste of their time " because my heart was artificially driven and felt I would never achieve any level of fitness. Another said I was nothing but a liability. But Steve was different and for once I had balance and consistency with an exercise regime. He wasn't put off by the prospect of training a heart patient, and in the process of working on my knees he began devising different exercise strategies that had the added benefit of improving my overall fitness. It was a natural progression from physio to coach, in fact, that's what I call Steve nowadays, " Coach ". It's a title and a role he has rightly earned.

Coach took me from mini-tramp, to stationary bike, before moving on to " real " running. Coach works out what my knees and joints can handle (and fixes any niggles), and my cardiologist and I work out what my heart can handle. It's a team effort.

I was only running for a short time before it became obvious that I wouldn't be able to run long distances continuously, not because of my knees, but because of my heart. Being non-physiologic, my heart cannot keep up with the requirements for running. The pacemaker can't make allowances for the physical demands required for more intense exercise. My heart can only do what the pacemaker tells it to do and the pacemaker doesn't really know how hard I am exercising or of any other physical demands required. It doesn't know if I'm walking up a hill or carrying a heavy load, it doesn't know if I'm sick or dehydrated, and these are the times that my cardiac output needs to increase. But being dependent on a pacemaker also means that I can have my heart rates, and the way my heart rate responds to activity, " programmed " or changed with the help of a computer.

My cardiologist and I have experimented with different pacemaker programs and different heart rate ranges in conjunction with various running strategies. If my heart rate is programmed too high it's great to run with, but too uncomfortable for normal, everyday activities (my heart pounds in my chest all day long and I get too tired), and if it's programmed too slow I get dizzy when I run .... so we have compromised with a slightly lower heart rate but coupled with a 2 or 3 minute jog/5 minute walk combination. My knees are happier with that option too, and it's better than not being able to run at all.

My cardiologist has warned me (repeatedly !!!!!!) that if

I push myself beyond my limitations I risk very serious heart damage. It's a warning I don't take lightly. For me, the New York City Marathon wasn't even about running or the finish line .... but about a better quality of life. Good health, endurance, being able to keep up with everyday life, fitness, and stamina were the things I really wanted, not necessarily becoming a marathon finisher. When I said I wanted to do the New York City Marathon, I actually meant "I want to get well". The words " marathon " and "wellness" all came to mean one and the same thing to me, and you can't be getting well if you're out killing yourself with a gruelling training program. I didn't make a move without medical advice.

Once it became clear that I wasn't going to be able to do a marathon the same way as most other athletes and would have to use walk/run intervals, my marathon goal also had to change. Some people aim for a time-limit goal for their first marathon, most just aim to finish. My goal became the start-line. I dared not dream for much more than that. There were just too many variables that I couldn't control. The start-line also represented hope and optimism, the things which were sadly lacking in my life at the time. To line up at a start-line represents a chance of finishing and that was symbolic of what my life is all about, ... a chance to dream.

So for over a year and a half, I just visualized the start line with all the hype and hoopla that the New York City Marathon is famous for, blending in anonymously with the 37,000 other runners ..... and just doing my best with what I had on the day. More importantly, I wasn't going to be watching from the sidelines like I had as a child, I wasn't going to be singled out because of my heart condition, I wasn't going to be a scorer or mascot .... I was going to be a part of the biggest marathon spectacle on Earth ..... and in the best physical shape of my life.

2004 became a year of firsts for me and I found myself doing things I had never even contemplated before. I appeared in a TV game show to try and win some extra cash for my New York trip. As my training progressed and my fitness improved, I participated in fun runs.   I was implanted with my 4th pacemaker which proved to be my best one yet.   Stories about a pacemaker patient training for the New York Marathon started appearing in newspapers. "Team Chooka" which initially consisted of Coach and my cardiologist, grew to also include a nutritionist, podiatrist, massage therapist, and a small group of some very special friends who became the official cheer squad, and of course, my mum.   At times it was overwhelming to have such a dedicated group of supporters. I found myself with a level of fitness I had never experienced before, and could not only work more than my usual hours during the week, but could also slot in my training, my appointments with the various "Team Chooka" members, and still have a very nice social life .... with energy to spare.   For the first time I had some spontaneity in my life.   I could go out whenever I pleased and not have to think too much about the physical toll it might possibly take.   My dream of better health and endurance was coming true.

The 2004 marathon far exceeded all my expectations ...... at least what I can remember of it.   I think I spent most of the 26 miles wide eyed and open mouthed, just gob smacked by it all.   I'd heard about the masses lining the streets, but nothing could have prepared me for the show that the New Yorkers put on.   Bands played, kids lined up to " high 5 " me, and millions screamed, clapped and cheered.   From the roar of the crowd, anyone would think I was a serious threat to the Kenyans.

Finishing the race in Central Park was just magic, and receiving my finisher's medal is something I'll always remember ! It was hard taking it all in .... that I had realized such a lofty goal, that 18 months of hard work had come to fruition.   The skills of my medical team, ' Coach Sandor ', and my amazing support crew had resulted in me crossing an official marathon finish-line despite my complex medical history.   An event many believed would never happen.

On my return home, I found myself with an even higher level of fitness of which I had never experienced before.   I not only felt fit, I felt super-human, and at one stage didn't even know that the strange but wonderful sensations I was feeling whenever I went for a training run was actually 'wellness'. It took some getting used to, everything seemed effortless. I felt so fit, and started to think that if I continued training, then who knows how much fitter I would become. I was also frightened that if I stopped training, then my health would revert back to what it once was ..... and I couldn't go back to living like THAT !

I quickly signed up for a second, and then a third New York Marathon. For my third marathon, Coach introduced me to an exercise physiologist named Simon Gellie. Simon devised a strength and conditioning program for me that not only resulted in far less injury and more efficient running form, but also a new walk/running interval for the race.

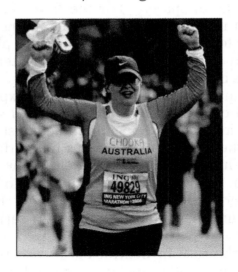

In 2006 I was able to do almost the entire marathon on intervals of 2 or so minutes of walking followed by 30 seconds of sprinting (and I mean SPRINTING). My heart rate monitor that I wear also has interval alarms to alert me when to start and stop running. It was an amazing experience to finish a race like that, with energy to spare and virtually injury-free, when just a few years before I was struggling to work a sedentary desk job.

In 2007 my cardiologist informed me that he felt it was no longer safe for me to continue participating in marathons, that he had reservations about the safety of doing such events with the particular heart condition I have and given the amount of time I had been pacemaker dependent. It's an opinion that I respect. I took up marathons to build a stronger healthier heart, and I had to give up marathons for the exact same reason .... to KEEP my stronger, healthier heart.

I don't run marathons anymore, but I have a marathon life-style, I still do 8-12 fun runs a year and love every minute of it. I am able to continue working in a job that I love, and still have the energy to enjoy a very full social life. I also became a volunteer for the Heart Foundation here in Melbourne, sharing my story at public speaking events to raise awareness of heart disease (particularly in women) and to raise funds for medical research. I am also writing my own book about my battery operated life, the ride I've been on for the last 45 years and the life-changing lessons I've learned along the way.

But most of all, I'm grateful for the experiences I've had and the people I've met, and the lessons I've learned. While I've been able to surround myself with positive, supportive friends and health professionals who were also invaluable sources of support, it hasn't always been that way. I've lost a few friends along this journey because they couldn't understand why I chose the path that I did, and there was no way I could make them understand.

I had some friends who judged what I was supposedly capable of and had opinions about what I should or should not attempt despite knowing almost nothing about my condition or what I had l experienced living as an invalid; they had no idea what it is like to live with the threat of having a heart history repeat itself all over again if I wasn't careful. I had friends who would not offer any words of encouragement or congratulations whenever I achieved a milestone. The one thing all of these friends had in common was that they all had so much potential to do more with their lives and for whatever reason, were not. I can only guess that seeing "someone like me" achieve such a lofty goal was too confronting for them and possibly invalidated any excuses they were making for themselves?

There were also doctors (not my primary care physicians) who didn't hesitate to tell me that they thought what I was doing was wrong and foolish and it literally broke my heart at times. My only answer to them is to look at the quality of life I'm leading today. My heart is in magnificent shape despite 29 years of total pacemaker dependency. Two months ago I was implanted with my 6th pacemaker and I am able to continue working a full-time job, enjoy shorter distance fun runs, able to take care of my elderly mother, and still have the energy and stamina for a very nice social life. This is why I undertook the marathon journey, to have more options in life. Mission accomplished if I say so myself!

Organisations such as ' Cardiac Athletes ' are so important. It's a place where there is so much support from people who are in the exact same boat. It's a place to find the information and resources to help you make informed decisions about your own health management or to steer you through the maze of confusion when the answers aren't always known. I didn't discover CA until relatively late in my marathon journey, how I wish I had discovered them sooner!!!

*(I am pleased to report as this manuscript goes to be published Chooka posted on Facebook that with her latest new Dual Sensor Pacemaker and company rep programming she has once again, after many years of being stuck at 90 beats per minute, managed to get her heart rate up into the 160's during a gym workout and is also once again enjoying the simple pleasures of sweating profusely and post exercise achy legs !)

CHAPTER 5

Tom P :

" I know I need to do the mileage, but I allow life to interrupt it. "

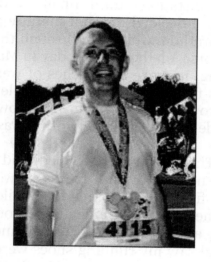

CARDIAC ATHLETE 5

First name: Tom
Country: USA
Diagnosis: Aortic Regurgitation; Coronary Artery Disease
Treatment: Bovine Aortic Valve Replacement; CABG x 1
Other facts: Medtronic Global Hero

I didn't begin running until moving to Buffalo in 1983. It was the beginning of the second running boom, and I had friends and co-workers who kept urging me to give running a try. I went to a week-long training program and couldn't stand the sitting all day, big meals, I needed to get moving, and a co-worker was running every morning before breakfast

..... how could I say no ? My co-worker ran with me, slowly, for 10 minutes and told me to turn around and head back as he ran off. After a week of this, I was hooked !

Buffalo has a great running community and there are races every weekend, and back then, everyone had free beer at the finish. I knew it was okay to drink after a race when the Sisters of Mercy, at the Kenmore Mercy Hospital 5k, were tapping the beer keg at 8:30 on a Sunday morning, in full habit ! I followed the usual mid-pack runner journey. I improved my 5k times until I plateaued, then started running longer distances, until finally I decided it was marathon time. I decided my first marathon would be the 1990 Buffalo marathon, which ran through the entire city, in a figure eight course, on the first Sunday in May.

That morning, I awoke to 6 inches of wet, sloppy snow, and the sky was full of more ! I was not letting this mess stop me. I drove to the start in downtown, and all the runners sat inside the Hilton Hotel until it was start time.

We walked to the start, and the gun sounded immediately. The snow never stopped, and because it was May, there were no plows on any trucks, so we just ran in the wet snow. My first marathon ended at mile 20. My wife and 3 children met me at that mile marker, outside a subway stop. As soon as she saw me, she demanded I stop. I looked down and saw my running shoes were all bloody. I started shivering uncontrollably. My first marathon, my first DNF. Not to worry though, I came back the next year and finished the same course in 4:14.

My running continued after moving to Syracuse, where I got to run with 8-10 co-workers every day at lunch time. I learned how great it was to have a group. No matter what the weather, no one wanted to be the wuss that did not show up for the run. Most, if not all, of the runners were faster than me, so once a week I would have to back off and recover with a slower run. But, I was never in better shape and it was most definitely from running hard often.

After finally finishing the marathon on my second attempt, I continued running marathons. I ran Buffalo again, qualifying for the 100th running of the Boston

Marathon in 1996. Then I ran London with Team Diabetes, raising money to fight a disease that has touched many friends and family. I ran other marathons: Marine Corps., Walt Disney World, then the Walt Disney World half (my first half) with many family and friends, my first attempt at coaching others into running. Then I ran the first Goofy challenge at Walt Disney World (where you run the half marathon on Saturday morning and then the full marathon on Sunday ... that's 39.9 miles on back to back days) ! I ran the inaugural Disneyland Half Marathon the same year.

In April of 2006, after finishing the Goofy Challenge, I went to my doctor to pick up my yearly allergy medication prescription. Upon listening to my chest, he mentioned my heart murmur, which we had always attributed to my distance running, was much louder. He ordered an echocardiogram immediately, which I had done later that same day. The technician was very nice and said I had one heck of an aortic valve leak ! To be honest, this didn't really bother me, and I kept running, as I was ramping up my training for the Utica Boilermaker 15k in July. That weekend was the annual Heart Run in Syracuse, which I did every year in honor of my father, who died in 1976 from his second heart attack. Back then, after his first heart attack in 1974, they didn't do any surgery, and basically put him on Coumadin and told him NOT to exert himself in any way. My father died when I was 21 years old.

Anyway, the weekend of the Heart Run in 2006, I ran 5 miles on Sunday morning. As I was finishing up my shower, the phone rang. It was my doctor, and he asked me what I thought was a funny question; " Have you been running ? " I answered of course I have, just finished 5 miles. He told me to stop right away due to the echocardiogram, I needed to see a cardiologist right away and he had already set up an appointment for me with a cardiologist.

My first ever visit to a cardiologist was not a good experience. This doctor had no use for runners and let me know it. He wanted to run a stress test and I agreed, but did not get a very good feeling from talking to him. As any runner would, I went to the stress test prepared to beat that damn treadmill. I changed into shorts, running shoes and tech t shirt (and I am so sure the doctor and nurses had never seen that before for a stress test !).

The stress test showed how bad the aortic valve was, and he predicted I would need surgery within six months or so. He said if I had to run, avoid hills, anything too long, and to not max out my heart rate (basically no racing, just running).

Afterwards, I began talking to anyone about heart issues, and found some recommendations for cardiologists from other weekend athletes like myself. I visited another cardiologist, who looked over my records, talked to me about running (he was a part time runner himself), and felt I should continue running. He said to listen to my body, and that if I paid attention, I would be able to tell him when it was time for the surgery to replace my valve. He let me train and run the Disneyland Half Marathon, which gave me both the inaugural Goofy Challenge and the inaugural Disneyland Half Marathon medal ! Now runners know what a big deal that is !

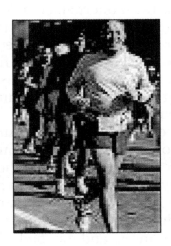

After finishing the half marathon in mid-September, I could hardly believe I had a heart problem. Sure my time was a little slow, but I did not race it, I just ran it. My training was easier than I had previously been using, so of course my time was slow.

Then, on Thanksgiving, a cold day in late November, I

went out for a quick and easy 3 miles to start the day. I felt very tired, and not quite right .... that's all I can call it. At the ¾ mile mark I had to stop and walk, and even then I could not really catch my breath. I decided to turn around and head home. I kept trying to run, but only went about 20-30 steps each time and had to stop and walk.

When I got home, I told my wife something was not right, that I was tired, but there was not pain or any other symptoms, but I should call the cardiologist on Friday. I took the first appointment I could, and stopped running all together until I could talk to the doctor. Funny thing was a neighbor had seen me running that Thanksgiving morning while he was driving down the road, and stopped to see if I was all right. He said he didn't really think it was me when he saw a runner on the side of the road, because I was going so slow and when he saw me, he said I did not look good.

When I went in to see the cardiologist, I told him my story about running on Thanksgiving, my wife added the part about my neighbor stopping his car to see if I was okay. My doctor got up and started walking out of the exam room. I asked where we were going, and he said, " Well, I told you your body would let you know when it was surgery time, and it just did, so let's set up the surgery ".

I started to panic. Up until now, it was just talk, and heck I was running up until a few days ago. Now it was serious. The doctor and I had previously talked about surgeons, so he already knew who to call to set up the office visit to discuss the surgery.

A few weeks later, I was in the surgeon's office. He briefly looked at my medical records, and we started to talk. He explained every aspect of the surgery and made me feel very at ease. I had chosen him because of his record (which was available from New York State on the internet), and recommendations from family and friends. He said my biggest decision was what type of valve I wanted, with the understanding he had the last say on what went into my chest based on what everything looked like when he got in there.

Now, I had been on www.Valvereplacement.org for months getting as much information as I could, and had acquired a lot of information on valve types. I really had not made any decisions, as both tissue and mechanical have good points and bad points. It really is a decision that you base on what you personally feel more comfortable with. Do you want a mechanical, which should last for your lifetime, but leaves you taking anti-coagulants the rest of your life along with the requisite testing that goes along with that. Then there are two types of tissue valves. The porcine vale is the actual aortic valve from a pig's heart. The bovine pericardial tissue valve is actually hand made from the pericardial tissue (the sack around the heart) from a cow.

While talking to the surgeon, he had a mechanical valve in his hand, slowly moving it back and forth and making it click. My wife asked if that was what it would sound like in my chest, and he said most likely it would. I then blurted out I wanted a tissue valve, and I knew he would like to use the Edwards bovine pericardial valve if possible. So we set the date for the surgery, January 27, 2007.

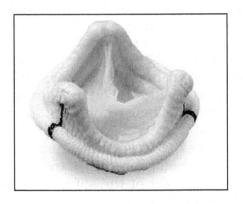

Image reproduced from:
http://www.heart-valve-surgery.com/heart-surgery-blog/2010/11/24/heart-valve-replacement-failure-aortic/

I had a heart catheterization for the day before surgery. My cardiologist did the cath, and found the left anterior descending artery partially blocked. We both agreed that while I was going to be wide open on the operating table, it might be a good time to get a bypass on that !

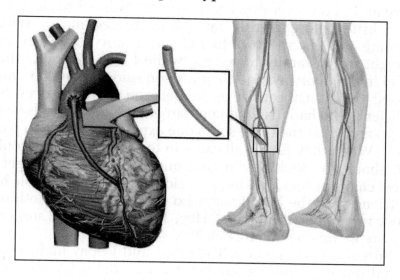

Illustration reproduced from:
http://en.wikipedia.org/wiki/Coronary_artery_bypass_surg ery

Surgery was at 7:30 the next morning so I got to spend that night in the hospital , on the heart floor, and talked with nurses and my roommate because I could not sleep.

The morning of surgery, my wife came to see me off. I remember waiting to go into the O.R. and talking with the man next to me who was a 80-something year old veterinarian who was still practicing part time, and was having a new aortic valve installed that day also. I remember being wheeled into the O.R. and sliding onto the table. Then they strapped my arms down and told me they would start some drugs. That's it ...

... Literally, the next second in my mind, I woke up in SICU, but couldn't open my eyes. I moved around, and remember the nurse talking in my ear that it was too soon, and I would be going back to sleep. The next time I woke up, same thing ...

The third time was a charm ... I woke up and had no breathing tube and could open my eyes. The nurse was right there and said everything was fine. She wanted to clean me up a little before getting my family to see me. While cleaning me up, she had to tell me a story. When she brought in my family to see me while I was still out, they stood in the doorway, and then my son said, " here I go " and passed out. Of course as he fell, he knocked over his girlfriend who had just had knee surgery. Now, my kids were 27, 30 and 33 at the time, so no one expected any one to pass out ! When they finally all came in to see me, all they could talk about was Nick passing out and how they had to get a wheel chair for him, and he got a ride out to the car, while his girlfriend with the bum knee, who took the hit, got nothing. I just remember thinking, " Hey, I just had heart surgery, why are we talking about Nick ?! "

Surgery was done on a Thursday, and Friday night I was moved down to the regular heart floor. Saturday morning brought doctors, nurses, helpers. I had the nurse write on the white board in my room all the things I had to accomplish to get out of the hospital: get the chest tubes removed, get the pacer wires out, walk the floor and also the stairs, pee on my own, and finally have a bowel movement !

By Saturday afternoon I had walked the floor, climbed the stairs, had my chest tubes out, had the pacer wires out, got the catheter out .... now it was just that darn bowel movement. By Saturday night, my nurse asked if I wanted some extra strong prune puree, he guaranteed it would get the bowels moving. By Sunday morning, he was right!

I went home Monday morning and continued recovery. I was given a basic walking program, where I walked around the house for 10, 15, 20 minutes, increasing slowly to 30 minutes in 2 weeks. After that I hit my treadmill (after all, it was February in Syracuse !). I increased my walking to one hour a day. Then twice a day, one hour at a time.

By the time I went back to my cardiologist for my 4 week check-up, he said I looked great and I asked if I could start running. He stated as long as my sternum was healed enough and didn't hurt, go for it ! So I started slowly, real slowly, as I was still on a number of drugs for recovery, including beta blockers that keep your heart rate low no matter what you try to do. At five weeks, I went back to my surgeon for a check-up and he was surprised I was already running ! He asked me to wait another week, as he felt more comfortable with me running at 6 weeks. So, being a good patient, I rested a week and started up again, even slower. My running during recovery was not a linear progression. Rather, I would run for a few weeks at the same pace, unable to improve at all. Then one day I would go out and BOOM, it was felt and I was a bit faster. Then, nothing for a few weeks, and BOOM, another jump in fitness.

Now, all along this journey I had been a regular on www.valvereplacement.org , and was interested especially in the active lifestyle forum where I read of other runners who had valves replaced and how their recovery went. Soon, one mentioned www.cardiacathletes.com , where heart patients with many different issues participated in various sports, but all recovered and helped each other in the process. So I joined up and found an extremely supportive group of people who understood the problems, concerns and issues with returning to (or starting up) athletic endeavors. I still find this site the most important part of my continuing recovery.

After recovering from surgery enough to get back into full training, I heard about **Medtronics Global Hero** program.

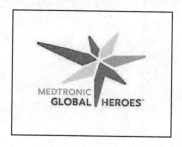

http://www.medtronic.com/globalheroes/

https://www.facebook.com/MedtronicGlobalHeroes

http://www.youtube.com/user/MedtronicGlobalHero

Medtronics is a medical device manufacturer in Minneapolis, and a major sponsor of the Twin Cities Marathon. Their Global Hero program picks individuals from among medical resumes sent to them, and invites them to Minneapolis to run either the 10 mile race, or the marathon, all expenses paid. Of course, I had to apply ! After submitting the application, I continued my training, and returned to the Utica 15k Boilermaker, finishing 20 minutes slower than the previous year. Soon after the race, I heard from Medtronics that I was accepted as a Global Hero, and could run the Twin Cities Marathon ! I had to get serious about training.

Also happening around this time, there was a group of runners on valvereplacement.org that started meeting up at races. The first year, 5 of them ran the marathon relay at Vermont City in Burlington. Although I had already been diagnosed, and told surgery was not far off, I did not join them because I thought it would be unfair as the rest had already had surgery and recovered.

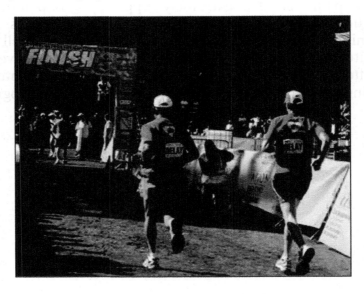

In 2007, they were meeting up for Akron Road Runner to run in relay teams. This year, more people were attending as the invitation was extended to Cardiac Athletes. So, I joined up, and in September, I ventured to Ohio and met an outstanding group of runners. We were hosted by Mark Siwik, who took care of preparations, making out the teams, getting the packets, hosting a brunch after the race so we could all meet and mingle some more. It was a weekend I will never forget. The camaraderie usually found among runners was amplified a thousand time over by the common heart issues as well as fondness for running. The weekend was truly a turning point in my recovery.

Just 5 days later, I was travelling to Minneapolis for the Twin Cities Marathon. My flight from Syracuse connected in Cleveland. As I waited at the gate, up walked Mark Siwik! He was also accepted as a Global Hero, and we would be travelling together ! We arrived in Minneapolis, and travelled to the host hotel.

The next day we were all given a tour of the Medtronics facility, met the officers of the company, and had a luncheon with employees. We met the other Global Heroes, who had differing medical devices, implanted defibrillators, deep brain stimulators, artificial heart valves, insulin pumps, pacemakers, but were runners ! We were given a bus tour of the marathon course, so those of us running the marathon would have a feel for the course.

Now, marathoners know how much we like to know the course, so now I knew we were being hosted by true runners!

Sunday morning, we were up at 6 a.m. to catch the bus (with the elite runners) to the start, and it was already 70 degrees ! In Minneapolis ! In October ! We arrived at the start at the Metrodome by 6:30. Now, usually it is good to be able to go into the dome to wait for the start, to stay warm. This day, I hung around outside as much as possible. The 10 mile race starts first, so I watched the start and then went to my corral. I was already sweating.

The race actually started a few minutes early, and we were off touring the city. The heat was already unbearable to me. Although the only medicine I was taking at this point after surgery was an aspirin and an ace inhibitor, I knew I was susceptible to the heat. The ace inhibitor keeps the blood vessels open, even though when I sweat and start to dehydrate, I need the vessels to constrict to keep my blood pressure up and not pass out. So, I was wary of the heat and took it easy. But by mile 10, I know I was in trouble. Water was pouring off the brim of my running hat, and it wasn't raining ! I was drenched from sweat.

The race had placed buses at each mile marker for people to drop out so as not to tax the medical facilities on the course. They had been announcing it every mile since mile 5. Despite their best efforts, the water stops were running out of water for those of us farther back. So coming up to mile 13, I decided it was time to stop and call it a race. This was my second DNF in my running career, and what hurt most was it was first attempt at the marathon post-surgery.

When I arrived back at the finish line area, I found I was the only one to drop out. I cheered the other runners home, but none of this made me feel any better. Later that day, I heard that they had closed the Chicago Marathon mid race due to the heat, and a few runners had died there. I also heard that they nearly cancelled the Twin Cities race. It had reached 80 degrees before the start, but it only got to 79 ! This race made me realize how important it was for me to now pay attention to my body, how I felt, how I was performing, and never assume I could handle anything. I was no longer the same person as before surgery. I could still run marathons, but I had to be smarter about it.

After that rocky start back to marathoning post-surgery, I continued to train, and finished the New York City marathon in 2008. I continued meeting up with the Cardiac Athletes every year. After Akron, I ran the half marathon at the Jersey Shore, ran on a marathon relay team at the Wineglass Marathon in upstate New York, and ran on a team at the Harrisburg marathon. Each year, our number of runners has grown, new people join us, and bring new experiences and energy to the group.

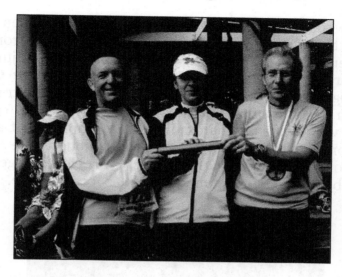

Three Cardiac Athlete relay team members holding the relay baton they handed to eachother during the race which carried the engraved name of their highly respected team mate 'Josh' who had sadly recently passed on. This was then presented to the deceased partner as a very touching souvenir of remembrance.

Along with these races, I had made a silent pledge to try and run the same races I had in 2006, the year leading up to my surgery. So, in 2009 I began to make plans for the Goofy Challenge and the Disneyland Half Marathon in 2010., and both would be their fifth anniversary of the race, so there would be special medals ! And, to add to the bling, Disney was awarding a special " coast-to-coast " medal for anyone who finished a race at Walk Disney World and a race in Anaheim in the same year ! Talk about a medal bonanza ! That sealed my decision. My training was going well, when in May I suffered a bit of a setback.   I was diagnosed with carcinosarcoma skin cancer. I was able to have it surgically removed with complete success.

In September, it was decided that I should undergo radiation treatments as the cancer I had was very rare.   I began treatment 5 days a week for six weeks. I was able to train through most of the treatments, until the last 2.   I became so tired that I could barely work, and then all I wanted to do was sleep. It took 2 weeks to recover from the treatments enough so I could start running again. I jumped head first back into my training schedule for the Goofy Challenge and never looked back. I do believe that training through the radiation treatments helped me. As cancer goes, I was better off than most of the people I met at the radiation treatment center. And to be honest, the whole cancer ordeal was not nearly as scary as the heart surgery, so this setback did not affect me as much as it could have.

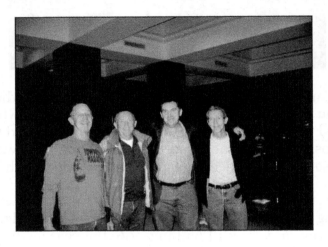

Harrisburg 2010, Lars finally meets some great guys ... who just happen to be Cardiac Athletes.

In January, 2010, I ran the 5th annual Goofy challenge, finishing both the half marathon and full marathon in the same weekend at Walt Disney World. Now, it was not without problems. It seems that weekend, Florida decided to set record low temperatures. Both races have a 6 a.m. start, and on Saturday it was snowing at the start ! It turned to sleet for the rest of the race.

At the finish, we were all cold, wet, and cold ! On Sunday morning it was 27 degrees at the start, and barely got above freezing at the finish. At all the water stops during the marathon, the road was covered with ice, and runners were falling.   Any spilled water from the cups instantly turned into ice on the roads.   My times were 10-20 minutes slower than in 2006, but I was happy to have conquered the challenge.

In September 2010, I travelled to Anaheim to run the fifth annual Disneyland Half Marathon.   It was great to be back there, and I ran about 10 minutes slower than in 2006. While I was in California, I was able to visit Edwards Lifesciences, where my artificial heart valve was made.   I was given an excellent tour that showed me all the steps that go into making my bovine pericardial tissue valve.   There was a museum display of the history of artificial heart valves which was very interesting as it showed how the valves have developed from very rudimentary to very sophisticated.   At the end, I was able to meet the people who actually made the very valve that was in my chest !   It was a very emotional moment.   I brought all my Disney race medals with me from over the years, and gave them to the people who's work had saved my life.   I have a picture of all of them with me, wearing the medals !

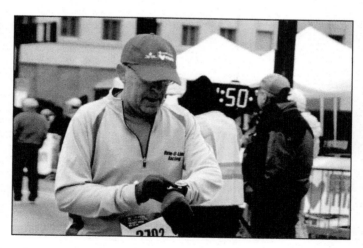

I continue to run, and race, and have come to terms with being slower than I was before surgery. I believe that I have a new appreciation for running, and find a camaraderie further back in the pack at a race that I didn't have when I was faster.   I no longer am a slave to a training schedule when training for a big race. I know I need to do the mileage, but I allow life to interrupt it. I just rearrange the training schedule around my personal life, and still accomplish my goals.

CHAPTER 6

Brad :

" OK Sir, you ARE having a heart attack. "

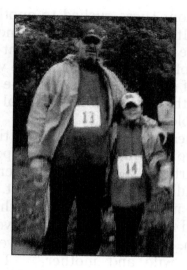

CARDIAC ATHLETE 6

First name: Brad
Forum name: "The New Me"
Country: USA
Diagnosis: Family History; Angina; Heart Attack
Treatment: Stent

It was the morning of December 15th, 2008 and I was blindsided by " OK Sir, you ARE having a heart attack ! " I don't know who that nurse was, but when she said those words, she did more to change my life than anyone else ever had. Those words sank into my being like a cold icicle and I began to shake, uncontrollably.

I looked past the foot of the ER bed at my wife, who was holding my 4 year old daughter. I could only catch glimpses of the panicked look on her face as bodies began to fill the room. I managed to get off our secret symbol using my fingers....1, 4, and 3...the number of letters in each word of "I Love You." That meant a great deal to me to get that message to her, because having lost my father at age 50 to a heart attack, I really didn't think I would make it through that day.

In short fashion, I was rushed to another hospital that had a Cath Lab. It was a bizarre trip for me, being inside an emergency vehicle as a victim, as I spent the previous 12 years as a police officer. Time and space were a blur and I soon found myself in the Cath Lab, with the physician having difficulty getting the Cath into my femoral artery because I was shaking so violently.

I remember hearing something about them sedating me and my next recollection was the tech pointing to a live picture of my heart and showing me the renewed blood flow after he successfully placed my new stent. I wasn't at all sure what this all meant at the time, but the relaxed pace of the people around me allowed me to believe that I might see the sun rise again. I was rolled to a recovery room, where I was met by my wife and mother. I was completely exhausted, most of all mentally. A nurse advised me that I was very lucky and that I appeared to suffer only minor damage to my heart muscle. I had a thousand questions and not one ounce of mental energy to entertain even one of them, I simply fell asleep.

I woke up, fully that is, in the ICU. Now what? How did I get to this point? I still laugh a little every time I see one of those statin drug commercials where the guy says " I couldn't believe it, a heart attack, at age 57." Well try it at age 41 if you want a real shocker ! I knew the family history, Dad at 50, his parents in their forties and my aunt at 48, heck, my older sister has had multiple heart attacks and is on oxygen, but the hard lesson is that knowing is not the same as experiencing.   Yes, I knew all this, but I still ate at McDonald's 2-3 times a week, never formally exercised and smoked for the past 20 years.   I just spent two days and an entire sleepless night chewing ant-acids for the terrible burning chest pain that could not be a heart attack, no way.

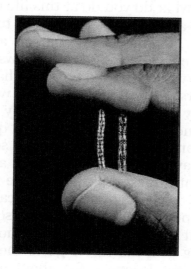

Stents. Image reproduced from: http://usatoday30.usatoday.com/news/health/2008-08-19-angioplasty-wrist_N.htm

On a funny side note to this disbelief of mine ... On that sleepless night before finally going to the ER in the morning, I figured, since I couldn't sleep, I would approach the wife for some intimacy.   Well, I was successful in my advances and afterward, I actually said to her (you can't make this stuff up) " Not bad for a guy who feels like he's having a heart attack, huh ? "   Thankfully, we are still able to laugh about that one.

I was living in a very typical, 40 something year old, mentality of immortality.   Walking blindly through what should have been an obvious, but too easy to ignore reality. Adding to my poor cardiac genetics was an incredible amount of stress.   Eighteen months before, I was forced to retire from my police career after two back surgeries, including a spinal fusion. We were struggling to survive, as I was unable to find a new job ... my world was crumbling and there were 3 young kids and a wife depending on me ... now this.

So now what, what do you do at this life changing fork in the road ? First and foremost, I wanted to live and for as long as possible. I am a strong person and usually very opinionated and educated about my views and decisions. The bad part here was that I had no idea what I was doing or what the best course of action would be. I was completely at the mercy of my doctors, who basically gave me good standard advice and told me to take it easy, quit smoking and take the medications they prescribed. And so home, I went.

Now some, maybe most people, put in a little effort and do mostly the right things, especially in the first few months post heart attack. I, on the other hand, became an overnight health fanatic. Apparently this really did scare me to death and I am so glad it did. The last puff of smoke I inhaled was just before getting into the car to go to the ER. I did use nicotine replacement lozenges for about a year, but have been nicotine free ever since. After examining and learning about my blood work, I decided that I was not going to eat saturated or hydrogenated fats, which is virtually impossible. Plenty of Omega3 fatty acids for my low HDL, fresh vegetables every day, Anti-oxidant rich foods, monitoring blood pressure daily, and the list goes on and on. Soon my blood work results were fantastic and my blood pressure was under control.

I had been walking my dog every night before the heart attack and resumed some walking almost immediately after. Started with a quarter mile and slowly worked my way back to the 2 miles I was doing before the heart attack.

Despite the new healthy lifestyle, all was not going well. Now the first month was great and I felt completely normal, with no ill effects that I could detect. But about five weeks after the event, I had that burning chest pain again. Panic quickly set in and I called my cardiologist, who I had only met once in the hospital. I guess I was demanding answers and wanted to know how I can tell if this is another heart attack. He really surprised and ticked me off with his cold hearted answer, " Go take your dog for a walk and if it gets worse, go to the ER." What ! Was he crazy !? I went to the ER and after several hours, I was released and nothing was found.

I had many difficulties and anxious ER trips over the next 6 months, only to find that I had acid reflux from some of my new medications. It was a bit more involved, but that's another story.

The important part of this story was my cardiologists advice, I hated him for that and even left him as a result of his callous directions. I later found out how valuable and important that advice would be. One night, after being tired of going to the ER only to feel embarrassed by the finding nothing wrong again, I went for that walk. I took my cell phone and my key fob with the nitro pills and I walked as fast as I could. Thirty minutes later, I was more confident about my physical well-being than I had been in many months. I did it, I exerted myself and found no increase in pain, and in fact I felt better. I provided myself with the proof I needed that I was not having another heart attack this time and for many times after that.

Naturally, I began to time my walks, in order to see if I was improving my physical well-being. Not long after, my competitive spirit kicked in and I started trying to beat my previous times. This led to short bits of jogging, a block or two during the whole walk at first. It was about this time that I saw my current cardiologist. When I told him what I had been doing for exercise, he quickly cautioned me and stated the following words, that still drive me to this day ...
"Don't push it and don't think you are going to run any marathons someday. " Ouch, that hurt ... he basically just told me that I was a cardiac cripple. If he knew me better, he probably would not have said that, because he lit my defiant fire. I really don't like being told what I can't do.

My next step, search the internet to see what I could find about post heart attack exercise. I Googled " how much running can I do after a heart attack ? " I found a myriad of sites and information and wandered into a site called **Cardiac Athletes**. " Bit of a play on words here " I thought ... Cardiac Athletes ? Oh did I hit the jackpot ! This place was filled with people just like me, people with cardiac illness that were pushing the limits and accomplishing truly ground-breaking things. This was the confidence builder I needed to go forth with my desire ... to prove my cardiologist wrong !

There really is nothing reckless going on at Cardiac Athletes. In my opinion, it is a gathering place for very brave souls, that are very much in tune with their health and conditions and are training and competing in a very smart fashion, all in the name of furthering the belief and understanding that exercise provides enormous benefits as a treatment for cardiac illness as well as a preventative measure. I didn't visit this website and suddenly start asking my heart to allow me to run five miles. What I did do, was realize that others have regained much of their athletic ability through proper training and monitoring of their heart conditions.

For me, it was the beginning of adding new, short running distances to my walk, until many months later when I was able to run 2.5 miles without a walking break. That led to adding distance, until September, 26, 2010, when I ran the first 5K race of my entire life, just 21 months after my heart attack. Just 21 months before, I was in such a deplorable condition, I honestly thought I was not going to make it through the day and now I was able to run 3.1 miles and do it faster than many of that days competitors that were much younger than me. I really did it, I really felt whole again, in control of my future again.

The improvement in my health and ability did not stop there. I continued to train and extend my distances and times. I never pushed beyond what felt comfortable, listening to my body as a guide to my limits. In November, I met with about fifty other Cardiac Athletes, at their yearly meeting, held at a running event. I joined 3 other amazing members in the form of a marathon relay team. As a new runner, they were gracious enough to give me the short leg of 4.6 miles. It seemed very long to me and I remember being very afraid of letting the others down, but the outpouring of support from my fellow Cardiac Athletes was incredible. We finished well, taking third place in the men's masters division. What a great feeling of accomplishment that was, to place in field of runners who were not former cardiac patients.

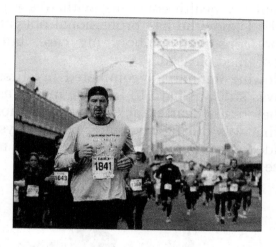

With the passage of time and continued training, the improvements continued. The following spring I ran my first 10K race, meeting a goal I had set of less than one hour. I wondered where this might lead and what my limits would be, if any. My fellow Cardiac Athletes were a constant source of knowledge, encouragement and inspiration. It wasn't long before I allowed a previously unimaginable goal into my plans, a half marathon. I was scared of it, but knew that completing it would bring me the ultimate feeling of vitality and confidence in my well-being, two things that the heart attack stripped from my mind. I signed up for my first half marathon, which was scheduled for September 16th, 2011, less than one year after my first 5K and less than 4 years after my heart attack. I followed a typical training program and felt fantastic on race morning, completing the race in 2hrs 11min 16sec. I cannot begin to express the value and importance this achievement held for me. I know it was also important for my family, because despite their steadfast support and encouragement, deep down I knew they were concerned about my heart health and the unknowns that come after a heart attack. I could see and feel the change in the attitudes of those around me. I showed them, as well as myself, that I was not a cardiac cripple. I was capable of physical tasks that I only dreamed about before the heart attack. I think we all breathed easier and allowed ourselves to relax about my health concerns, with was a huge stress relief for all. I know he has professional obligations to be cautious and conservative about my care, but even my cardiologist seemed pleased.

The following January, I completed my first 100 mile month. It was still was hard to imagine myself as a runner, just think, before my heart attack, I never ran more than 1.5 miles and that was during my yearly police physical. That spring, I added another half marathon and a 10 miler to my growing race bib and medal collection.

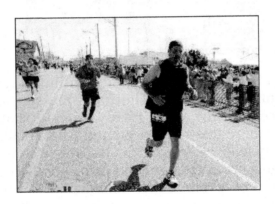

In the fall, I added my third and fastest half marathon at the Cardiac Athlete meeting in Baltimore. Spring of 2014 brought another 10 miler and my 4th half marathon, but it also brought my selection as a Medtronic Global Hero for the Fall 10 miler in the Twin Cities. I'm very excited and humbled by this honor. It is definitely a pinnacle moment in this journey and a very emotional one when I think of what went into getting to this point. Beyond Global heroes, there will be as much running and exercise as my body will allow and although there are no full marathons in my immediate future, it is very high on my bucket list.

All these post heart attack achievements meant a great deal to me and changed the perception of what a heart attack victim's life should be, for anyone that knew my situation. With my own health in check, I turned my attention to what became my greatest achievement. After my heart attack, or what many of us refer to as our "Wake Up Call," my focus was my family history, what went wrong for them and what can I do with that knowledge to increase my odds. The common issues I found were genetically low HDL, high blood sugar, high triglycerides and smoking. With dietary changes, medication, supplements and exercise, I was able to change these things to my favor. Now, I needed to break the chain, change the family history and do that by working with my children to increase their odds of a long and healthy life. My proudest and most important moment as a Cardiac Athlete was when my 10 year old daughter showed a desire to run a 5K race. I didn't have to beg her, preach to her or bribe her, I did it by example and that was a great feeling. It was the moment when I first felt that I broke that generational chain of setting the example of smoking, eating poorly and not exercising. It was the moment when I felt that I may have done the greatest thing I could for the future of my family, giving them a better chance of living long and healthy by showing them good habits rather than bad. I think giving them the memories of a father who ran 3-4 times a week, instead of a father that always had a cigarette hanging out of his mouth was the best way of giving them that chance. We trained and ran that 5K and several others in the year that followed. She still has interest in running and is already starting to think about longer distances.

My youngest daughter, the one seated on my wife's lap when I heard that I was having a heart attack, soon followed suit with her own 5k races. Now my wife has caught the running bug as well, running her first 10 miler and half marathon with me in the spring of 2014. I think it is very important to remember how are positive, healthy attitudes can project into the lives of those around us.

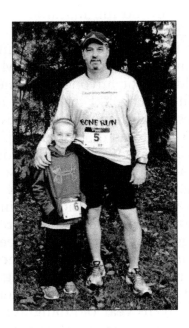

Cardiac Athletes also share an underlying, common mission. While we directly battle our personal issue and strive to inspire others, we also fight to change society's impression of a "cardiac cripple." It is an issue that many Cardiac Athletes face every day, the mindset that you are no longer capable of hard, physical activity, stressful situations and are now a fragile individual. It is the way others view, handle and trust your abilities. This is especially true in the workplace. I am one of many, who have had to hide their issue from the general public and workplace. While I am clearly more physically fit than many coworkers, it would be very detrimental to my employment if this issue was known. It is draining, demeaning and weighs heavily on one's life. Here I stand; strong, conquering major challenges and paving the way for others, yet these normally valuable traits in the workplace would be overshadowed by the misconceptions of my issue. This simply has to change; it is an antiquated, invalid mindset that has no place in our modern, medically technological world. When our hearts develop a problem, they can not only be repaired; they can heal and perhaps most importantly to this mindset...improve. We face a monumental task as Cardiac Athletes, we face a world that may not be ready for us, but one by one, event by event, we are changing their minds.

What did I learn from all this......It has been almost five years since that wakeup call and I've had plenty of time to reflect on what it has meant of this during all those runs. I know I am very lucky, not everyone can survive a heart attack and those that do may not find themselves in a condition that will allow them to exercise. I know now, just how precious life is. I look at everything differently. I no longer have the word "Someday" in my vocabulary, as in "Someday I'll do that." I know that I was living blindly before the heart attack, taking many things and time for granted. I now cherish things and think more deeply about them. I feel blessed to have the ability to inspire others and to do my part to break the mold of the "cardiac cripple" in our society. The list goes on, but overall, I would say that I have a new level of self-awareness.

Knowing what I know now, what advice would I give.....I would tell anyone who finds their self-facing recovery from a cardiac or other serious illness is that what seems like a curse at first, may in fact be a gift. While I have certainly, at times, felt the worst, gut wrenching, anguish as a result of the heart attack, I have also truly lived more in the past five years than I did in the 41 years before it. It took a lot to come to grips with my situation, but I now know that I would rather live the way I am now, than live blindly through an entire life without a wakeup call.

What message would I like to send.....I think my place as a Cardiac Athlete is to inspire those who are not athletes recovering from a cardiac issue, but those who were not athletic before their issue. I want those people to see that it doesn't have to ever be too late to become athletic. There are many, like me, who find themselves with cardiac issues as a result of an unhealthy lifestyle. In fact, it is probably the most common type of scenario leading to cardiac problems. But, it does not mean that you can't take control of your life, change your habits and live on as a healthy, active person. I know there are many people, just like me, waiting to be inspired, looking for many answers and needing guidance and direction. I know this is not for everyone, but if this sounds like the type of change you need, ask your doctor and if it feels right, start jogging a few blocks on your dog walks....you may just wind up with a great new life and a few medals too!

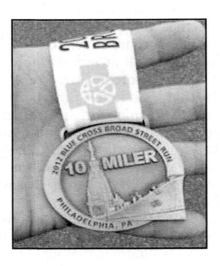

My first year was tough; I used to count each passing month as " Bonus Months ", as in extra months of life that technology gave me. Now, I don't celebrate the months. I'm now adding up my " Bonus Years ", as in the extra years I am getting because of perseverance with my new healthy lifestyle and becoming **" The New Me "**.

CHAPTER 7

Aimee :

"I have kids who need me. I'll have the surgery."

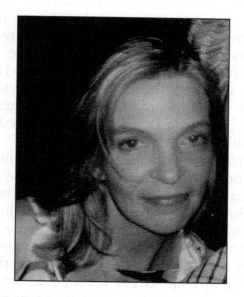

CARDIAC ATHLETE 7

First name: Aimee
Country: USA
Diagnosis: Aortic Regurgitation; Aortic Aneurysm
Treatment: Aorta and tissue Aortic Valve Replacement

Dec of 2009, I underwent the most in-depth, invasive battery of medical tests I'd ever experienced. I was a bone marrow match for someone stricken with cancer. As a donor, one must be perfectly healthy. Admittedly, I was a little worried.

What if the doctors found some terrible disease? What if I had cancer too, or my heart was failing? The donation coordinator assured me my fears were normal and if the doctors did find something wrong, I'd have the ability to treat it before it really harmed me. Advance warning can be a lifesaver.

I walked through the University of Michigan oncology unit to get one last physical check and the final decision from the doctors. They listened, poked, prodded, measured and poured over a thick file of test results.

Chest x-rays, heart monitors, blood tests, urine samples, mouth swabs, you name it every last bit of my body was checked and two female oncologists held the results in their hands. They looked me over, examine the results individually, came back in the room and looked at each other smiling. One turned toward me, smiled broadly and said, "You're really healthy aren't you? Younger than your biological age." And on Dec 15, 2009 I shared some of my good health with a sick stranger in need of it.

Dec 9, 2010 I was on a gurney after spending three days in the cardiothoracic intensive care unit at the University of Michigan. I was saying goodbye, possibly for the last time, to my family. How was I the picture of health just a year ago and on my deathbed now? It didn't make sense.

What I knew was sometime over the summer, exhaustion had overtaken me. One day, I fell asleep on the couch and could not bring myself to get up and do anything for 18 hours. I was training for a 5k and could never really build up to one. I always had to walk a bit, even when following a strict plan. I blamed my crazy work schedule, my lack of determination, anything but a physical problem.

When I went for a check-up and the doctor pressed the stethoscope to my heart, the answer was swirling around. I had a heart murmur. I was reassured it was no big deal, everyone has a murmur at one time or another. But, I needed to get it checked because mine was, "loud."

My Doctor scheduled me for an in office EKG on Friday. But something struck her as odd. A nurse called and told me the Doctor had changed her mind and she sent me for an emergency echo the Monday before my EKG.

I knew right away in the echo, something was wrong. During tests, a tech normally administers the test but says nothing. My tech asked me if I came in due to pain. When I told her I wasn't in any pain, her expression was pure shock and could not be hidden. "You're not in pain?" She remained silent for the rest of the echo, but I knew if I should be in pain, she had seen something. When she was done, rather than sending me on my way and telling me my doctor would call in a few days with results, she said she needed to get permission from the head cardiologist to see if I could leave.

My heart sunk. Something was horribly wrong with me. She came back, told me I could go home, but not to lift anything. I explained that I had to work on Wednesday and I lift things when I work. I thought I might need to get a note. She shook her head no, and said I would not be working on Wednesday. I would see a doctor before then.

I began to brace myself for the worst. I called my family to brace them as well. Everyone thought I was overreacting. Maybe it was nothing. But I knew with every bit of my being something bad was happening in my heart. I just had no idea how bad.

As I pulled the door to my house open, my cell phone rang. It was my doctor's office. When I answered my heart sunk again. It was not a nurse, as is standard protocol. It was my Doctor. I don't think my brain could process the information properly. I heard only bits of what she said. "Large Aortic Aneurysm. Don't drive. Get a ride. Go straight to the ER. there's a cardiothoracic surgical team waiting."

My second grader was about to come home from school. My eighth grader was upstairs sick. I couldn't be this sick, they needed me!

I started to weep a bit on the phone. My Doctor started to softly apologize like she was consoling someone at a funeral. "I'm sorry. I'm so sorry." I felt, at that moment, like it was my funeral. I immediately started making calls.

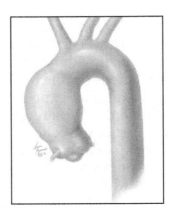

Illustration reproduced from:
http://www.ucaorta.org/ascending-aortic-aneurysms.html

I could not bring myself to tell my children. I knew facing them was going to be the hardest. I knew I wouldn't be able to stay strong. And I knew I had to.

I called my work first to let them know they needed to cover my shift. I started laughing through tears when the voice on the other end asked, "Well...do you think you'll make it in on Friday?" Then I began breaking the news to my family. One by one I called, staying calm and repeated the word aneurysm. My family has a history with aneurysms so there was no need to explain further. My Father had suffered a brain aneurysm when I was in second grade. We knew all too well that there was a very good chance I wouldn't survive. It almost seemed impossible that we would be lucky enough to have two aneurysm survivors in one family. My mind then focused on my children. I think in that moment I got angry at my body for being weak. I was mad on behalf of my children and I was ready to fight like Hell. They needed me. My mind shifted from fear and self-pity to fight. No way I was leaving my children this soon. No way.

When my ride arrived to take me to the hospital, I let him tell my little boys. We all hugged and I let my mind go to that place again. I wondered if it would be the last time I got to hug my children. As my oldest son began to softly cry, that fight bubbled up in me again. I laughed as if it was nothing and told him not to worry. I said I was a fighter and tried to reassure him there was no way I was going to die. After that, I refused to weep or feel sorry for myself. I was bracing for a fight and I only allowed myself to visualize winning.

I arrived at the hospital making inappropriate jokes. It was the only thing I could do to maintain composure. "Talk about a bleeding heart Liberal, huh?" I casually walked up to check in to the ER. "Hi, I'm Aimee Bingham and I have an aneurysm." I couldn't deny the seriousness at that point.

A flurry of activity surrounded me. Someone swooped in behind me with a wheel chair. Someone else shouted, "The aneurysm is here!" And before I could so much as give a birth date or the proper spelling of my name, I was rushed away.

I continued to act as if the response to my arrival was no big deal. "Wow, what great service! I've never had this short of a wait in the ER!" My mind was trying to deny the truth so that I could stay strong. But, I became somewhat of a carnival attraction with the staff. Doctors and nurses all wanted to be a part of my team. And when nobody was looking, they would sneak over to me, grab my hand and say a version of the same thing. "You are a miracle. You shouldn't have walked into the ER. You shouldn't be alive. It's amazing. I've never seen anything like it." I didn't tell my loved ones because I didn't want to scare them.

As luck would have it, or perhaps because I was a medical marvel, I got the very best heart surgeon the University of Michigan had to offer. I didn't know who he was at the time. But I could tell by the way the Doctors and nurses seemed to bow down before him, that I had received a revered and impressive surgeon. He walked in and normally confident doctors started to act like intimidated children. I had no idea people wait for months to see him. I was not aware other hospitals pattern their Cardiothoracic intensive care units after the one he developed for the University of Michigan. And I wouldn't know until later that he has the nation's largest practice treating aortic aneurysmal disease and valve repair. I could tell when a hush fell over a giddy crowd, he was something big: a Pavarotti amongst church choir singers. My friend is the former Dean of the Medical School's son. When he found out what was happening he sent a text. "Get Dr. Deeb. If you don't have him I'll call my Dad and make it happen."

Dr. Deeb walked in the room and exuded confidence. He did not mince words. My mind was trying hard to minimize what was happening. Dr. Deeb did not allow that luxury. "Do you know who John Ritter is?"

I nodded yes. My Mother and Sister were in the room with me. He looked at both of them and back at me. "Do you remember how he died ?" I did. I remember a still youngish man, in his 50's, looking pretty healthy, and then dropping dead on the set of his TV show. "You have John Ritter disease. If you don't have surgery and your aneurysm dissects, even in the hospital with me next to you, you will drop dead. I won't be able to save you."

My Sister and Mother started to cry. I swallowed hard and sent them out of the room. I could not afford weakness and their tears might allow my own to fall. I was not entertaining death, only survival. He went on to give statistics. If my aneurysm dissected my chance of survival was less than 5%. If I got the surgery my survival rate was 85%. He added, and I am paraphrasing with my overall good health and his ability, my chance for survival was really much higher. "I have kids who need me. I'll have the surgery." He nodded and said, "I think you made the right choice."

I really had no idea how bad things were for me. None. My mind was in complete, no time to die I have kids to raise, ignore, ignore, ignore mode.

A month after surgery, I met with a PA for a check-up. I think it hit me then, a full month after the ordeal. She looked at my MRI while I was in the room and her reaction told me. "I've worked for Dr. Deeb for 20 years and have never seen an aneurysm this big."

During the same check-up, a tech administering my echo

said she'd seen aneurysms that big. She was about a year from retiring. But she added they were always the ones that travelled down toward the stomach, never up toward the neck. She said sort of casually, maybe because I did survive, "I'm sure there have been aneurysms this big, but those people never made it to the hospital."

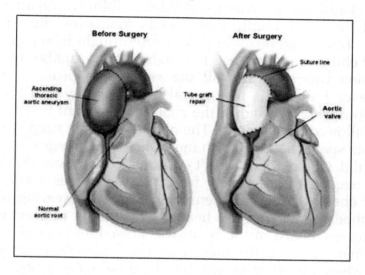

Image reproduced from:
http://www.heartosaurus.com/2010/09/what-is-ascending-aortic-aneurysm-in.html

How big was it? 7 centimeters. And on screen, in 3D, it looked like my artery had bulged out like a golf ball. It is why Dr. Deeb showed up to take the case. It is why people were grabbing me and telling me how miraculous it was I'd walked into the hospital. It's why the Tech asked me if I was in pain. The aneurysm was huge. Most arteries rupture before they stretch that far. I was a medical anomaly and based on everything we know about the heart, I should be dead. But there I sat in the ER, being ohhed and ahhed over by people who see terrible medical situations every day, cracking jokes and refusing to cry.

Just as my artery stretched beyond its limits to survive,

so too did my mind. I actually believed they were going to release me and schedule the surgery later. I was not released. Instead, I went straight to the Cardiothoracic Intensive Care Unit.

The people on my unit were 70 to 80 years old. The whole floor was quiet. I came in and shook everything up. At 35, I still had my parents, children, siblings, and an active social life. My family and friends took over the waiting room. Boxes and boxes of pizza were brought in and passed. Small children played tag. I brought chaos. And because my situation was so grave, all the rules were broken. I ate whatever I wanted. No special heart healthy diet for me. Children were allowed in the room. More than two visitors were allowed in the room. The night before my surgery three visitors spent the night with me. One of them was a 13 year-old child. One of them wasn't even related, but was a friend.

I needed to be anxiety free. So the nurses turned the other cheek when people entertained me by wearing blown up rubber gloves on their heads. They didn't redirect when the nurses' board in the room was erased and covered with drawings. In fact, the only time any redirection was given was when my visitors got too loud and disturbed other patients. And the one rule we were given was that my youngest son not walk down the hall where the man who had just received a heart transplant was recovering. The germ issue was dangerous for them both.

One woman, working the desk did try to make us follow the rules. She must have been informed, through orders from the great and powerful Dr. Deeb, that I was the exception. Because one day she stepped in and apologized, "I'm sorry. We just aren't used to this. Our patients aren't usually this young. They don't have so many family and friends. I'm not trying to be rude to anyone. I'm just a little overwhelmed."

The day of my surgery is a blur. I was constantly under the influence of strong anti-anxiety medication so my blood pressure and heart rate remained low. It left me smiling and fearless but foggy.

I remember the odd sensation of being in pre-op. A line

had been jabbed into my neck and I was being attached to different machines, once that was done my family was able to come in and say goodbye to me. It was a very odd experience because, in those moments just before what could be death, people are supposed to impart words of comfort or wisdom. But my mind was still in denial. I was not going to die so I wasn't going to say goodbye to anyone.

My Dad sternly warned me that the universe is only right when kids bury their parents, not the other way around. I could only impart that I would be at his funeral, sick as it sounds. My son begged me not to die on him. I with 100% confidence told him, no problem. I have this.

Before surgery I wanted to write each of my sons a letter, just in case. But writing it seemed like admitting that I was not going to make it. So I took the chance and left them without letters. I could not entertain my last goodbye, even for a second.

As soon as my family was gone I woke up. I was back in my room. But I was blind and could only make out the sun was shining in my eyes through the window. The same nurse was there from the day before so I did not realize I'd been out for 15 hours. I still thought it was the day before. And I was a little bewildered. Where did everyone go? I found out later what had happened.

I was supposed to wake up at 9 am. So the family and friends that sat through what must have been ten hours of torture waiting for word that I made it through surgery, were told to go home and get rest. They were allowed back to see me as I slept on life support, and then they went home.

Everyone was to return by 9 when I would be roused from my medically induced slumber. But it didn't work out that way. I woke up 3 hours early trying to get the tube out of my throat.

My ICU nurse told me I had a fighting spirit and that it would help my recovery. I am told when I woke the ICU staff erupted in applause and cheering. Dr. Deeb had worked some sort of medical magic. He had to replace ten inches of my aorta due to damage. And for what I believe is the first time ever, he was able to do that AND give me a tissue heart valve. Together, we made history.

Most people with the amount of damage I had end up with mechanical valves. But I was very young and mechanical valves can really change how a person lives their life. Tissue valves require less medication and regular monitoring. Dr. Deeb wanted me to live a normal life after surgery. He wasn't sure if he could do it, but he was going to try. I had no idea, when I woke, what I had inside keeping my blood going in the right direction. But what I had was a valve made from the tissue of a pig. I became even more of a medical marvel than when I walked into the ER.

When I tell people my story, the first question is always if I appreciate every moment because of it. Everyone wants a success like mine to have a beautiful happy ending. The truth of the matter is, when you have heart surgery, they tell you about all the physical systems and issues you will experience. The people in charge of care giving let you know how to care for your body. I was warned about what would happen to me mentally. But not nearly as much as I was told how to eat right how to care for my body. The reality of it was, my body made a full recovery very quickly. I was released from the hospital three days after I woke up from heart surgery. The most difficult part of my recovery was the subsequent emotional havoc it caused.

A year earlier I was labelled healthy, really healthy. There was no warning and further no reason anyone could find at the time. So I walked around every single day with the horrible fear that I was going to abruptly drop dead.

Uncontrollable thoughts would pop in my head. I would be shopping and think, "I'm just going to fall down dead right here in the produce section." A few weeks after my surgery, I had a dream I was trying to make plans with my friend and couldn't because her only free day was going to be the day of my funeral. I once woke up gasping for air around the same time because I had been dreaming I was drowning. I was haunted by the fact that my situation was rare and there was nothing to predict it, no way to change it, nothing I could take charge of myself to prevent it from happening again. I was thin, I had low blood pressure and my cholesterol was good. I didn't have a reason I could help control and that terrified me.

The thing that helped me stave off the demons in my mind was finding a group of people like me. I ran 5k's previous to heart surgery. But, due to my expanding heart and ruined aortic valve, I could never really build up endurance to run further or faster. My mind turned the idea of being able to run and being able to run even further than average healthy people, into me being normal again.

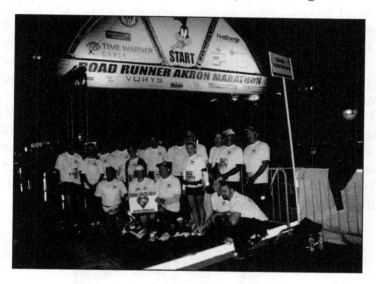

I found Cardiac Athletes online and saw all kinds of people with amazing comeback stories. I wanted one of my own. I literally started to run away from death, run away from bad dreams, run away from everything I'd been through. When I could finally run twelve miles without stopping and previously couldn't make three, I started to feel normal again. I started to feel like maybe I wasn't going to drop dead in the produce section.

Running made me feel better emotionally. It gave me a sense of power over my situation when I felt really powerless. I knew when my heart and lungs didn't prevent me from going the distance that I was still healthy in between checkups. I knew when I didn't hit the wall I'd been hitting with running before my surgery, I was really okay. I was going to make it. I was strong. After being a, "should have dropped dead already," patient, all I wanted was strength.

If I were to offer anything to someone just going through heart surgery it is this: take care of your mind as much as you take care of your body. Depression, anxiety, and even mental confusion are all very normal things to experience after heart surgery. The people around you mean well. But they want to hear you say every day is a gift. And the truth is, some days it won't seem that way. You might even have days that make you wonder why you survived. If you do get sad, the friends and family around you likely won't understand it. I am sure he meant well, but I had someone tell me to, "just get over it " because I'd survived.

It doesn't have to be that way. If you experience those feelings, know they are normal and know it does not make you weak to get help for it. A professional is far more prepared to handle what you're going through than your family and friends are. They went through it all with you and have their own set of emotions with which to deal.

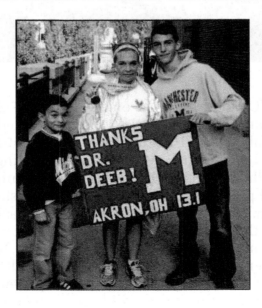

Strenuous (Doctor approved) activity is a great way to feel better. You can feel your body get stronger and the activity releases the good, happy chemicals in your brain. You are not a fragile ruined thing because you had open-heart surgery. You do have some control. And after what you've been through, being able to take charge is a great feeling.

Nine months after being lucky to be alive I crossed the finish line for my first half marathon. Never have I felt so empowered and in charge of my outcome than in that moment.

CHAPTER 8

Tom W :

" You've got a heart murmur ! "

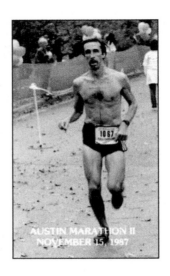

CARDIAC ATHLETE 8

First name: Tom
Country: USA
Diagnosis: Mitral Valve Regurgitation; Mitral Valve Prolapse
Treatment: Mitral Valve repair

My murmur

" You've got a heart murmur ! " I first heard this during a physical in my teen years. In later years, it would usually be the first thing a doctor would tell me when I received a physical exam. I know... I have a heart murmur.

A heart murmur, most specifically in my case a "mitral valve prolapse" means that one of my heart valves wasn't closing properly and was allowing some blood to regurgitate (flow backward) from my left ventricle to my left atrium, making a murmuring noise.

My heart murmur didn't stop me from running. I competed in high school and was captain of my college cross country team. I had to be a runner. I was too skinny and poorly coordinated to be successful in most sports, too tone deaf for music and too ugly for much of anything else.

My heart murmur served me well. During my draft physical, the doctor said, "We can't draft you, boy. You've got a bad heart murmur." Because of my heart murmur, I was able to miss the Vietnam War experience.

In bygone days, I placed first in my 35-39 age group at the 1987 Austin Marathon and in spite of my heart murmur I did pretty well in competitive running. I could usually place high in my age group (typically fourth in my age group when there were three awards). At my best, I've dipped under 3 hours in the marathon, one hour for 10 miles and 5 minutes for a mile. I've run the Boston Marathon and Pikes Peak Marathon and have completed Century (100 miles) bike rides. I won a few small races here and there.

Running has been and is a major part of my life for the past 48 years. Summing up my logged miles, I've run over 50,000 miles in those years and biked another 10,000. It's hard to imagine my life without running.

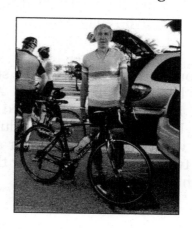

Surgery

"One of these days you're going to need surgery to repair that heart valve" was a typical bit of advice I'd get from doctors. In some ways, I looked forward to valve surgery. If my heart could become more efficient, maybe I could run faster.

Finally, in 2002 at the age of 52, my cardiologist said, "It's time to get your heart valve repaired." My heart was becoming enlarged and doctors warned of troubles. My wife and I researched the subject and found the best heart valve surgeon at one of the best clinics in the world. I had my mitral valve repaired. It was stitched up to close tighter and stop murmuring.

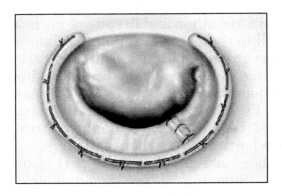

Illustration reproduced from:
http://my.clevelandclinic.org/heart/disorders/valve/mitral-valve-repair.aspx

There were some complications after surgery but after two months I was back running ... slowly. After 6 months I ran my first race. It was slow but I expected the road back to be long and hard. I was willing to pay my dues to come back. After 8 months I wasn't improving. After a year I stopped improving. After two years it became clear that the effects of aging are outweighing any recovery.

The Results

What was the net effect of the surgery on my running? In one quick procedure, heart surgery had reduced me from a 52 year old runner to someone who was shuffling along like a 65 year old. Two months before the surgery, I ran a marathon averaging in the 7:30 per mile range. After surgery, with an all out effort, I'm lucky to beat that time for a single mile. My surgery had cost me about 45-60 seconds per mile, compared with my pre-surgery times.

Before surgery, I was competitive in the 50 and over men's age group. Now, I compare my time with how I would have placed in the 50 and over WOMEN's category (and I seldom would win). In spite of my best efforts, I essentially went from being a runner to being a plodder.

I still go to races and see my friends and former rivals, however briefly, as they fade over the horizon once the gun goes off. I wouldn't see them again until the award ceremony when they were given the medals I wanted to compete for.

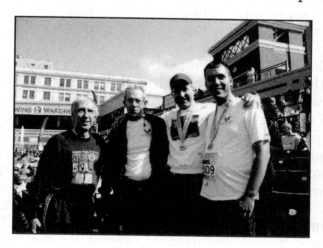

What could explain this drop in performance? I had the same legs, the same lungs, the same blood vessels, the same competitive attitude and the same training volume. The only thing that could explain this sudden drop in performance was the effect of the surgery.

But my mitral valve repair surgery was a "success". How could my performances get dramatically worse? I learned that "success" means different things to different people. To doctors, the disappearance of my murmur was indication of a success. To me, the drop in performance meant it was less than a complete success.

I had a lot of testing done and the answer became clear. Before surgery my ejection volume (the volume my heart produces on each beat) was 132 ml (although some of it was regurgitating). After surgery it was 85 ml. My heart simply wasn't pumping as much blood and it is blood that carries oxygen to the muscles. Without oxygen, my legs were tiring at a pace at which I could cruise comfortably a year earlier.

I had exercise treadmill test and spec imaging before and after surgery. Here are the results:

	Pre-surgery (2 months)	Post-surgery (8 months)
Ejection fraction %	48	49
Diastolic volume, ml	276	176
Systolic volume, ml	144	091
Ejection volume, ml	132	085

The key words in the report were "mitral valve stenosis". Due to the surgery, my mitral valve was narrowed beyond what it was originally. (NASCAR fans can relate to this in terms of running with a restrictor plate.) My mitral valve is choking me whenever I try to run hard.

By profession, I'm a hydraulic engineer so I could understand this. In engineer's terminology, I had positive displacement pump (my heart) with a throttled valve (mitral). In my job, I'd replace the valve, but that involves open heart surgery. Having gone through that once, I had no desire for a repeat performance, except for matters of life and death.

I've talked with any doctor who would listen, asking them about procedures to restore my heart pumping capacity, but I understand nothing short of open heart surgery is likely to correct my condition. Unless someone comes up with a new procedure to better open up my valve after valve repair surgery, as a runner, I needed to lower my sights.

Lesson Learned

My advice for athletes considering valve repair surgery is to make sure you warn your surgical team to "do no harm". A restrictive mitral valve may be better than a leaky valve. I'm not in a position to give medical advice but I can warn athletes to know what they are getting into.

The day before surgery my cardiologist and I discussed why I was having the surgery and the reason I gave was "To improve the quality of my life." The long term effect I can see from the surgery is a loss in the quality of my life, plus the surgery will probably prolong my death.

There is a saying, "When your only tool is a hammer, then everything looks like a nail." Doctors know how to repair heart murmurs, so they're more than happy to do it. They fixed mine. They don't know how to correct the resulting lower in pumping capacity. So, they aren't interested in talking about it.

Yes, the surgery didn't kill or cripple me. I still can function as a "normal human being", but, in some ways, I don't want to be a normal human being. I want to be a runner.

Doctors try to console me with, "At least you don't have that heart murmur anymore." There are days when I kind of miss my heart murmur.

Recent Times

Things aren't getting better with age. In the winter of 2012, I noticed I felt terrible when I tried to run, especially when I would hit a hill. My cardiologist checked it out and I had gone into afib (atrial fibrillation). Instead of going "lub-dub" the way it should, my heart was basically going "pfft-dub". During normal activity, I didn't notice it, except for a higher resting pulse, but when I tried to exert myself, my heart couldn't provide sufficient oxygen. I read that afib is not uncommon for people who had heart valve surgery.

After two months on meds, I underwent electrical cardioversion where they stop your heart and jump start it with electrical shocks to get it back into sinus rhythm. So far it's working. My cardiologist has me on a blood thinner (Xarelto) and beta blocker (Metoprolol) "for the rest of my life". The beta blocker isn't bad although it has probably slowed me down even further, but the blood thinner has turned me into a virtual hemophiliac who bleeds and bruises at the slightest provocation.

My latest adventure started summer 2012 with my routine checkup with my primary care doctor. After listening to my heart, he said, "We better run an EKG on you." (not a good sign.) The nurse ran it and brought in the senior nurse and they ran it again (not a good sign). Then they started moving the leads around and making sure they were connected right (not a good sign). My doctor looked at the EKG and said "We should put a Holter monitor on you." (not a good sign.)

I wore the monitor for a day. My primary care doctor, said "See your cardiologist" (not a good sign). I saw my cardiologist and his conclusion was, "Yeh you could go into afib at any time but keep on your meds with no restrictions." (phew).

Here is a summary of the findings. Maybe somebody can translate into English. "... evidence of a first degree AV block and probably a nonspecific intraventricular conduction defect ... rare unifocal PVC ... 17,826 APCs ... 4 runs of nonsustained SVT ... no major ST segment shifts ... isolated pauses ... most were less than 2 seconds ... no major arrhythmia."

AV block can be caused by beta blockers and he has me on a low dose now. Those APCs are, I believe, atrial premature contractions, which I understand are common, but one every 6 seconds or so sounds excessive. I think SVTs are supraventricular tachycardia, which I understand are a bit more serious.

My interpretation of all this is that my heart's electrical system is pretty messed up but not in an immediately life threatening way.

So I continue to run and bike and try to do the best I can. I think I'm alive today with a good quality of life because of my athletic endeavors. At 62, I ran a 1:54 half marathon and a 24:17 5K, nothing great but pretty satisfying for all I've been through. I still can take home age group awards at small races.

Meanwhile, I try to give back to the sport by serving on the Board of Directors of our local running club and maintenance person for our local rails-to-trails. I help out at running events when I can't run, due to my periodic injuries (don't get me started on injuries).

Cardiac Athletes

Finding the Cardiac Athletes web site has been a blessing. First, it pointed out to me what a whiner I am, complaining about my running results. When I compare what I've been through with the experiences of other members, I realize that most of the other members have been through a lot worse than me and I'm fortunate to be where I am at this point in my life. It turns out that in spite of my problems, I'm doing better than a lot of folks. I need to count my blessings.

Second, the American annual get-togethers organised by **H.E.A.R.T.** are a lot of fun.

http://heartorg.forumotion.com/

I participated in our marathon relay teams in the Wineglass Marathon in 2009, the Harrisburg Marathon in 2010 and the Akron Marathon in 2011. I had a great time at these events and look forward to doing more with the group. I'm proud to wear my Cardiac Athletes shirt.

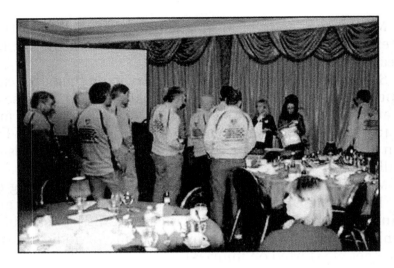

Third, I appreciate the support from the other cardiac athletes. Their stories of overcoming adversity are truly inspiring. I feel privileged to be among them and they are just nice people. I know Lars doesn't like the expression "cardiac cripple", but in a way we are crippled to some extent. But instead of taking things lying down, we are thumbing our noses at our problems and doing our best to overcome them. As one runner said at the 2009 meeting, "we are a life affirming group." It's great to be a member.

I live in Nanticoke, Pa. and have been running competitively since 1965. I am an engineer with Bentley Systems, Inc. and can be contacted on: Tom.Walski@Bentley.com

CHAPTER 9

Venkat :

" Do you not believe in miracles ? "

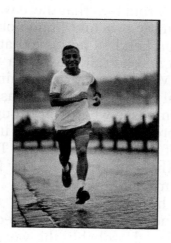

CARDIAC ATHLETE 9

First name: Venkat
Country: India
Diagnosis: Angina; Heart Attack
Treatment: Six Bypass Grafts

In Oct 2006 I was training to run the half marathon in the Standard Chartered Mumbai Marathon to be held in January 2007 when I felt myself unusually short of breath. I also had pain radiating, down my arm, my jaws ached. In short all the classical symptoms of an Angina of which I had read many, many times before.

I talked to my radiologist friend and told him about this and I also told him that I wanted to do a CT Angio to rule out any possibility.   He mockingly told me that since I seem to be having a fixation with Coronary Artery Disease, I might as well get the CT Angio done and rule out that possibility.

Two days later I was lying in the bed at a CT Angio center in Mumbai and I had driven down there on my own. After the test got over, I got up and dressed and went to meet the doctor. The doctor's face was quite ashen.

He made me sit down and asked me how I was feeling with apprehension and deep concern. He asked me what had brought me there, what was the incident and who else had come with me. I told him that there was no incident and that I had driven on my own and I had nobody else with me. He could not comprehend as he looked at my CT Angio on the monitor screen and he said there is a 100% block at the branch of the Left Main Artery. In his mind this indicated a massive Myocardial Infarction and he was wondering how I was so calm and composed when everything was awry.

But my story probably should begin in the year 1931 in my native village of Sedanipuram in the Thanjavur District of Tamil Naidu in the south of India. My father was born in 1929 and in 1931 my grandfather died.   My grandmother had told us that he was quite alright until one day he suddenly died and nobody knew why. Medical facilities then were not advanced and probably the word Coronary Artery Disease did not even exist in the dictionary then.

Skipping the decades, in 1980 my father's colleague one day came rushing home and told me that my father was in a taxicab and that there was something drastically wrong with him. I immediately rushed down to see what had happened and I found my father in the rear seat groaning and completely drenched in sweat.   I did not know what was happening, I took him to the Medical Dept. of Air India where he was employed and from there we rushed to the Cardiac Incentive Care Unit of a hospital. Soon words like cholesterol, cardiac disease, myocardial infarction, angina entered my vocabulary.

After discharge my father tried to manage the disease medically but by 1984 we discovered that he could not even climb the staircase of our two storey house.   A Coronary

Artery Bypass Graft (CABG, pronounced Cabbage) was in order and in those years in India such surgeries were rare and the failure rate were said to be 50%, which was not at all comforting.

Fortunately we could travel to London from India and he was operated in the Princess Grace hospital at Baker Street under the hands of a very capable cardiac surgeon. When he was discharged, I distinctly remember the advice of the nutritionist who told us all the dos and don'ts of following a heart healthy meal plan. We came back and my mom quickly saw that the kitchen and the entire household was heart friendly. I knew from that time that I was also genetically fated to suffer from Coronary Artery Disease.

A few years later when I got married and with new responsibilities felt that I must have a medical insurance. I took the policy coverage for what it would then cost to have a CABG in a good hospital. Amongst my friends I was one of them who had prudent eating habits. I never went out and ordered anything buttered. I was the one who rustled every one up to play soccer on the beach every Sunday. I did two or three treks every year. I was always a member of a gym and built a library of books on exercising.

From the age of 30, I stated doing annual medical check-ups. My triglycerides and lipids were always high and I continuously took efforts to control them by life style management and avoided medication. When a whole bunch of us turned 40 I booked a local hospital, to full capacity, and 30 of us went and got ourselves a complete medical check-up. None of us would have otherwise gone on our own and each of us discovered some medical issue or the other. I instantly became popular with my friends wives.

My own doctor advised me to start taking Statins but I told him that I will avoid medications and continue to be more intense in the discipline of my life style. I then took up running and made my gym visits even more regular.

In 1993 when I was about 36 years of age my younger brother came home one day removed his T-Shirt and collapsed on the spot. A massive first Cardiac Attack took him away from us. My mother who was at home could not

119

even comprehend what was happening and in front of her eyes he frothed in the mouth and passed away. It was yet another revelation that the killer disease could strike so swiftly and suddenly. As a family we only strengthened our discipline and became even more diligent in our diet and exercise routine.

And so it came to pass that I started running half marathons from the year 2004 and was thus training in October 2006.

My doctor who performed my CT Angio strongly advised me against driving on my own and going back home. He urged me to call a taxicab. I however drove back and met a cardiologist the same evening. I was issued a ' cease and desist ' order, from further physical activity. A blood thinner, a beta blocker, a blood pressure tablet and two statins were prescribed. I was also prescribed a 2D echo, a Nuclear imaging test and lastly a proper Angiogram.

It was clear that the heart was extensively diseased and there were multiple blocks all over. Up to 6 grafts were contemplated. And why did I survive in spite of the 100% block on the left main artery. Only because of the collaterals that had developed due to my regular exercise. Do you not believe in miracles ?

By the middle of December I completed all tests and soon met three leading cardiologists in order to settle the debate. All three looked at my history and the unanimous opinion was that I was a fit and proper candidate for a CABG.

Being an elective surgical patient, I had the luxury of planning my surgery according to my convenience. I thus arrived and walked in from the front door rather than being rushed in through the Emergency entrance. I chose the beginning of the month and also a weekend since it was logistically convenient for all.

Thus the morning of Saturday, 3rd February 2007 saw me getting up at 5.30a.m. My full body was shaved clean. I was wheeled through corridors as I admired the various types of light fittings on the ceilings. As soon as I entered a very cold room with very large bright lights, an injection was administered and I lost all consciousness.

When I first stirred in the ICU, I realized that there was the respirator pipe in my mouth and that my mouth was parched. My request for water was met with a dose of a drop or two, while I could have drunk a whole jug. I had so many wires running out of my body that I did not know where I ended and where the equipment began. I learnt that I had undergone a six way CABG and that I was in the Operation Theater for about seven hours.

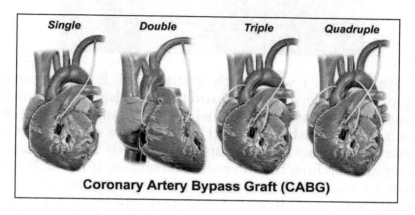

Single   Double   Triple   Quadruple

Coronary Artery Bypass Graft (CABG)

Illustration reproduced from:
http://en.wikipedia.org/wiki/File:Blausen_0152_CABG_All_.png

I was fortunate that my hospital Asian Heart had a tie up with Cleveland Clinic and the Cardiac Rehab there was world class. I followed every Rehab procedure to the T and my philosophy was I should have the best recovery and Rehab as was possible.

For three months I rehabilitated well and then soon started regaining my former athletic lifestyle. About six months after my surgery I went on a 3 hour hike which I did very comfortably. In the October of 2007, I ran a 10K distance and by Jan 2008, within 11 months of my surgery, I again ran the Half Marathon in Mumbai. I was featured on the front page of most dailies as the local hero.

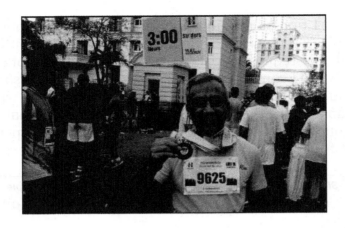

However as I was eagerly getting back into my former vigorous lifestyle, a lot of questions kept arising in my mind. I was taking a battery of medicines and I was not sure how much I could push myself. I was not sure of the effect of those medications on my running and newly mended heart. I kept on searching the Internet and consider it my lucky day when I found a link to Cardiac Athletes. My joy knew no bounds and I considered it a God given gift that I could join such a rare and exclusive community. I was warmly received like a family member. The bonding and the sense of camaraderie that prevails can only be experienced by those who have undergone similar tribulations in their own lives.

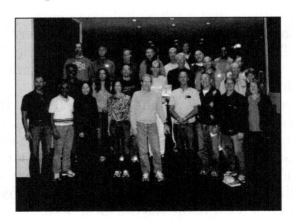

Cardiac Athletes at the H.E.A.R.T annual meeting
Baltimore, USA, 2012.

Today with the immense support and confidence that I have gained over the years by being a member of Cardiac Athletes, I have run over 75 Half Marathons. A distance that I love. In fact for the last three years I have been running a Half Marathon every single calendar month. An achievement that raises the eyebrows of those much younger and fitter than me.

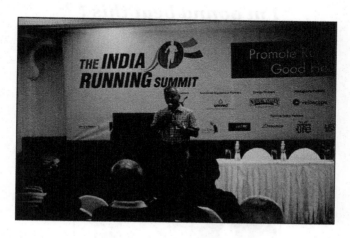

After selling my stake in the start-up that I founded, I have taken up the mission of 'Promoting Running for Gòod Health' under the name of **YouTooCanRun**. It is a social entrepreneurship and is intended to promote running so as to stave off lifestyle diseases.

https://youtoocanrun.com/

https://www.facebook.com/pages/You-Too-Can-Run-Sports-Management-P-Ltd/216193438522661

http://www.youtube.com/watch?v=NxjFZlnh6is

http://runnersforlife.com/page/heroes-of-running-p-venkatraman

All this could not be possible were it not for the encouraging team at Cardiac Athletes.

CHAPTER 10

Laura :

" I'm gonna beat this ! "

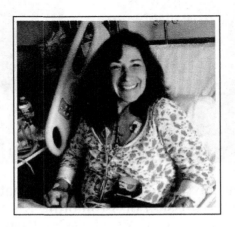

CARDIAC ATHLETE 10

First name: Laura
Country: USA
Diagnosis: Bicuspid Aortic Valve
Treatment: Tissue and Mechanical Aortic Valve Replacements

When bad news calls, this is a great, positive, uniquely human reaction.   But, what we don't know is just how many ways and over what expanse of time a person may have to " beat " something.   We aren't Rocky, we may not be Norma Rae, we can't be Scarlett O'Hara.   We are just who we are. A collection of experiences and knowledge, with an individual set of coping mechanisms. " Beating " anything to which you have no real control is a journey.

My journey began at birth. I was born with a bicuspid aortic valve. Now, back in 1958 there was no ultrasound imaging to confirm this and it was given a variety of vague names, which existed in the back of my mind as I did all the normal kid things, punctuated with yearly check-up visits to St Michaels Hospital in Newark, NJ.

I played tennis and captained my high school team, joined the rugby team in college and graduated to post college power lifting and bodybuilding. Eventually, I left behind any thought of congenital heart disease and moved to NYC, pursued a career, went back to school and became a Physical Therapist, got married and had children.

Fast forward to turning 40 and my yearly check-up. My GP heard the once faint, familiar murmur had grown louder. Consultation with the cardiologist led to a few tests and BAMM ! Vague congenital heart defect had a name. Bicuspid aortic valve with aortic aneurysm. This congenital defect is found mostly in men-but I always liked to be different. "Therefore", commanded my cardiologist, " no more power lifting. "

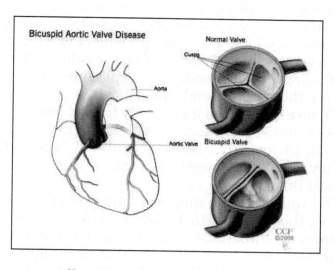

Illustration reproduced from:
http://my.clevelandclinic.org/heart/disorders/bicuspid_aor
tic_valve_disease.aspx

Weightlifting put too much pressure on the defective valve. Weightlifting had defined my life and who I was for nearly 20 years. I had to do something else and that something else was run and bike. It wasn't easy going aerobic from anaerobic but I slogged along.

I had a great new group of running and biking buddies and happily, but terribly slowly, raced duathlons, 5ks, half marathons 10Ks, bike tours and anything else that looked like fun. Heart disease wasn't so bad..

I was never fast, but about 2 years in, it was evident I was getting even slower. I reasoned that I was getting was older. After longer races I began to feel pretty sick, having to sleep for 2 hours afterwards, nauseous with post-race headaches. I kept it quiet and just assumed I wasn't in as good as shape as I should be. I needed to work harder, stop being such a slacker. My daughter, upon seeing me repeatedly head for the bed after a race said : " I don't think something can be good for you if it makes you feel this bad after " Smart ass kid ...

Forward to August 2004 check-up: My wonderful, funny compassionate cardiologist, Dr. Blick breaks the bad news: "Time is up, you need a valve replacement." I am 45 years old and although I knew this was possible, I was floored. But only for a short while. I wasn't afraid. Really. There is less than 3% mortality with aortic valve replacements.

I meet the surgeon and opted for a porcine valve so I wouldn't have to take coumadin. My friends have a party for me a couple days before surgery with lots of gag heart related gifts and much joviality. Humor has always been and always will be my best weapon against harm. I was ready. I was gonna beat this.

Until I woke up from surgery I can't explain just how bad I felt. In the giant CICU, I vaguely recall having the tube pulled from my throat and seeing my friends and family who were allowed a brief visit. I remember the unique, helpless feeling of throwing up (thank you allergy to general anesthesia) with a sternum, newly flayed and sewn shut with wire. Yeah, it's just as bad as it sounds. I had lost a lot of blood thanks to an accidental tearing of my heart wall during surgery and felt indescribably weak. The surgeon had warned me I would have more musculoskeletal pain since I had so much muscle mass. He wasn't kidding. I couldn't decide what hurt more, my chest, my upper back or my lower back. I couldn't walk 30ft without getting winded and exhausted. At one point, my hemoglobin at 7, just prior to a blood transfusion, I was sure I was dying and no one was brave enough to tell me.

It was a long haul. Walking up my driveway became a goal which took me two weeks to accomplish. Lifting my arms to wash my hair or put on a shirt hurt my shoulders and chest. Recovery was slow, so slow. I was dismayed.

Adding insult to injury, it hurt to laugh. My secret weapon was neutralized ! Damn, I thought I can beat this. I was weak. I couldn't lift a full tea kettle for weeks. What the hell ? No doctor, surgeon or medical journal told me how to get back to the athlete (however average) I left behind, I was a medical professional and I didn't know where to turn.

One night, depressed and feeling adrift I Googled valve replacements and athletes. Behold !!! **Valve Replacements.com** website appeared, proving there is truly a website for everyone. This was the discovery of a lifetime. People like me, athletes and regular folk, all in the same boat. We meet online, shared stories, made friends.

Eventually 5 of us struck up an online friendship and decided to do a relay marathon. Paul Hobbs hosted the first of what was to be many relay marathons. It was in Vermont. It was wonderful.

I remember sitting on Paul's kitchen floor with 4 other people with who I formed online friendships and we talked about how weird it was to actually see your heart beating through the skin for several months after surgery. We agreed there was such a thing as " pump head " (during open heart surgery, blood is directed away from your stopped heart through a Cardiopulmonary Bypass pump which oxygenates it and returns it to your vital organs. Patients agree it leaves one with memory loss and slow thinking for a little while post-surgery. Doctors, of course, disagree.)

Christina, Paul, Hugh, Mark and I formed an unbreakable bond. We did the marathon relay. We cheered, we hugged we laughed. We beat this thing !!!

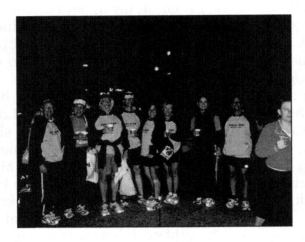

Time went by. Our Valve-o-line race team grew and we partnered with the group Cardiac Athletes. Five of us ran Vermont. Two years later, 25 of us did NJ State Marathon. It was like flowers growing in concrete, a phoenix rising from the ashes. We beat this thing.

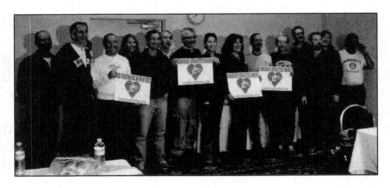

Until June 2011. Five years after surgery, I crossed the finish line at the Lava Man Triathlon in Lavalette, NJ. It was damn hot that day. I had a great swim and bike but fell apart on the run. Oh well. Believe me when I say I was always the happiest finisher in any race and had done many after my surgery.

That night my son and I stayed up late watching " Rudy. " My throat felt weird, almost like a buzzing feeling but I thought I was just a little dried out from the days heat.

I woke up around 2 am to a loud repetitive " squeak " "Ugh, now what's wrong with the air conditioner ? " I stood up and listened, ear towards the vent. Nothing. Then I realized the squeak was coming from me, from my chest, from my heart. Crap. Really ?

I did what anyone would do and Googled squeaking heart. It was not good news. Two days later Dr Blick looking as upset as I felt, told me the valve had failed. I needed another one and soon. The first person I called was my Valve-o-line buddy, Hugh. " I'm screwed, Hugh " I said (actually I said another word, but I don't think I can write that one). He agreed. We laughed.

Readers Digest version: I am finally, after many weeks wait, in the office of Dr. Leonard Girardi of Cornell Weil, NY Presbyterian Hospital. Dr Girardi is an expert in Marfans Syndrome and handles delicate, complicated heart surgeries. (No, I don't have Marfans). I was just a little alarmed my cardiologist insisted I see him. My wonderful friend Moira, accompanies me to my to my consult. Dr Girardi explains the surgery. I will have the valve, whose leaflet has partially torn away replaced. Had the leaflet completely torn away I would've died or had a massive stroke. Lucky me. He states he might have to rebuild the aorta and the aortic root, due to the proliferation of scar tissue attaching my heart and aorta to my sternum following the previous surgery. This is an unexpected twist and I am somewhat shell shocked. I try to remain optimistic. This man is the best there is for delicate, complicated heart surgeries. I feel pretty good about things.

Dr Girardi ends the conversation and schedules my surgery and stands up. He puts his hand on my shoulder and says " I am so sorry you have to go through this " Huh ? Wait, this is serious. I ask : Can I just sit here a minute ? " He nods, exits his office and I fall apart, alone in the office. This time, I am scared.

I get my Will revised, I organize all my good jewellery

and mementos, make sure each of my kids have complete photo albums of their formative years. I try not to freak out my wonderful ex-husband (who stood by my hospital bed through both surgeries) and all my exceptional family and friends. I don't tell many people because I don't want to talk about it. I keep working and making jokes because this is how I can get through each day successfully. I notice my hands and face begin to swell the last weeks prior to surgery and I can't walk up stairs or inclines without losing my breath.

Surgery time arrives In August 2011. My sister, Noreen, is once again on hospital sentry duty. My friends from college, Liz and Chris, visit the night before surgery along with my good friend Laurie and we laugh till we think we might pee ourselves. One of the mystified interns who comes to check me out pre op, jokingly asks if I am aware I am having heart surgery tomorrow.

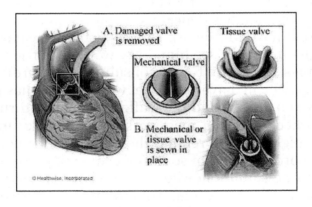

Illustration reproduced from:
http://media.radiosai.org/journals/Vol_06/01OCT08/09-healingtouch.htm

The next night, I wake up in the CICU yet again. This time they can't remove the breathing or " vent " tube. I am not able to breathe on my own. My hands are tied to the bed to insure I won't pull out the tube. I am wide awake and alert. I am trying not to panic. This is not easy to do, by the way, with a tube in the throat and hands tied to the bed. I get sick (again, thank you allergy to general anesthesia). Ah, there was that familiar chest flayed, tearing apart pain !

Proving wrong that things couldn't get any worse, the nurse begins to suction me through the tube to remove the mess.   I can best describe this as someone pulling on your lungs with a mini straw vacuum.   It is terrifying in the most visceral sense of the word.   Seeing the frantic look in my eyes, the nurse unties one of my hands so I can write and communicate.   I write " How long ? "   " About 4 hours, I'm sorry " she responds.   Desperate not to lose all sanity, I remember the advice my friend Joe gave to me prior to surgery: " If things get rough, just pretend each obstacle is a leg of the Iron Man race. It will be your Cardiac Iron Man "

I begin to swim.   Leg one of the Iron Man.   I close my eyes and turn my head, take an imaginary breath.   I picture myself moving thru Mirror Lake in Lake Placid.   ICU nurses have seen everything, but I bet this is the first time they saw someone swimming.

Five long hours later the tube comes out. No one got the plates of the truck that hit me.   Morphine makes me throw up more and we switch to percoset.   Thank you to the chemist who invented percoset. The nurses and doctors are extraordinary at NY Presbyterian.

The pain improves over the course of two days, except when the resident pulls out the chest tubes and heart lead wires ... " Just cough when I say go ... you won't feel a thing " Right.

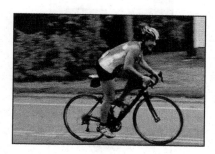

This time, it takes me much less time to recover.   This time the valve is the correct size and will stand up to the rigors of training.

My surgeon spent many hours artfully removing scar tissue which attached my aorta and heart to my sternum, insuring I wouldn't have what he termed a " mortal event " when my chest was sawed open. My surgeon is a superstar. Mick Jagger ain't got nothing on Leonard Girardi.

This time, for the first time ever, I feel really great when I finally progress to running and biking. THIS is what it feels like to have a normal functioning heart. The last surgery didn't make me feel this good. This valve, mechanical though it be, works perfectly. I am amazed. I have NEVER felt this good before.

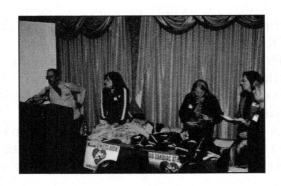

In November 2010, I meet my wonderful, supportive lifelong friends from all over the USA, England and Australia in Harrisburg, Pa for the relay of the Harrisburg Marathon. I run 4 miles, 3 months after surgery. It is my fastest 4 miles in my life.

" I beat this thing."

CHAPTER 11

Jeff ' LostViking ' :

" Back In Circulation "

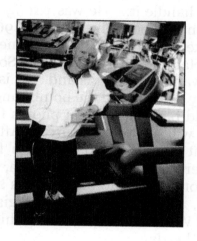

CARDIAC ATHLETE 11

First name: Jeff
Forum name: "LostViking"
Country: USA
Diagnosis: Coronary Artery Disease; Angina
Treatment: Three Bypass Grafts

Section 1a - Family History

" Wake him up momma, wake him up," my oldest sister pleaded. Pain etched her face " I wish I could sweetie," my mother replied.

I stood with my mother, brother, and two sisters, confined in a small viewing room, confused as to why daddy just lay there in the big wooden box. I was six-years-old. So began my personal battle with a thing called " heart disease." When you're six-years-old, daddy can throw a ball a mile, he can fix anything, and he can beat up anybody. But when my cousin Nellie came to our door that day in September all bets were off.

When Nellie came to the door she did so to tell us dad had suffered a heart attack in her bean field. She hired him after his employer let him go after learning of his heart condition, though she was reluctant to do so, but dad insisted he could handle it. He was wrong. He was forty-six-years-old when he died. The year was 1966.

My father, like so many of his era, joined the Army Air Corp after Pearl Harbor. He served in the South Pacific. As the marines advanced from island to island capturing airfields so did my dad, to load the bombs and belts of ammo on bombers. Old black and white photos from the islands are something I will always treasure. After the war dad came home, went to work, and started a family. In my neighborhood everybody was a war veteran, from the barber to the grocery store owner, to all the guys swigging beer at the bowling alley. They were heroes and giants to me. My interest in World War II took root during this time in my life and continues to this day.

Section 1b - Pre-Op Warning Signs

Back in 1972 I watched the summer Olympics and learned a new word; marathon. Frank Shorter won the gold medal for the U.S. and I remember the announcers talking about " the wall." The runners could hit " the wall," and will they be able to continue ? I was riveted to the television waiting to see the runners try and climb over some wall or physical barrier. Later, I learned of the physical demands of the race, and that " the wall " meant runners struggled to press on through fatigue. I wondered at the time if I could make it over " the wall " and decided to do a marathon someday to find out. Finally, in 1997 I did.

Yes, I made it over " the wall," but my knees were

strained from over-training and I wasn't happy with my finish time. I always felt I could do better, but to me marathons were like vasectomies; one was enough for any man. Before that, I'd done some weight-lifting and an occasional organized run to stay in shape. That and trying to eat healthy, I thought, would keep me far away from heart disease. When I began training for another marathon I took my time building up a broad mileage base, hitting nine miles in late March of 2005. I then began building up toward the thirteen mile benchmark I'd set for myself.

One day in April of 2005 I went for a four mile run in the morning. The air was a little cool and as I ran I had a cold sensation in my windpipe. After the run I felt a little more fatigued than usual and also a little nauseous. I walked around for a bit and the ill feeling passed, as did the cold windpipe sensation. A few days later I went running again and felt the same coldness in my windpipe accompanied with some tingling in my forearms. At that point I walked for a while then finally jogged home. Three days later I had a six mile run planned and wanted to see how I felt at that point as I wanted to make up for a missed running session that week. " How I felt " would change my life forever. The cold windpipe sensation hit me hard at one mile along with very tight forearms. I walked back home, puzzled as to why this kept happening to me. At my wife's urging I made an appointment with my doctor.

Section 2 - Diagnosis

A stress test was scheduled at the Oregon Heart and Vascular Institute on Friday afternoon. I was shot full of radioactive dye and put on a treadmill. When my symptoms reappeared they put me on a table and took pictures of my heart that revealed a blocked coronary artery. The bottom line of the test was sobering; heart disease. I was shocked, afraid, and filled with dread. Heart disease had become the bully of my life and just wouldn't leave me alone. Growing up, I soaked up every article or program on the subject so that it wouldn't happen to me. Now, here I was with a wife and two kids, facing the same possible fate as my dad.

An angiogram was scheduled for Saturday morning with the idea of a stent or even angioplasty as a remedy for my blocked coronary artery. When the time finally came for the angiogram I was ready to get fixed and get on with my life. However, the worst was yet to come; my blockage was located in a fork of my artery which meant open heart surgery. There would be no easy way out for me.

Section 3 - Mental State

After Nellie left our house that September day my sister called my mom at work to tell her what had happened. I was left out of the loop until she got home. All I knew was my brother seemed to be in shock and my sister kept crying. I was standing by the front door when mom got home. I will always remember her putting a hand to my cheek and saying " poor Jeff doesn't have a dad." None of the other kids were singled out this way, and I was too young to understand her statement could have been impulsive. But right then and there I became different from everyone else in the world. Everyone else had a dad and I didn't. Let the pity party begin. I used it as a crutch for many years when things didn't go my way. I blamed life, God, and anything else for my troubles. I know now that others had it worse growing up, but at the time I felt like the unluckiest kid around.

The news that I would have open heart surgery stunned Carol and I. I wanted to live, to beat heart disease; therefore I chose to be optimistic that my upcoming procedure could put the question of, " Will it happen to me too ? " behind me. I've always had an interest in fitness and exercise, and tried to eat healthy, in the hope that I wouldn't follow in the footsteps of my father. The cardiologist told me that's what probably kept me alive, otherwise I could have been a statistic of heart disease too. The fact that I was diagnosed and had surgery scheduled within four days of each other meant I wouldn't have time to sit and dwell on my situation as some I know had, I would get it over with quickly.

Section 4 - Procedure

The cardiac surgeon briefed us on my upcoming surgery and said I would have a Cardiac Arterial Bypass Graft, or CABG. In this procedure the blocked area would be bypassed using the radial artery from my left arm along with the mammary artery in my chest. The instructional video was a little vague on the whole procedure, and I remember sitting in my physicians waiting room a week after being discharged from the hospital, looking in a magazine. I opened it up to a story on open heart surgery and was stopped dead in my tracks. The lead picture was of a surgery in progress, with the chest cavity spread open with a metal contraption and rubber-gloved hands reaching in. " There's no way that happened to me," I said to myself, but it really did. I have the scars to prove it.

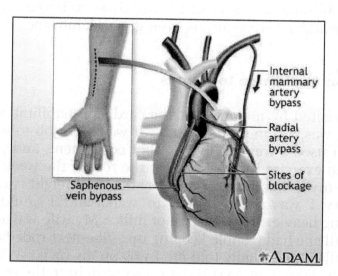

Illustration reproduced from:
http://www.mybwmc.org/library/3/100190

Section 5 - Recovery and Insights

I awoke in I.C.U. which I've always considered crucial to my recovery, with chest tubes and a catheter. Nurses helped me to my feet when I was awake and alert enough, to aid in circulation and to help me get my bearings. I was in a lot of pain but I was alive. I had gone through major invasive surgery and I was alive-with no complications I might add. I knew that for the most part, the things I couldn't control were behind me, and now it would be up to me to follow the instructions of the medical and rehabilitation staff in order to get back into the mainstream of life. Heart disease took a shot at me and I had survived.

Growing up fatherless had put a chip on my shoulder and gave me drive and determination to be better then the next person, but I never knew at what. I saw a movie once, as a kid, about a war veteran that had to recover from his wounds and get back into society. I always wondered if I could go through something like that, and here was my chance to find out. I wanted the tubes out of my chest so I could walk on my own and get stronger, recover, get back into society.

Section 6 - Return to Sports

I was visited by members of the cardiac rehabilitation staff while I was still in the hospital. It was their job to monitor me as I used a treadmill, and other equipment, and provide me with exercise instructions for the rest of the week once I began my rehabilitation. For the first eight weeks of recovery I was only allowed to walk, and I couldn't lift anything heavier than a gallon of milk. My wife walked with me until she had trouble keeping up. She next rode her bike as I walked and finally told me I was on my own. When my surgeon cleared me to run again I went right to the track and ran three miles.

I must say the rehab staff was a little taken aback at this news and I was told to pace myself. When I would report to rehab and crank up the treadmill to jog on it, I was looked at by the other patients as a freak of nature. One time, I felt something over my shoulder and looked back to see an elderly gentleman staring at me as if he'd seen a ghost. "No-one runs in rehab" seemed to be the other patients' attitude and limitations, but I was on a mission. I'd always felt different than everybody else and was about to prove it.

On the Monday of week twelve I officially graduated from cardiac rehab. That day, one of the staff asked if I still wanted to run the marathon I'd been training for. He told me that with three more months of rehab he could at least get me to the starting line of a November marathon. I was told that to their knowledge, no one had run a marathon seven months after open heart surgery. As a textbook overachiever I was very interested in this news, and decided to take them up on their offer.

The highlight of my comeback came seven months and two days after my surgery when I ran the Seattle Marathon, and set a personal best time. At the time of my diagnosis, the cardiologists told me I wouldn't be running any marathons for quite a while, " maybe next year." Sorry doctors, but I had to prove you wrong. By the way, I had just turned forty-six, the age of my father when he died.

Section 7 - Finding Cardiac Athletes

After I ran the marathon I became a Heart to Heart volunteer at my hospital. I made weekly visits to the cardiac care ward, checking on post-op heart patients and sharing my recovery story with them. When I saw how my recovery boosted the morale of the patients I looked for other things to do to keep raising the bar of cardiac recovery. Triathlons came into the picture, and in early 2006 I added swimming and cycling to my running routine. I completed a handful of triathlons in 2006 including a 70.3 mile event.

I joined a website devoted to triathletes, and one day in 2009 I received a message from another member, Grayg8r. He asked if I'd ever heard of a website called " Cardiac Athletes." I checked it out immediately and knew I'd found a home.

I'm extremely competitive, and in the races I entered I again felt separated from everyone else.   I never used my surgery as a crutch, but there was no " open heart surgery survivor " age group category.   I wondered how the faster athletes would fare if they'd been opened up too.   It would be interesting to me to see how heart surgery might change their race outcomes.   I wondered, " What if this Olympic Athlete had to have heart surgery ? " " How would he compare with his old self ? "   I might not ever know.   But I do know that with Cardiac Athletes I'm among my own kind.

Section 8 - Meeting Up

Greyg8r, aka Richard, came to my home town on business 2010.   We got together for a run and dinner.   It was fun comparing " war stories " and simple things like heart rates. In November of 2010 my wife Carol and I travelled to Harrisburg, Pennsylvania for the annual Cardiac Athletes " Heart Run."

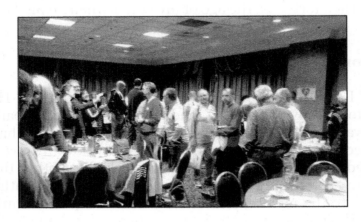

I was simply amazed at how I felt so at home with everyone even though I'd just met them.   Here was a room full of people who understood me, for the most part, and what I'd gone through.   I imagine it would be like travelling in a foreign country and not being understood by the local populace, and suddenly, here comes a group of people that speak my language. We were like-minded type-A heart patients who were out to change the world. It meant so much to me that I volunteered to help plan and execute the 2011 event.

Section 9 - Sporting Achievements

It's interesting to me that I had the Cardiac Athlete mind-set before I knew the others existed. Once I completed rehab, started running again, and completed the marathon seven months after surgery I looked for other things to do to "raise the bar" of cardiac recovery. I never ask for special treatment due to my " condition " because I don't feel I have one. What I do have is a positive attitude and the will to achieve, to get back into life and motivate others. The only limitations I feel I have are those I place upon myself. With that in mind let me list my accomplishments since my triple bypass in April of 2005:

2005

April 25
Open heart surgery and triple vessel bypass.

November 27
Seven months and two days after heart surgery, ran the Seattle Marathon in 4:23 breaking my previous marathon time by thirty-one minutes.

2006

April 23
Albany Sprint Triathlon.

May 20
Lebanon Sprint Triathlon.

June 24
Completed Pacific Crest Half Ironman Triathlon. 70.3 miles.

July 3
93 mile bike ride from Eugene, Oregon to Waldport, Oregon
6 hours 33 minutes.

August 12
Mid-Summer Sprint Triathlon.

September 10
Lincoln City Sprint Triathlon.

2007

April 7
Beaver Freezer Sprint Triathlon, Corvallis Oregon

April 29
New P.R. in Eugene half-marathon 1:54:42

May 26
Longest bike ride to date-102 miles

June 24
Ironman Coeur d'Alene in 15:56:16. That's 15 hours folks!

July 29
Mid-Summer Olympic Triathlon, Fairview, Oregon.

October 7
Completed the Portland Marathon.

2008

May 5
Ran Eugene Marathon in 4:29:37 in preparation for the
Ironman event in June

May 17
Rode bike from Castle Rock, Washington to the Johnstone
Observatory at Mt. St. Helens. A distance of 52 miles.
Starting altitude 250 feet. Ending altitude 4200 feet

May 25
Duck Bill Thrill Olympic Distance triathlon, Fall Creek,
Oregon

June 22
Ironman Coeur d'Alene. New PR 15:13:38

August 16
14 mile Hardesty Hard Core trail run, Hardesty Mountain

2009

May 5
Eugene Half-Marathon.

Aug 16
Completed the Ironman Lake Stevens 70.3 mile triathlon.

Nov 15
I swam fifty minutes (1.2 miles) in Kailua Bay, rode fifty
miles on the Queen K Highway, and ran fifty minutes from
the Natural Energy Labs back to Kona, Hawaii all to declare
myself fifty-years-old.

2010

January
Continued wear-testing Brooks running shoes. Current shoe-
Trance 10

January 4
Begin training for upcoming season

May
Upgraded to the Garmin 310XT heart rate monitor

May 2
Complete Eugene Half-Marathon in 1:58:23. New personal best time.

May 27
Spoke to the seniors group at Fairfield Baptist Church

June 23
Spoke to the "Young at Heart" group luncheon

June 27
Completed 3rd Ironman Triathlon in Coeur d'Alene, Idaho

July 5
Training continues for the 5k "Warrior Dash" and Harrisburg Marathon in Harrisburg, Pennsylvania

August
Shot commercial and interview for Peace Health "Amazing Medical" campaign.

September 11
Took second place in age group in the "Warrior Dash."

October 16
5k run

November 14
Ran lead leg on one of the Cardiac Athletes relay teams in the Harrisburg Marathon, in Harrisburg, Pennsylvania.

All told I've completed 4 marathons, 3 half-marathons, 1-14 mile trail run, 2-5k runs, 1 Warrior Dash obstacle course, 1-10k run, 3 Ironman 140.6 mile triathlons, 2- 70.3 mile half-Ironman triathlons, 2 Olympic distance triathlons, and 5 Sprint triathlons.

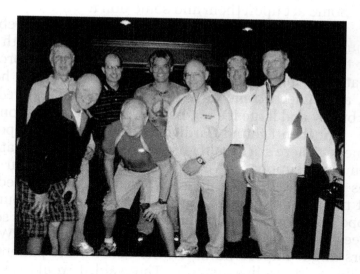

Jeff with other Cardiac Athlete buddies.

Section 10 - Giving Back

One afternoon I was returning home from a run and saw my wife walking down the street. She told me she was going to a yard sale so I went with her. I rummaged through some books and spotted one titled " I Dare You." Thumbing through it I could tell it was a motivational book written in 1958. Actually, the copy I held was the seventeenth edition. The author was William H. Danforth, founder of the Ralston Purina Company. I thought it would be fun to read how people were motivated " back then." It turned out to be something of a life changing book, for in it Mr. Danforth wrote *" Our most valuable possessions are those which can be shared without lessening; those which, when shared, multiply. Our least valuable possessions are those which, when divided, are diminished. "* I consider my story one of my greatest assets. I've seen tragedy turned around just by sharing with people. I became a volunteer to share with people lying in the very bed I once was in. Some hear my words and some don't. Some act upon them and some don't.

I designed and launched my own website, www.jumpstartmyheart.org , after my surgery, with the intent to offer information on heart disease and to provide motivation to anyone that visited my site. I had high hopes for it, and indeed some have seen it and even ordered my book, but by and large it's not been everything I envisioned it to be. But then I found Cardiac Athletes, and many people like me. There's a wealth of information there that one person can't supply. We Cardiac Athletes have our own stories of success in the midst of tragedy that, singled out might not add up to much, but collectively offer a mountain of hope to people. I truly believe we are, in a sense, "pioneers" in cardiac recovery, as Lars calls us. Where doctors might impose limits on the usual heart patient, we say " I'm going to live again." That said, I would say to a heart patient, " I dare you to get back into the world, scars and all."

The true measure of success is the ratio between what you could have been and what you are. I once was shy, scared, and lacking in confidence, but once I awoke from heart surgery I was a changed man. Heart disease doesn't take weekends off and neither should we. Where once I sat at the back of the room, I now want to be the key-note speaker. I've had the opportunity to speak on a handful of occasions, and though I'm not a trained orator I know I have a message.

Each time I speak I get better, but I don't worry about if I'm the best they've ever heard. My message far outweighs the fear I may feel standing up there and that's the key to continued growth and success - " Those who dare not, do not."

Long ago, I had a dream of being involved in the world of fitness, so much so that I even applied at the local health club. Unbeknownst to me they called my house to say I was hired but my mom intercepted the call. She told them no, that I was going to keep my job at the drug store. I was crushed. A normal person would have called the gym to tell them yes, I would quit the drug store, but not me. There was no fight in me and so I let my mom steal my dream.

After my surgery, friends would talk to me about fitness, or their aches and pains as if I were a doctor. One day in 2010 I remembered my dream of being involved in the world of fitness. So, I weighed my options and decided I would study to be a personal trainer through the American College of Sports Medicine. ACSM degrees were what all the techs in cardiac rehab had and I figured ACSM must be the best.

I began studying in earnest and in May of 2011 I went to the University of Oregon testing department and took my test. The worst part about it was the " submit test " screen. Thirty-three years earlier I had a dream and now I was one click away from realizing it. I took a breath and clicked the submit button. The computer gave me my score and I had passed !

I now tell people I waited over thirty years to fulfil my dream and that if they don't get what they are after in a short period of time just keep after it. I started my own business, **" My Trainer Jeff LLC "** and have been training clients for nearly two years.

http://mytrainerjeff.com/

https://www.facebook.com/pages/My-Trainer-Jeff-LLC/217238548455986

https://personaltrainercentral.com/trainers/profile.plx?ID=3341

http://www.youtube.com/watch?v=6lj5jtbm9SQ

http://www.youtube.com/watch?v=L_Nie3Y4XaU

http://www.cardiacathletes.com/resources-for-cardiac-athletes.php

I recall watching Jack Lalanne on television when I was a boy and a seed was planted then.   Now, it was finally starting to sprout.

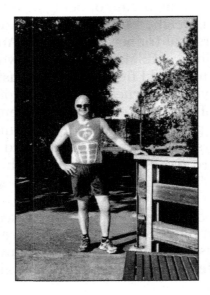

It seemed like most of the people I worked with had issues I had to work around.   Things like arthritis, high blood pressure, hip replacement, knee replacements.   I decided I wasn't going to be training the beautiful people and so filled out a stack of forms to become a Medicare service provider.   I really hope it's what launches me into full time fitness training.   I still speak on occasion and would like to do more of that someday.   I put a class together and I teach it at my local park and rec centers.

My message is " **Be Fit For Life** " and I'm living proof it works.

CHAPTER 12

Jack ' SumoRunner ' :

" I was not going to be a sedentary type any longer."

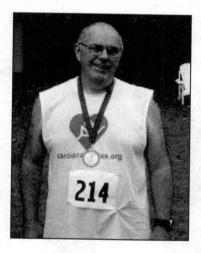

CARDIAC ATHLETE 12

First name: Jack
Forum name: "SumoRunner"
Country: USA
Diagnosis: Rheumatic Fever; Aortic Regurgitation
Treatment: Aortic Valve Replacement

I'm Jack Berkery, known online as Sumo Runner, a heavyweight for a distance runner and consequently a somewhat slow one, but I make up in enthusiasm what I lack in speed. I didn't give myself that moniker, rather it was bestowed on me by a colleague more than 20 years ago who was always amazed at how well I ran "for a big guy". At the time of this writing I'm 63 years old, a semi-retired software engineer, husband for 42 years, father of four and grandfather of three. I live in upstate New York where summer is too short, winters are way too long, but the climate for running is superb.

I had an artificial aortic valve replacement in 1991 which may be among the oldest of the Cardiac Athletes devices or procedures, making me truly a pioneer in this endeavor. I had a heart valve defect since early childhood. Damaged by Rheumatic Fever at the age of 5 and again at 10, the heart murmur as it was always called kept me out of sports, the military and most any type of exertion for the first couple decades of my life.

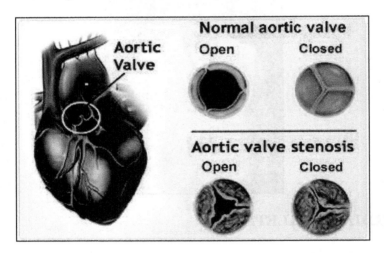

Illustration reproduced from:
http://www.medindia.net/patients/patientinfo/aortic-valve-stenosis.htm

The first time I encountered limitations was in 1963 at age 15 when I tried to go out for the high school cross country team. The sports team doctor shunted me aside and said no competitive sports, ever. It was assumed in those days that such heart problems could only get worse, so the prescription was to take it easy for the rest of your, perhaps short, life.   I can remember a conversation between the family doctor and my mother where he told her I could live a normal life until sometime in my 40s but thereafter things could get dicey.   No, it wasn't upsetting at all. To a ten year old, 40 is so ancient as to be beyond comprehension.   He was right since it did begin to fail at age 42 and he was wrong since by that time there were options that made it not at all dicey.

After high school, at age 18 I was called up in the draft as the Viet Nam war raged and they needed tens of thousands of new recruits each month.   At the initial physical I was actually passed and expected to be sworn in any day.   The selective service physical was a cattle call with hundreds of young men being shuttled through several examination rooms and given only a very cursory examination, so it was easy for a thing like that to get missed on the initial exam. More or less walking through the door constituted acceptance.   Little did I know though, that my own family doctor sat on the local draft review board.   The moment he saw my name, I got a 4F classification, unfit for military duty.   I guess since a few of my friends later came home with scars, missing parts or in body bags, that was somewhat fortunate, but getting an official US Government designation as unfit is damaging to a young man's ego.   It weighed heavily on my psyche thereafter.   I still have that draft card somewhere, could never bring myself to throw it away.

Another odd thing that was attempted in the 1950s and 60s was penicillin prophylaxis.   That was a regimen of taking a tablet or two each day the way so many now take an aspirin a day to ward off evil spirits.   It turned out that was the wrong type of drug to use for that purpose.   In effect, what they were doing was using me and so many others as incubators for penicillin resistant bacteria.   I tried explaining to my doctor a few times that whenever I went off the drug for more than a couple days I would get terribly ill. Coincidence, he'd say.   I stayed on that regimen until perhaps 1970 or 71.   The year I stopped altogether I was sick repeatedly for months, nothing serious, just a series of nasty colds and flu's.

Somewhere around that same time the medical community came to the realization that even defective hearts could benefit from a good workout. I don't remember when I heard about that and I'm certain no one told me to revise the ' take it easy for life strategy '. I simply decided at some point that I was not going to be a sedentary type any longer. Exactly when I began to run on a regular basis escapes me now. I have memories of running around the neighborhood after moving to a new home in 1973. I also recall, in one of those famous ' where were you when ' moments, that I was just returning from a run when I found out President Richard Nixon was resigning. That was August of 1974. Running was an on again, off again thing for a few years and I wouldn't have called myself a real runner until I entered my first race in 1978.

1978 changed everything. I had turned 30 and finally I was no longer the sickly weakling I had been forced to be as a youth. I could work out as well as anyone. By then of course my doctor was well aware of and approved of the exercise, which was more than running. It was also daily sit-ups, push-ups, cycling and occasional light weight lifting. Mostly running though. I just took to it like fish to water. It turns out that I have poor strength, very little speed but stamina to beat the band. Being sedentary through the teens and twenties I never knew what type of athletics I might be cut out for. At age 30 I discovered it.

That year was the 100th anniversary of the company where I worked and there were many different celebrations. Among them was a fitness challenge, a jog-a-thon, not a high intensity or high mileage thing, just a challenge to get in shape by the fall when they scheduled a 10K road race. I started keeping a running log and averaged just over 3 miles a day which as it turns out is still about the same amount I continue to run today. Over a span of decades though, it accumulates to some fairly impressive numbers. The logs which I continue to keep and still retain now total over 34,000 miles. The circumference of the earth being a mere 25,000 makes it sound even more significant. All on what most distance runners consider very modest training.

That first race was a onetime only event which was never repeated but the second one I entered, a 15K in November is still quite popular and my favorite because I have now done it 27 times. That's the accomplishment that I'm most proud of, simply being able to make it to the starting line that many years, the majority of which were after the heart surgery. Many more followed of course. I've never been a marathoner, but prefer to train for a good hard mile on the track or 5K road races. I've done hundreds of races in these 5 decades and continue doing sometimes 30 or more a year. No marathons though. The reason for that was early on, when I first began getting in shape, my wife who is a far greater worry wart than most made me promise to avoid marathons. I kept my word and have been quite happy not to subject myself to that abuse.

As a stocky guy I've never been an especially fast runner, never broke the 6 minute barrier for the mile, never faster than 20 minutes for a 5K, but I was consistent throughout my 30s and into the early 40s. One particularly eventful stretch was from 40 to 41 when I ran several all-time personal bests at distances between 2 Km and 15 Km. There were never any age group awards, the local talent was far too deep for me to penetrate that far up in the pack but I was ecstatic to continue to run PR's into my 40s. There was a 43:04 10K and a 67:03 15K, times I'd give me eye teeth for these days and most 40-somethings would consider very respectable. I was on a tear for those two years, training and racing at peak performance and feeling superbly fit, strong and confident. Then it all came crashing down.

1990, age 42, at the top of my game, I had done all the right training, performed well in all the right tune-up races. I was primed for my favorite 15K which was by then my 10th time in that race and expecting to be able to at least match the previous year's personal best of 67 minutes. Oh, it began fine with a pace close to 7 minutes per mile through the first four and just over 35 minutes at mile 5. Everything was working, flowing smoothly, but by the time I reached mile 6 I was carrying a piano on my back.

The last third of the race became a hard slog and I

finished several minutes slower than anticipated. Just having one bad race wasn't the issue though. That happens from time to time for any number of reasons. I simply could not recover from it. The rule of thumb for recovering from a hard race effort is that it should take about 1 day per mile raced before you feel up to 100% again. For a 15K that should be 9 or 10 days, but I did not feel normal after two weeks, three weeks, a month, just tired and washed out from even a short easy run. That's when I made an appointment with my Cardiologist.

I had been seeing this doctor for many years and we had discussed the fact that I'd eventually need a valve replacement, but it was always far off in the indefinite future. He said more than once, "You'll know when it's time before I will." It was time. You know, the brain is an odd thing. It can be aware of an impending situation for 30 years and have been presented with all the facts well in advance but until it's time to face the action, nothing registers in a serious way. This was as if it was the first time I had to deal with the eventuality of life changing open heart surgery. The leakage and back pressure from the damaged valve had increased to a dangerous level, significant enough that it could fail in the near future. Even if I were to return to a sedentary life, it was probably good for only 4 or 5 more years. I was told to stop running until the surgery could be scheduled, which I did, mostly. That was a year of anxiety and apprehension. The surgery was scheduled for July and this was only January. I had way too much time to think about it. It was a year I'd rather forget.

I didn't run for the next 7 months but stayed in shaped by power walking for 3 to 4 miles a day, but I did run a mile the day before the operation. Just one. Just in case it was my last. I had no idea whether I'd ever be able to return to it and wanted to remind myself of what, I don't know. Perhaps I was saying "Wait here, I'll be right back as soon as I can".

The procedure was uneventful as far as I knew. Being so highly drugged there was little realization of the impending situation. What I remember from that day was telling the

OR staff I wanted all my blood back. Those were the days when there was a danger of the blood supply being tainted with HIV. There were no reliable tests for it then, so it was advised if you were strong enough, to put away your own blood to be re-transfused after surgery. I was able to put up 4 pints in 4 weeks and still had the strength to run that one mile. That was one benefit of a healthy lifestyle I had never figured on. So, upon being wheeled into the OR all I could think to say was give it back. They did.

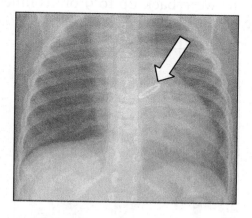

X-ray image showing sewing ring of aortic valve replacement. Reproduced from:
https://www.bcm.edu/departments/radiology/cases/pediatr ic/text/8j1A.htm

The recovery went fairly well, or so it seemed. I was walking a mile every day from the first day I came home, eventually working up to 3 miles after a month. I felt well enough to return to work at 4 weeks but waited the requisite 6 because that was the time my employer had allotted. It was also at 6 weeks that I tried running again. I didn't make it as far as 100 meters before gasping for breath. It didn't progress much beyond that for the next several days. Explaining this to the Cardiologist a bit later, he expressed no surprise. "It's because they collapsed one of your lungs in surgery." What? Wait, no one told me that before. I was operating on reduced power for 6 weeks and no one had warned me of it. " Oh, it'll re-inflate in time. What you need to do is keep running and that'll bring it back faster. "

It was another full 6 weeks before I could finish a whole mile non-stop and every step of it, every day was a struggle. That piano was still weighing me down. Once I reached that point though, I knew everything was going to be all right eventually. I ran a 3 mile race on January 1, 1992 to start a comeback 5 months post-op. By the following summer the weekly long runs were back up to 9 or 10 miles and I even ran a 10K race on the track.

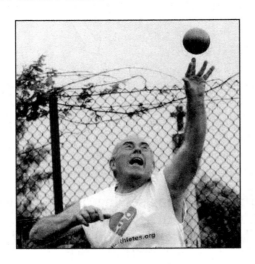

In July, 1992, almost a full year post-op I was interviewed and filmed for a commercial for Power Bars at a US Corporate Athletics Association track and field meet in Irvine CA. I was there running the 5K for the company team and no one had ever heard of a runner returning to the sport after serious open heart surgery. It was such a rarity in those days that the meet directors sent the film crew to find me and film me running around the track. The interview never made it anywhere, not on TV or in print I suspect because nobody was certain that what I was doing was medically safe or even advisable. And it was unique as far as I knew. There was no world wide web back then. The Internet was small and accessible to only universities and research institutions. I had been on line for several years by then and I was well acquainted with the Usenet news groups that existed. I searched in vain for others in the same position finding one or two contacts but each of us felt we were an experiment of one.

Oh wait, perhaps I should explain about my presence on the early Internet. I was the first online running coach, once billing myself as "The Common Sense Coach" in a pre-Sumo Runner incarnation. Since I worked at a corporate laboratory as a computer scientist, I had access to the Internet from the mid-80s, a time when one could actually count the number of computers attached world-wide and even map out where they were located. The primary method of communication was called Usenet. It was the precursor of the common web forum used for all sorts of special interests today. At first, under the recreational headings, we runners could only post notes to the misc. fitness group. There wasn't a running-only news group. That one forum received postings by footballers, weight lifters, cyclists, you name it and they all constantly argued over whether the other sports had any right to be on what they considered their turf.

By about 1990 several of us decided to split off a separate rec.running news group. There may have been a couple dozen at most in the beginning but it grew quickly. I wrote large portions of the original FAQ, distilling discussions we had rehashed many times on the misc.fitness forum as well as from personal experiences. I also offered my services as a running coach, advising people all over the net by email. I corresponded in that way for the next 5 or 6 years with all types from the absolute beginner to top class marathoners. All of which is to say, I was well known across the net and all were aware of my impending heart surgery. Had there been any other runners anywhere who had returned to competition after aortic valve replacement or any other procedure, I would have been put in touch with them. I was all alone.

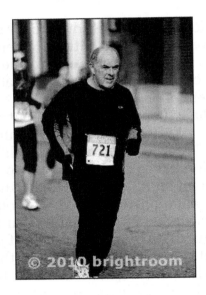

The problem with being a pioneer is that there is no road map to tell you which way to go, no trail blazed through the wilderness, no bridges across the rivers. Each direction one takes could lead to grand new vistas or disaster. You never know until rounding the next bend. I tended thereafter to be very conservative in my approach to training and racing and always had the nagging feeling that what I was doing could be, shall we say, a game changer. I continued training about the same 1000 miles per year as previously but seldom trained or raced hard. I entered about a dozen races the year after the surgery and every year following, give or take a few. The one I most wanted to return to was the one that threw me, the November 15K where I struggled so badly. I had to show that beast I wouldn't back down. I've now run it 27 times, 10 before the valve replacement, 17 since. I think, just maybe, I've made my point. But I was still alone, still uneasy, still searching for others in the same boat, still uncertain of what or how much I could do.

Fifteen years later, fifteen thousand miles later, a couple hundred races later, having passed through the 40s and then 50s, I found what I had been looking for. Throughout that time I had been writing frequently for the local road runners club newsletter. I wrote race reports, human interest stories, humor, training and racing advice, perhaps 50 or 60 articles on all things running. I also wrote about my experience as a post-heart surgery runner in the months immediately following the surgery and then a retrospective at 5 years, then 10, then 15 to let everyone know what was possible, that valve replacement wasn't limiting, but I never found the kindred spirits I searched for so vainly since 1991.

I don't remember how I found it or what made me go look for it after all that time, but some time in 2007 I was surfing the web and happened upon a forum especially for discussing valve replacement. These were people who understood all I went through, all I wanted to know and I could give them the benefit of my long experience as well. And there was even some discussion of running and fitness where one of the guys told me there was another forum a bit more hard edged called **CardiacAthletes.com** . Those were really my kind of people. Those were the ones I had been looking for all these 15 years.

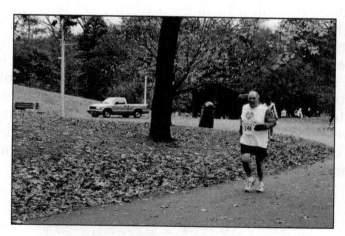

In 2007 I got a new attitude. I dropped 40 lbs and started training seriously again even returning to doing intervals on a track. I ran with renewed vigor and enthusiasm. Now approaching 60 I was under no delusion that I could return to the competitive shape I was in at 40, but it was worth the effort to see how much could be regained. The biggest change though, was that I stopped viewing myself as being handicapped. I stopped thinking of myself as a cardiac patient, as damaged goods, as limited by my affliction. I had no affliction any longer. It had been fixed and that was something I failed to grasp all those many years. Now I was an athlete lining up against other athletes in a test of abilities. I may not have been an elite, but I was there to compete and that's what I did for the first time in a long time.

The most pleasant surprise came in May of 2008. As a newly minted 60 year old I ran yet another 5K road race. With over 300 such races in my past and never a trophy at any age, I left before the awards were announced as usual. Later the race management emailed me that an age group trophy was mine for the taking. Who, me ? You can't be serious. He wasn't kidding. That was the first of 5 or 6 that year, a couple 1st place, a couple 2nd and 3rd, and more the year after that and the year after that. I haven't become so jaded as to be blasé about receiving a trophy and hope I never do. It's still a thrill even when I get one merely for being the third of three. You see, by this age much of the competition has fallen by the wayside. So many runners who were my betters through 4 decades are now no longer racing, some not even running any longer. The number of entrants over 60 are a small portion of the field but I'm proud to have lasted this long, to be able to toe the line one more year and give it my all. There's a great deal to be said about outliving the competition. This is, after all, an endurance sport.

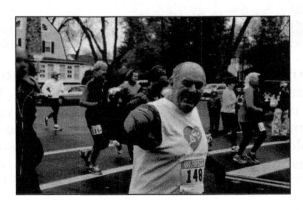

CHAPTER 13

Alan ' OldStarter ' :

"I will never forget her fist in my groin !"

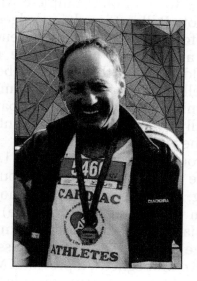

CARDIAC ATHLETE 13

First name: Alan
Forum name: "OldStarter"
Country: Australia
Diagnosis: CVD; Dilated Cardiomyopathy; AFib.
Treatment: Two Bypass Grafts

My name is Alan (aka Old Starter on the forum), I'm 56 years of age and I'm yet another Virgo with a heart history. Strange that. I'm a bit of an imposter really as my points of difference are I'm not really an athlete in the true sense of the word and I'm not an Alpha personality.

I reside in Ballarat, within Victoria, the Southern-most state of Australia. Ballarat is a rural city, located an hour from our State's capital Melbourne and working its way towards a population of 100,000 people. It's more like a big country town really, having been originally settled as a gold mining Mecca in 1837. We have many historically important houses and buildings in Ballarat that are part of our rich heritage as well as proudly boasting a number of major tourist destinations, including Sovereign Hill, a re-creation of the gold mining town of old, complete with gold panning and mining to boot. Ballarat is acknowledged as the home of the Aussie spirit for which our nation is renowned. Back in 1854 there was an uprising between the miners and the soldiers (minefield police of the day) that became known as the Eureka Rebellion. The flag that the miners chose has become the symbol for many other battles that have followed, especially by the Union movement against various employers over the years.

Our city surrounds a very pretty lake, Lake Wendouree, that is the home of many recreational pursuits including rowing, yachting, hockey, cycling (no, not on water but around the 6km perimeter of the Lake) and of course running, particularly long distance running. Ballarat has spawned a large number of world-class long distance runners with Steve Moneghetti, a previous Marathon winner at World's best level being our city's most lauded athlete. The running track around the lake has been named in honour of Steve, who now approaching 50, is still winning races in various veterans' meets and state-wide against all comers. And he's a real good bloke to boot ... a wonderful ambassador for our fair city.

Our climate varies from rain, drizzle and the occasional snow flurry with winter temperatures mostly between -3? and 10 or 12?C. Summer on the other hand brings temperatures into the 30s and occasionally low 40s C just to test us. Autumn is the best time of the year with sun-filled days and cloud-streaked skies and mild balmy temperatures.

Our landscape is one of rolling green hills, spotted with age old eucalypt trees,(interspersed with imported

Californian pine plantations) that managed to escape the wrath of the miners who raped and pillaged the forests in pursuit of wooden props for the myriad of deep mines and firewood to feed the boilers and to keep them warm and toasty. Ballarat reaches out to flat plains to the north and west, and to the East the volcanic hills that the first Irish immigrants prized so greatly to grow their precious potatoes. Enough of romancing the stone, it's time to pass on my cardiac experience thus far.

My cardiac resume consists of suffering from dilated cardiomyopathy that apparently arrived as a result of a viral infection at an undetermined time in days gone by. Some 18 months ago I had a successful, thank goodness, double bypass procedure to counter blockages in two of my heart's arteries that were discovered soon after my cardiomyopathy was diagnosed.

My life is of a typical Australian working class man. I am married to a wonderful lady who goes by the name of Arlene. We're proudly coming up to our thirtieth wedding anniversary later this year. We're as different as cheese and chalk; however as they always say, opposites attract. We have four living children, having lost our first, Jordan to a cardiac problem at two days of age. Our girls Eden and Tarlea are 25 and 23 respectively and our two boys, Jake and Jesse bring up the rear at 21 and 19. We're very proud of our children and their achievements too, along with our strong sense of family.

I work as a workplace instructor (teacher) in the forestry industry, leading a busy and somewhat transient work life covering a wide expanse of three states of Australia, being Victoria, South Australia and New South Wales.

As I admitted earlier I must admit right up front that I'm somewhat of an imposter as a Cardiac Athlete. My running style has been likened to that of an uncoordinated wombat and my swimming style to that of my dear mother's kitchen processor in overdrive. But, I love running as I call it, however others, including our eldest son Jake refer to it as fast plodding. I was never blessed with a great deal of athletic ability as a child, but could somehow manage to transport a discus a fairly reasonable distance. Exercise was never really my thing. Prior to beginning running I had been a 16 year smoker, with high cholesterol, often eating poorly and working silly hours in various forms of self-employment. So what prompted my change of direction you say? Quite strange really!

Around five or six years ago I had a motor vehicle accident in my wife's four wheel drive. The car initially collided with a kangaroo, closely followed by a tree and then a concrete culvert. No major injuries, I walked away thanking my lucky stars. A couple of weeks later my life turned for the worse. I had ruptured two discs in my neck as a result of the accident and had to wait quite a while before I was able to have surgery to repair the trouble. All I could bear to do was sit and whine about the pain, taking relief from increasing amounts of food and my weight ballooned to just under 100 kg. I had never been that big and it sure didn't feel comfortable, so after the operation I started walking in an all-out effort to lose weight.

My weight loss theory has always revolved around sweat, so I began to run fifty metres and walk fifty metres to work up a sweat and hopefully lose weight. Then it became running one hundred metres and walking one hundred metres and so on. A little internet research helped me to start a campaign to visit the aforementioned Lake Wendouree and to run five hundred metres and walk five hundred metres. What a feeling of elation it was the day when I circumnavigated the lake running non-stop for the very first time. I was over the moon. Right there and then my life changed.

Soon after I heard of a half marathon, the Medi Marathon that was going to take place in four or five months to raise money for medical research here in Ballarat. Could I do it ? What the hell I would give it a shot. No plan whatsoever I took to the road, running 3 or 4 mornings (five kilometres at a time) before work and a long run (12 or so kilometres) on the weekend. I built the k's up, too quickly at times, but once I knew that I could run thirty kilometres once, I could do it for the big day too. And I did ! Slowly, but

I did it. I was hooked. A marathon then became my next quest; however I learnt all about Ilio Tibial Band Syndrome and had an arthroscope to repair knee injuries I had succumbed to soon after.

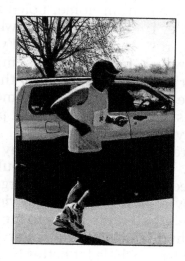

I bounced back and ran other events. Whilst preparing for the next Medi Marathon I fell ill to what I thought, (and so did my GP) was a bout of bronchitis, which was nothing new for me in Spring. Several courses of medication later the symptoms became worse. Coughing became incessant, especially late at night and exercise lost its appeal. Mowing the lawn became a painful and breathless experience and while running my first ten km race accompanied by both my sons, pondered whether my age was catching up with me, just like my wife had always told me. I really struggled to make the distance.

It was around this time that I followed a thread on an Australian running forum concerning one of the athletes who had been through a cardiac event. That person turned out to be Craig aka Bellthorpe. He was keeping everyone up to date with his recovery from a CABG procedure and most importantly of his goal to return to running at his earliest possible opportunity. You couldn't help but admire his attitude and fortitude. His story truly inspired me. I swear it was only a matter of a few days later when my own challenges arrived. Fate plays a strange hand sometimes doesn't it ?

One Tuesday night (October 20, 2009) soon after my life was to change once again. However not for the better I might add. I was away from home, holed up in a motel in Shepparton a smaller rural Victorian city when my coughing and breathlessness rose to a new level. I've never suffered from asthma, however I thought this must be exercise-induced asthma or similar. Best to go to the local hospital I thought, but where was it ? I wasn't at home in Ballarat now so I needed to consult the map in the local phone book, but I couldn't read it, my vision was fuzzy.

Gasping to breathe I reached for my cell phone and capitulated, I felt, by dialling for an ambulance. Boy am I glad I did ! Subsequent entry to the emergency department and assessment by a local physician provided answers that were foreign to me. It all came home to me when I managed to pass litres of fluid from my body after injections by the doctors. Boy did I feel a whole lot better !

Next morning a visiting technician did an ultra sound assessment of my heart and it was here I first learned of the dilated cardiomyopathy.

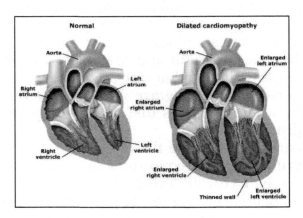

Illustration reproduced from:
http://www.rayur.com/cardiomyopathy-definition-causes-symptoms-diagnosis-complication-and-treatment.html

That was a reality check for sure. How could that be ? I was arguably fitter than I had ever been in my life. Yes, some of that was true, but it also became apparent that other things were starting to catch up with me. Hypertension and moderately high cholesterol readings came home to roost. Around twelve years ago I was struck down with pericarditis also. A nasty infection around my heart which may have initiated it I thought.

A few days later I returned home to Ballarat with my wife, accompanied by strict doctors' instructions to see a cardiologist as soon as possible. But I didn't even reach the appointment date as what seemed to be frequent late night visits to the emergency department of the hospital, hastened by blood pressure which was going through the roof and breathlessness which was scaring me to the back teeth.

After being admitted to hospital following another one of my late night events I had further tests, blood tests, ultrasounds and pen-ultimately an angiogram sealed my fate (October 29, 2009), all within just a few days. Needle after needle and the experience of my first angiogram tested my resilience. The pain of being on my back for two hours following the angiogram prepared me for the pain ahead. Luckily I was a long-term blood donor, so needles don't really faze me. The diagnosis had it that the left main artery in my heart was kinked along with a 50-60% blockage and the right coronary artery was also blocked to a lesser degree. What with this and the cardiomyopathy it felt like my life as I had known it was being stolen away by some greater power. And that thought was not good, that's for sure.

The propensity for rising fluid levels in my lungs worsened to the point that a phone call was made to the Alfred Hospital in Melbourne to discuss 'my case'. The person consulted was the head of the heart transplant team at the hospital and my head was spinning. Could it be that bad ? It sounded like fait accompli to me. All over red rover! My days were threatened, seriously.

That just didn't seem fair as I had a lot more living to do. Or was I just being a drama queen ? What of my wife and children ? Who would provide, who would advise ? Who would play Dad ? No sooner was it than I had a date and a time for a double bypass operation at the Alfred hospital. On Friday all arrangements were made for me to be admitted on Monday and operated on Tuesday morning. When the reality hit and I became increasingly anxious I distinctly remember my Coronary Care nurse Laura telling me that the CABG procedure was a good thing as it "Sure beats the hell out of the alternative". I will never forget her fist in my groin post angiogram and that poignant advice.

No time for reading the books that prepared you for the experience. The postman wouldn't make it in time before I was Melbourne bound. What a shock it had become. Thinking too much only made it worse. Luckily for me my wife was right by my side and we shed shared tears together as the time neared to leave home and to have the operation. Being a fairly emotional person at the best of times I farewelled our Ballarat-based children, choking up as I did so. I hugged them tighter than ever asking our eldest son Jake to take care of things if the unthinkable happened. Or was I being a drama queen ? My resolve was being tested yet again. I knew what depression felt like, as the Black Dog had bitten once or twice a few years back. But several things helped me to stay focussed. A wonderful loving wife and family, a really great mate (thanks Al2) and some sage advice from a bloke whom I had recently read about on a running website, telling of his experience of a cardiac event and bypass procedure. That person was Craig (or aka Bellthorpe) as the Cardiac Athlete community knows him. His staunch determination and fearsome resolve to return to running at the earliest possible safe opportunity inspired me. Just knowing what to expect was a huge relief. He was absolutely honest and called it exactly as it was. It helped me to mentally prepare my own strategy, to know what to expect and to set goals. A bit of a bucket list as some people say.

I would have to say that the best advice Craig gave me was the existence of the Cardiac Athletes website. It was an unbelievable feeling to read about all the CA community and their achievements. There seemed to be a common thread that bound these people together and it was with this belief that I too could dream to run again once my cardiac plumbing system was fixed. I spent hours and hours on the forum in the next few days desperate for more information. Arlene loves to call me 'do it to death Al' and boy did I do that. I have no doubt that the CA website was the major reason why I was able to maintain a positive outlook for the near future as I too wanted more than anything to survive and then to become a bona fide Cardiac Athlete.

To Lars I must offer heartfelt thanks for what he did for me and everyone else by creating and maintaining this wonderful site. I commend it to anyone who strives to maintain or return to active exercise whilst living with or having experienced a cardiac issue. All the various 'pillars of support' amongst the CA community are wonderful people too who continue to amaze me with their knowledge and ability to inspire others with their athletic achievements and attitude to their ongoing health challenges. When I had a bad day I disciplined myself by thinking of various CA members and how they would approach my situation. This always lifted me and stopped me falling into a depression chasm. To each and every one I owe a great deal of thanks. Their medicine was the best of all.

Monday soon rolled around as we walked into the foyer of the Alfred I struggled to climb the couple of steps. There was no going back now. I had to have this operation and it had to do me.

Late that day the surgeons came to meet and greet, informing me about all and sundry of the operation. I was feeling increasingly nervous, however once again, the more I learned the more comfortable I became with trusting my life to both of these men and their team. Their credentials were impeccable, one being a transplant specialist and the other his protégé I assumed, both extensively qualified and both excellent communicators at my level. I needed to feel 100% confident in them and I was.

I had an eerie experience after the surgeons left. Beyond the curtain in the bed next door was a Greek lady who was going through a similar experience to myself, albeit a few days later. The doctors were breaking the news to her that she needed a bypass procedure also and she was having trouble accepting the fact that she had no option other than to have the operation as soon as possible. In fact she was first cab off the rank next morning. She was in shock big time and I felt fortunate that at least I'd had three days to accept the news. Both her and her husband lost tears. How similar we were even though we didn't know one another from a bar of soap.

After our respective spouses left I offered her my best wishes and explained that both of us were going through the same thing on the same day; tomorrow. This helped both of us to prepare. And you know what; neither of us saw one another's faces. I often wonder how she fared ? As good as my experience I hope.

I spent Monday night (November 23rd 2009) peering out my hospital window watching the emergency helicopters come and go ferrying their life-threatened occupants to a safe haven. My roommate was a nice young bloke who had been in hospital for many, many months following an horrendous motor vehicle accident. He too inspired me with his never-say-die attitude, an infectious laugh, his wonderful relationship with all the doctors and nurses and a smile that never left his face. Little or no sleep didn't seem to matter.

The big day had arrived (Tuesday 24th November). It wasn't long before I was visited by a Hannibal Lector lookalike whose near blunt razor shore me from neck to toe. And I'm reasonably hirsute so that was a real experience too. Then followed an anti-germicidal shower and soon the call came. I was conveyed to the prep room to be readied for anaesthesia where a busy scene greeted me. The anaesthetist introduced himself and explained all the pertinent details. He was around my vintage and professed a love of all things mechanical, Beach Boys music, a life-long love of surfing and 20 plus years experience with cardiac procedures. Boy was I in luck. Anyone who had those qualifications had to be a good bloke didn't he ? He offered a little certain something to help calm my nerves, and I thought what the hell. And that was it ! I had been conned. And what a great con it was. No visions of HUGE needles, no countdowns, no nothing. I was out to it.

My next memory was somewhat blurred, where I could hear my wife talking, apparently to a doctor and a nurse in the recovery area of the Intensive Care Department. I drifted in and out, hearing my wife and eldest daughter crying at one stage. All I remember was the nurse telling her that they would put me out to it for a bit longer as I was bleeding a bit more than they would have liked.

Next awakening a day later was a nurse requesting that I wake up. It was hard work this waking up business. Wires and pipes in and out of me from all angles and directions, machines going beep, beep, beep and chiming infrequently. Lights flashing and people around me in all directions. By my side there was Arlene. You beauty I thought. I was alive. Thanks boss, I owe you a big one for this. Everything from here on in was up to me. A rather curiously angled bed supported me. Uncomfortable or what, and then it hit me. An oversize pipe down my windpipe, another pipe in my groin, wire and pipes emanating from and going into my neck and chest.

When I moved the first time the pain from my chest hit me. Just like Craig had advised me. He told me you will feel like you've been hit by a *!/?@ Kenworth truck, and boy was he right. Talking of Craig he was the first phone call I received post-op and it was great therapy. Just remembering what he had achieved motivated me no end.

The next thirty six hours were spent with nurses watching me like a hawk. The doctors were there all the way, especially when I experienced my first couple of bouts of Atrial Fibrillation. What the hell was my heart doing ? Had they given me someone else's heart when I was unaware ? My heart rate had always been around 40 beats per minute and now it was running turbocharged and wanted to jump out through my back. Ugh, I didn't like this. I felt like panic was setting in, but Malcolm my nurse told me that I wasn't allowed to panic on Wednesdays. It would have to wait till tomorrow. He explained that they were going to give me a drug that would ward off this problem and what was involved. Boy was he professional. Whenever the bells and whistles would go off he was right there. The man in command for whom I am very grateful.

I was very glad to leave intensive care a day later bound for the wards (Thursday 26th November). The nursing staff warned me that post-op depression was an almost universal part of the recovery process. I remember thinking how wondrous that would be ... not ! My own experience with depression some six or seven years previously brought me to a low of a very different kind. I struggled for quite some time to understand what was going on in my head and in my body. It was not a nice feeling to be out of control. Life's ups and downs in the past brought with them a range of emotions and challenges, but never, ever had I been out of control. It was always me steering the ship and I distinctly remember being very angry with the medical world for making me suffer depression once again. Or that's how I justified it at the time anyway. But then it dawned on me. No longer was depression a foreign feeling. I knew what its onset felt like and my strategy was to get prepared before it hit.

This approach was to stand me in good stead when the Black Dog arrived. First I had a real good blubber and got that out of the way first. There was only one opportunity to do it and I wouldn't allow the depression to drag me down that path again. But I needed to do it. Then it was time to regard each new step as one step closer to running. I continually reminded myself of how lucky I was to be alive and to have such a wonderful, loving wife and family. It was my responsibility to dig deep and get on top of this situation and send the Black Dog packing.

When any negative thoughts entered my head I denied them from taking over. This was my life and I was in command. Not some pharmacological concoction sending my hormones into a downward spiral again. Forward two steps and back one, but it was always in the forward direction.

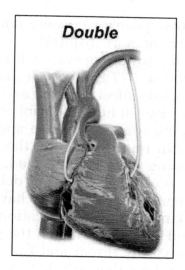

Illustration of double CABG reproduced from:
http://en.wikipedia.org/wiki/File:Blausen_0152_CABG_All_.png

Things began to return closer to normal as pipe by pipe, wire by wire everything was removed. I progressed from one ward to the next as the days wore on. I met different people along the way, some of whom utterly amazed me. One such angel was a lovely lady who of 82 who was recovering from a triple bypass and a wonderful person she was. Her husband a spritely 86 years young had the same procedure three years previously and returned to playing golf soon after, reducing his handicap by two post op. Another was a little girl, 22 or 23 years of age who was awaiting a heart transplant. She brought tears to my eyes. She was the same age as our girls and I couldn't help thinking about what life had dealt her. Hardly fair, no doubt. She had the most remarkable and prolific array of monitors and IVs I've ever seen around her bed. Her operation was scheduled for the day after I met her and yet again I often think of her.

One bloke was back in for his third valve replacement in six months and a brighter person you wouldn't meet, even when infection set in the last time. It helped me to meet these incredibly gutsy people who were far worse off than I and that was a source of more inspiration.

Unfortunately my wound opened a little when a sneeze caught me unawares. That was a 'most unpleasant' experience. A low grade infection set in and this necessitated staying a few extra days in hospital prior to returning home to Ballarat. Sleeping was a challenge and I found myself waking up every hour on the hour. In the past my wife has accused me of sleeping like the living dead, so discontinuous sleep was not only foreign it was entirely debilitating.

My bed mate next door and I were having competitions about who was taking the most medication. But he won as he was diabetic and I'm not. I hated the gross amounts of penicillin going down my throat and the nausea it caused. The nurses convinced me that pain killing medication was a very necessary part of the healing process. I tried to avoid them where possible, but eventually their advice made sense to me. Their advice was that if the body was busy coping with pain there was no time for it to work on healing. Oxycodone and other opioids did not agree with me, so I opted for less intrusive alternatives and a heavy regime of paracetamol. The whole experience taught me a lot about pain and the need for an increased pain threshold. Certainly the experience is one of short term pain for long term gain. Just like my old geography teacher taught me in secondary school. One thing I did learn was that you need meds and the right meds for you.

By now I was accustomed to using the belt at the base of the bed to lift myself up, in addition to walking around the ward and beyond as much as possible. The breathing exercises were yet another 'unique experience'. Gee it was hard work and my body's propensity to overheat at the earliest opportunity seemed to make it even more challenging. It seemed that my body's systems were all more than a little confused following such a major disturbance.

Food was a chore for the first couple of weeks and not enjoyable at all. My heart rate was starting to stabilise and settle back down, much to the pleasure of the medicos. The physio classes were my godsend as my inner exercise self was getting a very small dose of endorphins at last. The energy levels were low, a lot lower than I was used to, but I was on the improve.

Next the doctors allowed me to go downstairs to the cafe for a coffee and to go outside in the sun using monitoring devices to track me. Ah, little bit by little bit. I looked across the road to Fawkner Park a beautiful community park populated by a community of majestic oaks accompanied by a carpet of lush green grass some 2.7 km in perimeter. Running, or rather the possibility of it first firmly re-entered my mind front and centre right there and then. I'm still to go back and do a 'quick' half dozen laps around there, but I will. It's on the list you see !

Before leaving The Alfred the doctors arranged for me to speak to a nurse who specialised in cardiomyopathy patient support. Her advice was that I would have to make a major lifestyle adjustment, to strictly manage my diet and fluid intake and to accept that cardiomyopathy meant that I probably wouldn't work again and may have to accept that heart transplant may be in my future. Her attitude wasn't condescending, rather empathic, however I hadn't written myself off quite yet and when I asked her if and when I could go back to running I'll never forget the look on her face. I'm sure she felt I was having delusions of grandeur. Can't wait till I go back to run Fawkner Park and hopefully she will be still working at the Alfred.

All the way Arlene was right by my side day in day out. Our eldest daughter Eden was there too. How fortunate I am! Our 3 other children and their respective partners had visited by now and once over the initial shock were glad to see my progress each time they came. My brother-in-law bet me a 6 pack of Crown Lager beer that I couldn't ride my bicycle the 50kms from my house to his before my first anniversary. That was just what I needed. Another box to tick, you beauty.

When it was finally time to go home (Saturday 5th December) I was more excited than I care to mention. I won't forget the feeling of elation when I walked back inside our house. I was home, and collapsed into bed straight away as fatigue set in. The walk to the car and the trip home (one and a half hours) wore me down incredibly. Once home I settled in and thanked my lucky stars yet again.

Compiling my 'to do' list in hospital gave me something to think about and to establish a series of priorities. The whole program focussed on being able to run a lap of my Lake Wendouree in the next six months. It all began with the first home adventure which was to walk to the letter box and back. A whole 25 meters. Once, twice and thrice. Then up to the next block and back. Next I attacked a walk around the block; four or five hundred metres. Hard yakka ! Hard yakka ! The legs were moving. The better I felt the better I slept. The sleep deprivation and constant waking from the pain during each night, usually from the vein harvest site in my left leg was draining.

Just as I turned the corner the AF returned a couple of times. This necessitated Warfarin therapy and more blood tests. It really spooked me and a couple of late night visits to the emergency department brought back old memories. Just as soon as it arrived it was gone. My heart rate settled even further and I looked forward to starting the cardiac rehab program, soon. Interestingly my diary entry of Saturday 12th December says "feeling better now and it's starting to show according to other people. They say I have colour in my face again." The next night was my first night of uninterrupted sleep. Hallelujah !

One change that required an adjustment has been the amount of medication I have to take particularly to offset the cardiomyopathy. This includes a beta blocker, a calcium channel blocker, a diuretic, an ace inhibitor, a statin and aspirin. My normally low heart rate 40 to 45 BPM means that my cardiologist worries more than he should about the possibility of my heart throwing off clots again. However, I'm comfortable to take his advice as he knows a lot more about it than I ever will. If that means taking all these pills until I shuffle off at 80 years, 47 days of age so be it I say.

Also, a friend recommended that I take Co-Enzyme Q10 and I started taking it too after being cleared by the surgeon and my cardiologist. My wife will tell you it has a placebo effect, but all I know is there was no looking back now once I took it. My chest wound was healing well now. In fact the leg wound took longer to heal than the chest. I told myself that the more I could move, the more oxygen was going to be pumped around my body. And the more oxygen that was being pumped around would hasten the healing. That was my theory anyway.

By this time I was itching to start the cardiac rehabilitation program, but unfortunately the protocols and paperwork were mixed up and I had to wait another week or two. In my mind cardiac rehab attendance was a no brainer. If I wanted to get better, the sooner I got back on the bike the sooner I could run. Some people are very negative about fronting up for the program. That didn't even enter my mind. Curiosity was killing the cat and the sooner it happened the sooner I would know what was expected of me. Walking twice a day now and for increasingly longer distances up to 3kms.

When the first rehab class arrived (Friday 18th December) I fronted up to the rehabilitation centre and almost felt like the baby of the class. Other than one young lady I was the baby of the class at 54. There was a broad spectrum of people, by age, by gender, by condition, by pre-op or post-op, by motivation, by attitude. One bloke that comes to mind was eight months post bypass when he completed the program and told me he didn't know why he bothered doing the program. After all, he said, he didn't feel any better whatsoever. He only turned up one day a week for one hour and exercised as little as was possible. I shook my head and rolled my eyes as he told me he was going to start smoking again. He thought he may as well enjoy the rest of his life. I ask you, what an attitude ! All those resources, all the surgeons, doctors and nurses blood sweat and tears were about to go down the gurgler. What a fool. His entire operation was very heavily subsidised by the wonderful health care scheme we have in Australia. He was a taxpayer's loss too. By contrast there were two sixty year olds waiting for lung transplants. Wheeling their oxygen trolleys beside them, gasping deeply every second breath their efforts on the exercise bikes and other machines were to be admired.

Strangely enough up until that time I can't recall ever going to a gym in my life. I remembered looking around the room and spying a variety of equipment. The leg press machine appealed, as did the various types of exercise bikes, however it was the prospect of being able to work my way back to running on the treadmill that really turned my crank. Doing a few laps of the corridor during the first session gave me a starting point of where I was at in terms of fitness. Twenty laps and I was ready to have a little lie down; well almost. How quickly had my fitness been decimated; amazing ? It was back to climbing the mountain all over again.

Diet, psych and physio education sessions were interspersed with gym sessions in the rehab program. As each session came and went the weights on the machines went up, the time on the bikes increased and the number of step-ups and corridor laps climbed. Aah ! The endorphins were returning. How good was life again ? I'll never forget the look on the therapist when I broke out into a slow jog on the treadmill. She had told me about her hypertension the week previous, so I thought it best to advise her to take it easy, to sit down and take a deep breath. Her answer was to strap a monitor onto me, to be sure, to be sure. I didn't mind as the sweat started and I had ticked my first box. Boy was I a happy camper ?

Come graduation day and a tear crept into my eye. I wished everyone all the best for the future and the 'lung transplant twins' all the best for their ops. Only a few weeks ago (July 2011) I saw Charlie (one of the boys) and his new lungs were working a treat. He had been unwell for many, many years and it warmed my heart to see him so well. Boy, were we lucky boys or what ?

Following the 6 week check up with my surgeon I tried my hand at running. Very, very slowly ! Oh boy that was a new experience. Not the running so much but running on a hard surface made it more painful I think. I did make sure that I cleared it with the surgeon first, after complimenting him on his beautiful Mercedes coupe. He did advise me to check with my cardiologist too. When that time arrived he was very wary about allowing me. But I ran. From that point on when I see him I keep him up to date with what I've been up to and about the CA website too !

From here on in I took it back to the days when I first started running by combining a walk 150 metres with a 150 run and doing this around the Lake (6km). Aahh it felt good to be back on the track, even though my calf gave me curry after each run.

Next step was to return to work on Monday Feb 8, albeit on a part-time basis: three mornings and/or afternoons a week working up to full-time within four weeks. The energy supply was still down and I fell into bed each night, asleep within seconds it seemed. There was some under-estimation on my behalf about the amount of sleep I needed as I normally sleep around 6 hours a night but found 7 to 8 hours to be a must at this point.

March and I was back at work full-time and walking and running every day before or after work, 3 kms building up to 6kms, slowly, very slowly. The confidence was building and I remember pushing the envelope one day down on the beach at Warrnambool by tackling quite a steep hill three times. Boy was I weary and hell it felt good. I had turned the corner and running was no longer painful as it had been up until this point. The only discomfort was from my left calf where the surgeon had intervened or should that be intervened ? The bicycle was my next challenge even though I felt physically capable, the thought of falling off and bleeding to death due to the blood thinners didn't enthuse me. Well would you believe it was the thought of grazed knees and elbows ? My first ride was a leisurely flat ride of 58 kms and once again I slept very well that night.

Now that I was back exercising and feeling increasingly stronger and 'normal' it was time to have a go at my first event. Mothers' Day sees fun runs held everywhere in Victoria as a fundraiser for breast cancer research. Our eldest son Jake was keen to help the old boy get to the finish line too. Prior to completing this event (10Kms) I distinctly remember challenging myself to push 'it' again. I hit the exercise bike one night with the brake cranked up at 20+kph for an hour, jumped off, took my blood pressure and pulse straight away (153/83 and 117BPM) and next day ran 12 kms around Lake Wendouree as 'fast' as I could plod. This wasn't long after I had a post-op review with my surgeon and the past 6 months started to fade into the past. Just as it was in the first few days following the surgery every day was a small improvement.

Crossing the finish line on Mothers' Day (Sunday 9th May 2010 – 23+ weeks post op) brought a tear to my eye when I hugged Jake. It really was elation and a sense of achievement. How fortunate had I been when I looked around me at what seemed to be quite a few ladies, many of whom were a lot younger than me, wearing scarves to cover up the effects of chemotherapy.

Since then I have run in a few other events and have actually recorded better times than prior to the bypass; even faster plodding. The only major difference being now is that I do have days where for no apparent reason I get the stops and starts and need to walk. But that's ok just as my Coronary Care Nurse Laura told me "It sure beats the alternative".

A special post-op event was my first year's anniversary. It really was a special feeling to look back at where I was 365 days previously and where I had progressed to. So you ask, how did I celebrate ? Ran a lap of Lake Wendouree that's how ! Would you have expected anything else ?

So what haven't I done to date ? I haven't met any of the Cardiac Athletes in person that's what. That goal should be achieved later this year I hope. It would be very nice to attend one of the CA meetings in the future. Arlene and I would like to travel across the big pond next year to USA and that would be the ideal opportunity to tick this box wouldn't it ?

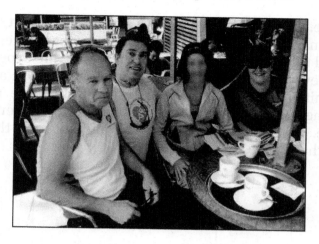

Now he has.

I've recently purchased a near-new classic mountain bike and aim to restore it back to its original livery soon. Then I'll invite my mate AL2 to tag along and we will have a crack at a few weekend tours around our beautiful countryside. Each year Victoria has the Great Victorian bike ride for 3 to 8 days around different regions of our beautiful State. That would be worth doing too. My aging knees will probably mean that more and more bicycling will eventually take over from running; but that's ok. My opportunity to run a marathon has probably passed me by, dang frazzle, but a half marathon will definitely be on the cards sometime in the near future. Need to revisit the Alfred before Christmas to run Fawkner Park too. Shee, there's a lot to live for isn't there ?

Aside from exercise I would like to become involved in helping out the cardiac cause somehow in my community. Options might include visiting cardiac patients in hospital, raising money for defibrillators for community groups and addressing different groups about my cardiac experience. Who knows ? I'm sure I'll know when the right opportunity arrives.

My future goals include celebrating my 60th birthday, enjoying semi-retirement, getting to know, play with and run around with all my grandchildren when they arrive and dreaming now, to live to 80 not out, accompanied all the way by Arlene. Boy it's good to be alive and dream isn't it?

In conclusion, can I say to any other cardiac patients who may read this and the many more interesting life experiences and achievements than mine in this book that you are only truly limited in life by yourself. Hopefully there may be something in my ramblings that will be of benefit to someone. I trust that every one of you will have the good fortune that I have had so far.

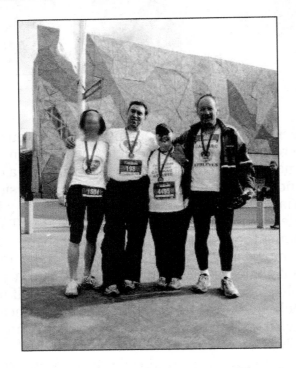

Growing Cardiac Athletes Team Victoria.

CHAPTER 14

' BillCobit ' :

" From ICU to Ironman "

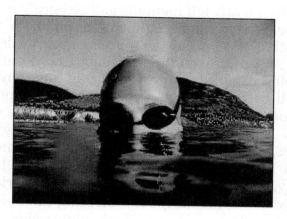

CARDIAC ATHLETE 14

First name: Bill
Forum name: "BillCobit "
Country: USA
Diagnosis: Endocarditis; Mitral Valve Prolapse
Treatment: Mitral Valve Repair

One Saturday afternoon I decided to inflate the tyres on an old bicycle I had, and I went for a ride. I hadn't been on a bicycle in years, but I was in an agitated, grumpy mood and needed to blow off some steam. I rode twelve miles and returned home with spent legs. I had made two observations: 1) the exercise and fresh air was invigorating and boosted my mood; 2) I was in poor physical shape. I slept fitfully that night and felt motivated to ride again. Within a short time, I found myself looking forward to cycling opportunities and I became creative at fitting them into my busy schedule. I was in my late 30's and had a demanding job that involved frequent business travel.

My irregular schedule and personal circumstances hadn't been conducive to physical recreation pursuits, and I had succumbed to inertia for several years. Although I had no health problems related to my lifestyle, "all work and no play" had made me the proverbial dull boy. I had been preoccupied with job-related challenges, didn't sleep very well, and I frequently felt mentally and physically tired.

Exercise started to become my mechanism for stress relief. Initially, I enjoyed the exercise buzz while I was on the bike. As I increased the frequency and duration of my rides, I felt sustained improvement in my physical and mental well-being. I lost some weight, I slept better, I thought more clearly, and I dealt more effectively with work challenges. I was hooked. I upgraded to a new bike and bought a resistance trainer for winter and night-time use.

Due to schedule limitations, I mostly rode by myself. Periodically, I was able to ride with a long-time friend of the same age who was similarly rediscovering the enjoyment of recreational cycling. As we both approached our 40th birthdays, we discussed the idea of a cycling tour. We contemplated something memorable and challenging that would be a final conquest before succumbing to the physical decline of "old age." We planned a cycling trip to Cape Breton Island, Nova Scotia, including the famed Cabot Trail that followed dramatic coastal mountains and provided spectacular scenery.

I trained for several months to prepare myself for the trip, which was as challenging and memorable as we had anticipated. It felt great to have set and achieved an ambitious goal, and I wanted more of that gratifying experience. The idea that this had been a final challenge before turning forty was dismissed, and we promptly began planning the next year's tour, which took us through the Adirondack Mountains in upstate New York. The tradition of an annual bike tour had been established.

I had never been much of a runner, but one winter I

decided to add jogging to my exercise regimen for some relief to the monotony of the bike trainer. It was much slower going and more effort than I had recalled from my mid-twenties, but I attributed that entirely to age. I nevertheless continued, deciding that it was good cross-training.

The following summer, I decided to participate in a short-course triathlon. I enjoyed cycling, my running distances had improved, and I had been a competitive swimmer in my youth. After a few weeks of swimming practice, I was ready to go. I had a decent swim and was predictably dropped on my fat tire bike. I was, however quite struck by my poor running. I was huffing with the elderly and overweight participants, while others effortlessly passed. Despite my decidedly uncompetitive performance, I enjoyed the event and planned to return the following year. I liked the festive, energetic atmosphere as well as the personal challenge.

I visited a new doctor for a routine physical exam, expecting the usual unremarkable result. As soon as he placed the stethoscope on my chest, he asked about the history related to my noisy heart valve. I explained that I'd been advised of mitral valve prolapse and a clinically insignificant murmur about fifteen years earlier. He shook his head. This was no routine murmur. It was indicative of clinically significant valve dysfunction. I'd had no previous encounter with the physician, and I wondered if his assessment was correct.

Follow-up with a cardiologist indicated a leaking mitral valve. I was advised by the cardiologist that I'd probably need surgery at some point in the future. I began asking questions about the likely cause, disease progression and the point at which I might need surgery. I had apparently exhausted my allotment of his time, as he expressed annoyance with my questions. He didn't "have a crystal ball," told me we could "discuss surgery when you can no longer ride a bike" and abruptly left the examination room. I don't know if I was more stunned by the diagnosis or by the doctor's curt indifference, but I left the visit feeling angry, confused and a bit frightened.

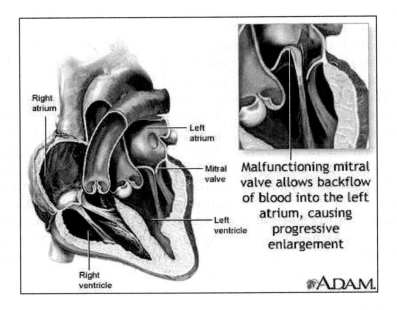

Illustration reproduced from:
http://www.walgreens.com/marketing/library/contents.htm
l?docid=000180&doctype=1

A few days later, I requested the report from my echocardiogram, planning to take it to a cardiologist who would treat me with a bit more respect and compassion. I began my own research into heart valve disease. My study quickly led me to the recollection of a "mystery illness" I'd had during the winter after the Cape Breton trip. For approximately one month, I had suffered fever, body aches, fatigue and periodic drenching night sweats. Repeated clinic visits had not identified the underlying cause. Bacterial infection was suspected but not confirmed. A few courses of antibiotics had been prescribed without any apparent affect. Shortly before an appointment with an infectious disease specialist, my symptoms abated. I cancelled the appointment, believing that my situation had resolved. I felt a bit run down over the next few months but felt like I was back to normal when spring arrived.

In retrospect, I suspected that I had suffered bacterial endocarditis, a potentially life-threatening infection of the inner lining of my heart. I compared my echocardiogram report with established professional guidelines and realized that my first cardiologist had given me bad guidance. Based on my physical heart dimensions and degree of mitral regurgitation, it appeared that surgery was indicated sooner rather than later. In fact, waiting until I could "no longer ride a bike" would likely be a point at which I would have irreversible heart failure, and surgery would be of no help. I concluded that credentials alone could not be relied upon and I resolved to thoroughly qualify the next cardiologist I engaged.

I called several cardiology practices, explaining to desk receptionists that I was seeking a cardiologist knowledgeable of valve disease who could provide me with some personalized care in context of my lifestyle and exercise habits and help me reconcile prior guidance with what I had learned from my own research. I could almost hear eyeballs rolling at the other end of the telephone line as the idea of an amateur internet cardiologist was being processed.

I had a different experience when I contacted a university-affiliated cardiology practice. "I think we have the perfect cardiologist for you," the desk receptionist said. Indeed, she was correct; the cardiologist was thorough, knowledgeable and respectful. As a medical school professor, he appreciated my research efforts and my desire to take an informed, active role in the management of my condition. A middle-aged Cardiac Athlete was a bit of an oddity to him. I was perplexed by my poor running ability while he viewed me as someone who could do what most patients in my condition could not. Conventional medical logic was that I was asymptomatic. We weren't quite sure how to sort all of that out. He conducted a stress echocardiogram to view my heart motion under exercise conditions. He observed some irregular heart motion and was concerned that I might have had a heart attack. I was restricted from all exercise until an angiogram could be scheduled.

Up to that point, I had accepted my circumstances fairly well, but being cut off from activities that had become such an integral part of my life was troubling. Fortunately, subsequent blood testing revealed a favorable lipid profile, and my coronary arteries were deemed clear when the angiogram was conducted. I was cleared for all activities and scheduled for a follow-up examination in six months. I resumed cycling, participated in two more triathlons and enjoyed a late summer bicycle tour in Virginia's Blue Ridge Mountains.

My next examination revealed some additional heart enlargement, and my cardiologist referred me to a university hospital surgeon to discuss surgery. I knew that mitral valve repair was preferable to valve replacement, and I had hoped that I was a candidate for repair. The surgeon explained that the extent of valve damage and the fact that both valve leaflets were involved suggested that repair was not a likely option. I was not ready to accept that opinion. I also was not ready to have the surgery performed at the university hospital. My research taught me that valve repairs could be technically complex, and that the skill of the surgeon was a critical success factor for a favorable outcome. The university hospital was well-known for bypass surgery, but that is very different from a valve procedure. The Cleveland Clinic was widely regarded as the top hospital for valve surgery, so I turned my attention there.

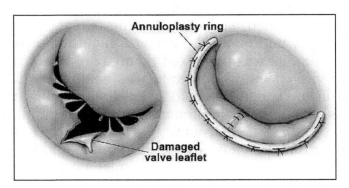

Illustration reproduced from:
http://nursingcrib.com/category/nursing-care-plan/

Surgeons and their specialties are profiled on the Cleveland Clinic web site. I prowled the Internet to find additional information about the skill and reputation of the mitral valve specialists. I was favorably impressed when I visited the Cardiothoracic Surgery Network website and learned that they were renowned experts who instructed other cardiac surgeons. They were also authors of numerous journal articles and cardiac surgery text books. I chose Dr. Marc Gillinov at the Cleveland Clinic as my surgeon and scheduled a surgery date shortly after the Christmas holiday.

I was a bit intimidated by the idea of having such major surgery so far from my home, but I quickly put those concerns aside once I began the planning process. The Cleveland Clinic serves patients from all over the world and has a well-organized program for patients who need to travel. Once I had made my choice, I was a bit surprised by my own peace of mind. I was ready to put the valve problem behind me and resume a normal and active life. I began thinking positive thoughts about returning to cycling and triathlon the following summer.

On the day of my surgery, I recall a deep breath from the gas mask, a few episodes of post-operative semi-consciousness, and then finally awakening to realize I was alive and had successfully made it through valve repair surgery. The diagnosis of bacterial endocarditis had been confirmed. It was the middle of the night and after visiting hours. My body was full of tubes and wires. My kind and attentive nurse (Heather, my guardian angel) offered morphine, and I accepted, quickly drifting back to unconsciousness.

Sometime later I awoke again. I was in miserable physical condition but in a very positive emotional state. Perhaps due to the combined influence of a motivational story I had read and the morphine, I began thinking ambitious and audacious thoughts. I had cycled the challenging roads around Lake Placid, New York, and began to visualize completing the Lake Placid

Ironman triathlon with my rebuilt engine. I had never attempted anything involving that level of challenge but it was very intriguing. In my mind I planned a three year journey to recover and work up to the required distance.

My wife arrived the next morning as soon as visiting hours resumed. When she had last seen me, I was agitated, disoriented and incoherent. She was relieved to see that I was awake and in good spirits but horrified by my ridiculous recovery goal. I couldn't lift my arms, but I was talking about completing a 2.4 mile swim, a 112 mile bike ride through the Adirondacks, and a 26.2 mile run. She took comfort in the prospect of more rational thought once I metabolized the drugs. That was not to be however, and a couple of days later I was still committed to the idea.

A very nice gentleman representing a heart patient support organization visited me while I was in the hospital. I believe he approached me in a manner that was appropriate for the typical patient in my position, but in light of my aspirations, his demeanor struck me as that of a funeral director. He explained how his organization offered sympathetic support and "hope" for cardiac patients. Hope is a good thing. Certainly, hopelessness is a very bad thing. However, given my frame of mind, I was not interested in laying around "hoping" for something; I was planning my journey to an Ironman. I had more than hope, I had a goal. It was kind of him to visit me, and I told him so, but I was glad when he left. After a few days of recovery I was discharged and returned home.

A week later, I made a planned postoperative visit with a new cardiologist who was closer to my home than the university. I asked about the possibility of running a short-course triathlon in five months. He was somewhat surprised that I was thinking such thoughts, but told me that it was indeed within the realm of possibility if I had a good recovery. I was giddy, but that feeling quickly passed.

Later that day, I developed a fever and other symptoms reminiscent of my endocarditis. My new cardiologist had me admitted to a local hospital where I began aggressive intravenous antibiotic therapy. A blood test indicated infection. The hospital cardiology staff suspected an infected valve and probable reoperation to install an artificial valve. I was devastated. I had been positive and motivated, but the prospect of reoperation and the artificial valve I sought to avoid was very demoralizing. To my great relief, a transesophageal echocardiogram showed no indication of valve infection. Wherever the bugs were, they weren't busy colonizing on my remodelled heart valve. After four days in the hospital, I was discharged again to return home with no further complication.

I was feeling well enough to become restless in between my frequent naps. My wife asked if I wanted to get out of the house, and I suggested we go browse at the bike store. There was an excellent deal on a road bike from the prior model year. I concluded it would be suitable for the longer triathlon distances I was contemplating and decided to buy it. The salesman offered to put it on a wind trainer so I could spin the cranks and confirm the fit, but I declined. He was somewhat bewildered, but he had no idea that I struggled to walk and had a two-piece sternum held together with surgical wire. I was in no condition to climb onto a bike. We took the bike home with us, and I began to look forward to riding it in the spring.

I began a cardiac rehabilitation program at a local hospital but was soon dismissed when I demonstrated the ability to exercise without untoward effect. I began walking a couple of times a day. It was exhausting at first, but I gradually developed stamina over the period of a few weeks. When I was cleared for driving, I returned to work. Although I had a desk job, I also found that exhausting for the first few days. I gradually settled into an exercise routine that took me from walking to jogging, a bit of swimming and some indoor riding. I had lost about 15 pounds after surgery, but my bodyweight was returning to normal as my appetite returned. By the time spring arrived, I was training outdoors and looking forward to my first postoperative triathlon, even though I felt a bit underpowered.

That first sprint-distance race was quite a struggle for me. By the time I got to the run, I felt terrible and succumbed to several walking intervals in an attempt to get my heart rate under control. I finished, but I was disappointed. A second event a month later (six months after surgery) was not any more successful. I started to doubt my ability to fulfil my goal of completing an Ironman in the future. The third event of the season was my first Olympic distance event, seven months after surgery. I didn't feel great, but it was a marked improvement over the prior two events.

Eight months after surgery it was time for the annual bike trip with my cycling buddy. I wasn't sure about my ability, but we decided to try it, and agreed we would rest whenever I needed it. I voted to return to the Adirondacks with the ulterior motive of incorporating a loop on the Ironman bike course. My friend was agreeable, and we had a very nice four day ride through the region. My performance was better than I expected, and I finally felt like I was headed toward a full recovery. The Ironman course was demanding, but with additional training, I could envision myself completing two loops for the required 112 miles.

The following summer I completed a half-iron triathlon, consistent with my three year plan to take on the Ironman. I felt fine during the event, but it was evident that my cardiovascular capacity was no better than it was prior to the surgery. I had been cautioned that I might not experience a performance increase, but I had planned to prove otherwise. It had been 18 months since my surgery, and I concluded that I had reached full recovery. My operation had been a success: the valve did not leak, my heart had returned to normal dimensions, I was stable and did not require any medications, but I still performed like a "heart patient." That was disappointing, but not much of a consideration in the overall scheme of life. I began calculating how slowly I could swim, bike and run during the Ironman race without being disqualified. I would finish close to the bike and marathon cut-off times, but I would make it if I could approximate my half-iron pace. The goal was still alive, but I began adjusting my performance expectations.

The third summer after my surgery I registered for the

next year's Lake Placid Ironman. Later that season, I completed a three quarter-iron distance race. I was slow but managed a pace that would suffice for completing the full distance. I had a little less than a year until I attempted to make good my vow to complete the Ironman.

It was a beautiful day in the High Peaks region of the Adirondack Mountains. The sun was climbing over the eastern slopes as I trod water in my wetsuit and awaited the cannon shot that would start the race. I contemplated where I had come from and what I was about to do.

Preparing for an Ironman does not involve a trial run of the full 140.6 miles. I was relying on faith that dutiful adherence to my training plan had adequately prepared me to survive the day. I swam well and struggled on the demanding bike course. My marathon didn't much resemble running, but I was determined to finish after having poured over three years of physical and emotional energy into the goal. I had imagined my moment of personal triumph would be crossing the finish line, but it came when I was only about 10 miles into the marathon, alternately walking and shuffling.

I looked up and saw the ski jumps from the 1980 Olympics with the sun dropping toward the horizon. It was a postcard image. At that moment, I was struck by the idea that three years earlier I was almost dead, but now I wasn't, and I was on my way to completing an Ironman! I expected to finish, but even if I did not, I could take satisfaction in how far I had come since setting my goal in the cardiac ICU.

I reflected on how much I enjoyed watching my children grow, the wonderful times I'd had with my wife, the great friends I had made. My vain pursuit was also a celebration of life. I was euphoric. That feeling passed, and I realized once again how exhausted I was. I kept pressing on and ultimately finished well after dark to the cheers of my family and a few friends. It had been a fantastic day. My cycling buddy had made the trip to Lake Placid to cheer me on. He congratulated me, then paid me a compliment that I will always remember. "Over the years" he said, "I have watched you get knocked down, only to get up, reinvent yourself, and do something against the odds. I think that's your defining character attribute. " I liked that. I decided that day that I would start thinking of myself as the guy who always got up, not the guy who got knocked down. I would focus not on what I had been, but on what I could still become. I couldn't go back in time, I couldn't undo anything to change the past, I couldn't restore my youth, but I could always be the guy who kept getting up. I decided that was a healthy and helpful way to look at my circumstances.

Over the next few years I completed the Lake Placid event two more times. Along the way, I became involved with the "Cardiac Athletes" community. It was wonderful to interact with people who were engaged in sport despite the challenges of heart disease. I wished I'd had the support of that warm, friendly community when I was facing heart surgery and during my rehabilitation. Nevertheless, I found tremendous educational and social value in my participation.

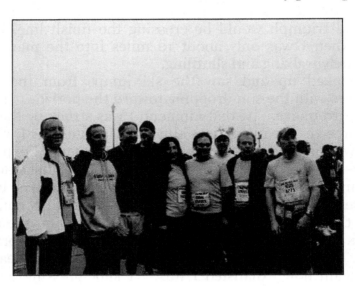

I've been fortunate enough to participate in some of the regional sport events hosted by group members, at which there is a wonderful sense of camaraderie and positive energy. I was especially touched when two members of the group made the trip to Lake Placid to cheer me on in my third Ironman event. It was an extraordinary gesture, but certainly not out of character for the closely-knit Cardiac Athletes community. I continue to enjoy my recreational sport pursuit, and my enjoyment is enhanced by being able to share my enthusiasm and reciprocal support with other community members. I will share some of my personal thoughts and perspective in the spirit that others may find them useful to their personal situations:

1. If you were an athlete prior to development of your heart condition, recognize that your reality has changed. Don't focus on what you may have lost; take advantage of the ability you have. Were you previously one of the world's premier athletes in your chosen sport? If not, you were just a guy or lady who was enjoying your sport to the best of your ability. There were plenty of people who were more successful than you were. Your performance may have diminished, but realize that things haven't changed much in the big scheme of recreational sport, and there is really no reason to miss the enjoyment of participation. If you formerly disparaged the efforts and results of people who performed as you now do, forgive yourself your previous conceit and insensitivity. Life teaches us lessons, and you've learned one more. Gaining empathy is good, and in that respect you have improved. Engage your new-and-improved self in the support and friendship of less talented athletes whom you may not have associated with before. You will find those experiences and relationships fulfilling.

2. If you were not an athlete prior to your diagnosis or treatment, but you want to reinvent yourself, realize that you may be atypical but you are certainly not alone. Find your way to others who have made the transition you are contemplating, utilizing social networking sites as useful tools. You may be facing uncertainty, but there are others who can encourage and guide you. You may be heading into territory that is unknown to you, but is not unfamiliar to others. You will find kind strangers who want you to succeed; they will encourage you when you are demoralized, they will cheer you when you are pursuing a goal, and they will share your joy when you achieve.

3. Educate yourself on your heart condition. That may seem daunting, but there are wonderful internet-based resources that can make you quite knowledgeable, which is a requirement for becoming your own advocate. You will learn that there are some scientific "absolutes" related to heart disease and physical activity, but there are also vast areas of grey. Having an appreciation for these will enable you to locate and work with responsible health practitioners who can support your interests.

4. Set goals that are challenging but realistic within the constraints of your medical condition. As in other aspects of life, the definition of "success" is the achievement of chosen goals. Being successful is enjoyable and gratifying. It can be particularly helpful to have a goal when you are facing a low point, such as a surgical intervention or the imposition of an activity restriction. Think about possibilities, and set out to do something you've never considered before. The journey to the goal will motivate and inspire you, and will lead you to experiences that enrich your life.

5. Don't underestimate the power of your support for others. You will encounter other "survivors" who have heart disease or who are overcoming or battling other serious health issues. You may not have walked in their shoes, but your own determination and success, however modest, can be an inspiration to others. Encourage others and celebrate their success.

CHAPTER 15

Sandy ' Scvb13 ' :

" You never know when your ticket will be called "

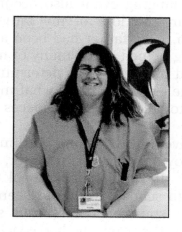

CARDIAC ATHLETE 15

First name: Sandy
Forum name: "scvb13 "
Country: USA
Diagnosis: Congenital Anomalous Right Coronary Artery
Treatment: One Bypass Graft

On Friday, March 13, 1970 I entered this world ... this should have been an ominous sign, being born on Friday the 13th. However, I'm not superstitious but after what I've been through it makes me wonder !   To truly understand the significance of my heart problem it's important to understand where I came from as a person and an athlete.

I started competitive sports at age 7, playing soccer for

my local competitive team. It was there that I found that I thrived on pushing myself to the limits. I also met many lifelong friends on those teams. I credit my second coach with instilling that deep drive and competitiveness in me as he pushed us in ways we never thought possible. We ran and trained for hours on end to the point of exhaustion yet we kept coming back for more. I was at my happiest when I was testing just how far I could push myself. As under 10 soccer players it wasn't uncommon for us to run 3 miles before and another 3 miles after a 2 hour soccer practice !

Another life changing event also occurred shortly after my freshman year, the loss of my father to a ruptured cerebral aneurysm. My father had been a huge part of my athletic life, having helped coach many of my softball teams, etc. It was at that moment I was determined to never have to rely on someone else after I saw what my mom had to go through trying to pick up the pieces financially and otherwise.

I took this drive and discipline with me throughout my athletic career enjoying a successful soccer, softball, and later volleyball career. It was in high school that I discovered volleyball, our high school coach had seen me at a softball all-star game the summer before and suggested to my brother I try out for the team (he had coached my brother in water polo many years before). I was flattered so I thought I'd give it a try. I was hooked. I played every chance I got and started playing year round my freshman year. I made varsity as a sophomore and had an amazing time playing on both my high school and club teams, again, making many lifelong friends. I wasn't highly recruited out of high school so I decided to continue playing for our local community college which was one of the top-ranked teams in California at the time. This is where I really feel I blossomed as a player..

Again, we were tested mentally and physically in ways I never thought possible. We endured 8-hour practices during double days, hours of being pushed and yelled at to be our best, yet we kept coming back for more. It takes a special type of athlete to handle this stress and my teammates and I thrived on it. We went on to finish as state runner-ups in California both years, and, although we didn't win state championships we still proved to ourselves that we could do almost anything we set out to do !

I was recruited by several schools after my two years at De Anza and chose West Texas A&M University to continue my volleyball career at. I arrived in the grassy high plains of West Texas in early August to meet my coach and teammates. I remember driving into the Panhandle and thinking, " this certainly isn't like California ". I was excited about the possibilities but also frightened as I'd never been away from home. Once my teammates and I stepped on the court and started to mesh as a team and as friends it was clear we had great potential. Each and every one of us set aside our individual needs to become part of something bigger, a team.

We endured hours upon hours of practice, weight training, studying films, etc. But, in the end, it was all worth it as we walked away with West Texas' first Div. II National Volleyball Championship in December of 1990.

We had an amazing run that year and the feeling of accomplishing a dream is like no other. Once the shock and awe started to wear off I think each of us understood that we had accomplished something very special and that we may never experience anything like that again.

The summer after that first year at WT brought many changes. We found out while on summer break that our beloved coach was moving on to a Div. I job and we were devastated. We arrived at campus in July to work camps but still didn't have a new coach lined up. In fact, here we were, National Champions and we didn't get a new coach until two weeks before the season started ! Also, because our school dropped the football program for that year due to financial constraints we were forced to become independent and were not affiliated with any league. We already had two strikes against us yet we were determined to make the most of it. We had lost our senior leadership and now there were only two seniors, myself, and another.

In many ways, I look upon that season as an even bigger

accomplishment because it seems we had so many strikes against us starting out. But, again, we put in countless hours of hard work and it paid off as we went on to win a second National Championship with our new coaching staff.

After those two wonderful years at WT, I continued to fuel my competitive drive by moving back to California to attend nursing school while playing on a competitive women's club team and trying new sports like triathlons and running. I am not a natural runner or swimmer but I enjoyed doing both sprint and Olympic triathlons for many summers during my 20s.

In 1999 I married my husband and also started graduate school for nursing. Another challenge. It was at this time that I stopped playing volleyball due to time constraints and the physical toll it was taking on my body due to chronic injuries (back, shoulder, knees). Thus, I began a decade of new and different challenges.

On October 1st, 2000, I went to work after spending the weekend moving with a " side cramp ". After working all day with progressively worsening pain my co-worker and other assistant manager drove me to Kaiser where it was determined I had appendicitis. Later that night, after working a full shift at the VA I was taken to what would become my first of many surgeries over the past 10 years. My husband dubbed me a " lemon " jokingly, but, boy he had no idea at that time !

Six months later I underwent bilateral fasciotomies for compartment syndrome in both calves caused by running. This is a very rare condition but can be caused when the muscles grow beyond what the fascia can handle. Go figure, it happened to me. But, once this was fixed I was able to begin working out again and even ran a 5K 10 days post-op ! I had my active life back, or so I thought.

A year later, as I was walking up the stairs to work, I felt a pop in my knee and it gave out. Another injury. This was the knee that I had torn my posterior cruciate ligament in during my volleyball days at De Anza. A few months of limping around with a brace and I was back in for arthroscopic knee surgery. Three years, three surgeries ...

this decade wasn't looking too good !

I was finally back on track and even did a triathlon in the summer of '04, although, I had a poor performance.   I chalked it up to inadequate training, although in hindsight there were other factors.

I became a mother in 2005, a life changing moment that I am so thankful for.   On Sept. 15, 2005 my husband and I welcomed our son into this world.   He has been our joy ever since.   I endured a very difficult pregnancy and birth and after seeing just how difficult it is to raise a child we both decided one was enough.   Little did I know that decision probably saved my life !

During my pregnancy I had several episodes of severe chest pain and mid-scapular pain.   My doctor and nurse practitioner chalked it up to GERD and possibly gall bladder disease.   I was told to re-evaluate it after my son was born if it returned.   We were on vacation at our condo in Palm Springs when my son was 8 months old when it returned with a vengeance.   We had eaten at one of our favorite BBQ restaurants there and about 4 hours after dinner the pain and vomiting started.   Luckily my mom was with us and she drove me to the hospital in the middle of the night.   They worked up my heart but everything was negative so they sent me on my way.

Two days later, when we were home, I had another episode and this time drove myself to Kaiser in the middle of the night.   They did an ultrasound and found that I had an inflamed gallbladder. I was scheduled for surgery six weeks later (they wanted to give it time to calm down).   Now I really was looking like a lemon ... in six years I was on my fourth surgery !

The next four years went by with various challenges of balancing work, raising a child, as well as some weird health symptoms (" heartburn ", frequent sinus infections, etc.). It seemed I could never get fit and no matter how hard I tried working out was always difficult.   I chalked it up to being overweight, out of shape, etc.   Well, clearly that wasn't the case as you'll see.

Twelve days after my 40th birthday, my life drastically

changed as I underwent emergency open heart surgery in the unit where I work.   Never in a million years did I think this could happen to me, yet it did.   Here's a look back on that day and how I started my full circle journey.   I am the assistant nurse manager in a very busy ICU at a large VA Hospital.

The date was Wednesday, March 24, 2010... it started out as any other workday early in the morning.   I remember waking up, showering, but feeling completely wiped out, absolutely exhausted.   I'd just turned 40, 12 days prior and was chalking the exhaustion up to a busy schedule.   What else could it be ?   Aren't all moms who work full-time exhausted ?   More on that later.   I had even posted on my Facebook page that I felt like a zombie.   As fate would have it, it's a good thing I went into work.

It was another busy day in the ICU when I arrived at work at 0720.   We had a full house and were expecting one open heart surgery patient at around noon.   Odd in that we don't usually have heart patients scheduled on Wednesdays so that means this case was fairly urgent.   After report, I started on my usual charge nurse paperwork and the unit was running smoothly.   As the assistant nurse manager, it's usually my role to be in charge and I also have admin time each week to complete other responsibilities such as scheduling, meetings, audits, etc.   It makes for a busy job but at least I don't get bored !

Each morning we have a bed meeting at 0900 with all the charge nurses and the bed control nurse to ensure the patients flow through the hospital smoothly.   This is our time to let everyone know how many patients can transfer out of our unit and how many beds we have available.   On this particular morning we started off with only a code bed but had several patients ready for transfer.   This is pretty typical for us.

After the meeting I started having chest pain, or "heartburn" as I thought it was.   I told my manager I was having heartburn and had my morning snack, figuring it would help if I had some food in my stomach.   It didn't.

I went back to the unit and continued to work for the

next hour and a half, progressively feeling worse. I don't know how to describe it except I was wiped out and had chest pain. I finally told one of my co-workers and she checked my pulse and immediately told me to go lay down in our empty room, the code bed. She's a very experienced nurse so I figured I better listen to her. She told me my HR was irregular and the next thing I know is I'm being hooked up to an EKG and our ICU Attending is in the room with me, along with a couple of nurses. I was feeling progressively worse, sweating, nauseated, and the pain was getting worse so they gave me a nitro tablet for under my tongue. Woo wee what a feeling that was, I got very lightheaded and had a bad headache ... but ... it helped the chest pain so I knew this was real.

At first we were talking about me driving to Kaiser (where my insurance is), but I knew at that point it wasn't safe to be in a car. Our doctor started an IV on me and got our cardiologist in to see me. She took one look at the EKG and told me this was real and I was not going to Kaiser but that I needed to get a cardiac catheterization ASAP as my EKG was showing some ST elevation in the inferior leads, the sign of a heart attack.

Holy Cow ! A cardiac cath ? A zillion thoughts were going through my mind ... I'm 40 years old with a 4 year old at home, this can't be happening ! I was terrified and started to cry.

By now there were three of our doctors in with me all working on stabilizing me, along with my own nurses. " Ok " I said, let's do it. I then figured I better go to the restroom because I was going to have to be flat on my back for several hours and God forbid I use a bedpan ! As it turns out, that was the least of my worries, but more on that later !

I got up to use the toilet in the room and at this point I didn't even care who saw me or that there was a camera watching my every move. On the way back to bed I started feeling even worse and started vomiting. My staff were preparing me for transport to the cath lab while I was puking my brains out. Once I got to the cath lab I was given Compazine for the vomiting, Fentanyl, and Versed to calm down. I'd also had several nitro tabs by now. I was happy to see two of my friends as my cath lab nurses and I know the doctor is one of the best.

I think I slept through most of my cath and woke up to find my husband and the cardiologist showing me the video and explaining how I had an extremely rare coronary artery anomaly. My right coronary artery was just a branch of my left anterior descending artery and was kinked and stenosed. Essentially, I was born with only a single coronary artery, a left main that had several branches feeding my entire heart.

At first the cardiologist thought it was something that could be treated with medications, but the next thing I knew is our cardiac surgeon was in the room telling me I needed coronary artery bypass surgery and quickly ! What ???? I told him, " you are bullshitting me ". But, he clearly wasn't. He looked very stressed and had me sign the consent right on the cath table. He explained that it wasn't safe for me to go by ambulance and asked if I minded if he did the surgery. Minded ? Of course not ! I know he is one of the best and I couldn't think of a better place to be with familiar faces everywhere.

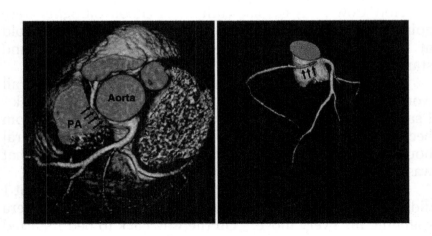

Images reproduced from:
http://www.ncbi.nlm.nih.gov/pmc/articles/PMC2771782/figure/F3/

After that they decided to do a 3D CT scan of my heart to verify that the coronary artery was, indeed, running under the aorta and pulmonary artery (essentially causing mechanical obstruction). I had received a lot of medications by this time and I don't know how long we had to wait for the CT scanner but it was a while. They also gave me several doses of beta blockers to try and slow my HR down as it was too fast to get a good scan.

Finally, the CT scan was completed and I was wheeled up to the Intermediate ICU where my husband works (he's a nurse also). I remember seeing my son in the elevator and daddy holding him and he looked very frightened. They checked me into my room and the cath lab nurse who had stayed by my side all day took out my sheath. She had to apply pressure on my groin for quite some time but I'm not sure how long.

That night in the ICU I was pretty much a fog ... I didn't sleep much but I also don't remember much until my husband came back at 0600 to visit. He hadn't slept much either in anticipation of my surgery. I do remember borrowing a laptop computer and posting on Facebook that I was taking my last sip of Gatorade before being NPO after midnight.

My surgery was scheduled for around 10:30-11 am, they had to do a case before me and then the OR would be ready. Our wonderful anesthesiologist came in to see me and told me he was assigned to the case and would I mind ? Of course not, he is awesome and very experienced.

Another anesthesiologist friend was also going to stay in the room and help. Wow, who gets two attending anesthesiologists ? I knew I was in good hands with people I trusted and that are like family.

The cardiac fellow also came to see me and asked how I was doing. " Nervous " I replied while trying to keep a brave face. He laughed and said he was probably more nervous because there were 50+ nurses upstairs that would kill him if anything happened to me ! Ha ! Two more of my best friends and co-workers stopped by right before their shift started and they were clearly upset but were trying to be brave. By this point I was mentally prepared for what needed to be done.

A few more hours went by and the OR staff showed up to wheel me to the OR ... haven't I seen this with patients a hundred times ? Now it was me ! I kissed my husband good bye and into the OR holding area I went. More familiar faces, my friend, a CRNA was starting an IV across the room and the OR nurse checking me in is an old friend as well. My anesthesiologist came to see me and ... that's all I really remember until later that night !

I was in surgery for about four hours and had a one vessel bypass. Of course I don't remember anything but I do remember waking up to people cheering for me and encouraging me to " open my eyes ". All I remember thinking is ... " leave me alone, can't you see I'm sleeping ? ". When I finally did open my eyes I saw a large group of our nursing staff standing around me and they were about to extubate me. The RT told me to take a deep breath and the next thing I know the tube is out. No pain, no discomfort, not what I had imagined at all after seeing it hundreds of times ! Phew ! I also remember thinking, " gee, my chest doesn't hurt too bad " ... well, that thought was short lived once the anesthetic and pain meds wore off !

I spent six days in the hospital after surgery, under the excellent care of staff and physicians in my own unit. The experience was the most challenging thing I've gone through mentally and physically but I've gone on to make a full recovery, even running a 5K six months postop !

I feel that this has made me a better nurse as I truly have a first hand perspective of what our heart patients experience. It has also helped me to slow down and smell the roses in life as you never really understand how precious it is until you experience something like this.

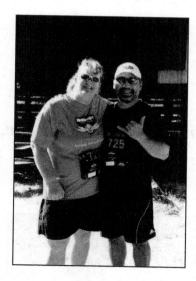

Since surgery, I've accomplished one of my goals of completing an obstacle course run by finishing the Gladiator Rock N Run, San Jose in 1 hour 38 minutes on a tough 4-mile hilly course. In addition, my son and I completed our first turkey trot together, the Silicon Valley Turkey Trot 2012. I continue to work fulltime in the ICU at the VA Palo Alto and spend my free time enjoying life with my wonderful family as you never know when your ticket will be called !

CHAPTER 16

Joe :

" If the training didn't kill me, the race certainly would "

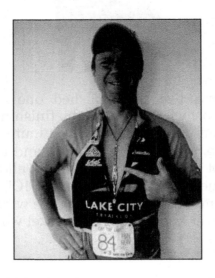

CARDIAC ATHLETE 16

First name: Joe
Country: USA
Diagnosis: Congenital Bicuspid Aortic Valve
Treatment: Tissue Aortic Valve Replacement

It was June of 2008 and I hadn't done any running in years. The last time I was on a bike was 20 years ago, and I couldn't swim without the aid of fins.   So what was tugging at me to enter an Ironman triathlon that warm June afternoon ?   I was sitting on the running leg of the Ford Ironman in Coeur d'Alene Idaho cheering on my neighbour who was doing his first IM (Iron Man – an ultra-long triathlon). Watching the athletes race past I felt an incredible urge to get out of my chair and run with them. Running has always been my passion but I had never actually been in or seen a race before. It was so inspiring to me to see those people competing. I was drawn in and bit with the IM bug !

My neighbour's wife warned me that IM training is like a second job and that I would never see my family. Despite that, and the fact that I had a chronic undiagnosed shoulder problem that prevented me from raising my arms above my head, I determined that I would someday run this race.

The next day, as my training began, there were several issues that needed to be dealt with. First I needed a bike and boy had they gone up in price over the past 20 years ! I headed to the bike shop with credit card in hand and took care of the bike issue.

I also needed to learn how to swim and with my shoulder issues that wouldn't be easy. My neighbour started giving me swimming lessons which, almost miraculously, cured me of my 15 years of shoulder pain. But I still had one more major issue to deal with.

My wife and I had discussed the fact that my heart rate became extremely high whenever I worked out. She felt we needed to find out why and I promised her I would take care of it. My plan in regard to the high HR was to procrastinate, which seems to be what I do the best. But my wife was persistent so I went to see my GP doctor. When I told him about it, he actually told me I was wrong. Your heart rate can't be that high he told me. I don't see him anymore.

My wife reminded me that our neighbor is a cardiologist so I called him, told him my concerns, and ended up scheduling an appointment with him for a stress echocardiogram. Upon my arrival the technician hooked me up to the various machines and gave me a run down on how the appointment would go so I would know what to expect.

As we began the test, I started to get the feeling that something was not right as we started to deviate from the itinerary he had laid out. More and more people started coming into the room, talking with a strange medical jargon that I would soon learn myself. I heard them mention something about a *'bicuspid aortic valve '* and thank goodness I am familiar with cars or I would not have known what any of those three words meant at the time ! *Valves* I know about. When they are bad in your vehicles engine, your car does not perform correctly and they need to be replaced. I would soon learn the same applied to the valves of the human heart.

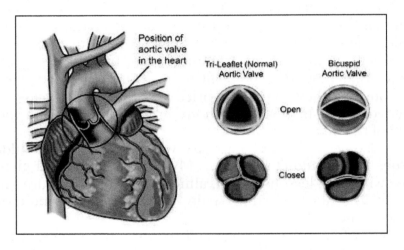

Illustration reproduced from:
http://www.valleyheartandvascular.com/Thoracic-Aneurysm-Program/Bicuspid-Aortic-Valve-(BAV).aspx

At the end of the test I was ushered, nervous and sweaty from the treadmill, in to see my cardiologist. He explained that a normal aortic valve has three cusps that open with each heartbeat to allow oxygenated blood to flow out from the heart to the body. Two of the three cusps in my heart were connected, a heart defect that I was born with and had lived with all my life. What that means is that the opening is much smaller and over time the valve develops " stenosis " it becomes stiff allowing even less blood to be pumped out from the heart making my heart work very hard to meet the oxygen demands of my body.

He told me that only 2% of the population has heart defects but that of those, mine was the most common. I never knew how useless statistics could be until they were in reference to me that day.

I asked him if I could continue my Ironman training and he told me "absolutely not !" He said that if the training didn't kill me, the race certainly would. He then told me " No " to marathons as well and suddenly I found myself negotiating with him. I asked, " but what if the course is very flat and I run slow ? " He shook his head. " How about a half marathon under the same circumstances ? " I pleaded. Reluctantly, he said that it would probably be ok. I had many more questions but with my head in a fog, I headed out to the parking lot, got in my truck, and wept.

I was told that my defective valve would probably last the rest of my life but I should probably ratchet down the workouts even more which I did with great reluctance.

Over the next year I worked to come to grips with my condition and found that I could still do sprint distance triathlons. I found it amusing that they called these short triathlons " Tinman " distance and it was just another way I associated with the Tinman from the Wizard of Oz. All he wanted was a heart.

I could still work out, but my heart regulated the intensity at which I could exert myself. If I pushed too hard, my legs would run out of oxygen and slow down. There was nothing I could do about it, my heart was in control. I could ride my bike on the flats at 22mph all day long, but try to bump it up even ½ mph and the legs would get that feeling and then slow down.

I read every article I could on how to be a better athlete but it soon became apparent that hardly any of it pertained to me with my condition. I was on my own and had to become a student of my own body and how it worked and reacted to certain things. I felt like I was reinventing the wheel.

A year after my diagnosis, I had another echo and was told that I would most likely need valve replacement surgery in 3 to 5 years. That was indeed unnerving considering my first diagnosis.

Several months later, in November of 2010, I was doing a turkey trot run with my Tri club when after about a half mile, I felt my legs starting to get numb. The feeling raced up my body towards my head until I finally had to stop. The feeling went away quite fast so I continued on with the run. After another 100 yards the same thing happened again.

The smart thing to do at that point would have been to slowly walk back to the start but I have never been accused of being all that smart so I finished the 6 mile run without further incidence and called my cardiologist about a week later. He told me that if this sort of thing kept happening, I should let him know.

Over the next couple of months, it did happen again a few more times and finally, at the end of January 2011, he told me I should either stop doing everything, or get the valve replaced. In my world, " everything " meant no swimming, biking, running, cutting wood, hiking or hunting. Incredibly, his recommendation was to put off the operation as long as possible which was, in his opinion, one to 3 more years. That's an awfully long time to sit on the couch I thought so I immediately scheduled an appointment with the surgeon.

Reality hit home for me when I found out that picking which valve to use was, like I had read somewhere, " an ugly flip of the coin." My surgeon told me that he would recommend a tissue valve for me but that a mechanical valve, which would require me to take blood thinners the rest of my life, would also be fine ... unless, as he put it " you juggle chainsaws for a living ". We both got a good chuckle when I reminded him that although I don't juggle them, I do use chainsaws frequently, and I also make knives for a living. Tissue valve it is !

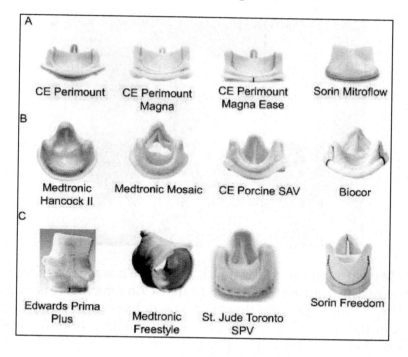

Image reproduced from:
http://interventions.onlinejacc.org/article.aspx?articleid=11
12587

The next question he asked me was when I wanted it done. I asked him if he had any plans for that afternoon and the operation was scheduled for a week later.

I guess the story of my experiences would not be complete without a blow by blow of the week I spent in the ICU but there was so much that went on during that time, and so much of it that needs to be forgotten so I'll only share one story about the hospital stay.

Going in I had an unusual philosophy about the whole ordeal that lay before me. My part was relatively easy. I would be under a little stress until they put me into a coma for the operation. Once I was under, I would be oblivious to everything going on. I would either wake up and see my wife or never wake up. Pretty easy job for me.

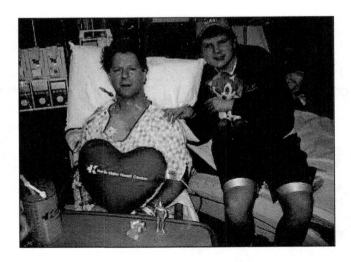

My wife, on the other hand, would be a wreck, pacing the floor of the waiting room for hours. Considering this ahead of time, I arranged for flowers to be delivered to her while I was in the operating room. They came with a note from me telling her to " Trust the Great Physician ". We both knew that God had us in his hands and whatever the outcome, He would still be there for us.

As I write this, I am 4 months post operation and looking forward to my favorite " Tinman " distance sprint triathlon a month away and my first Olympic distance Tri in August. I have already noticed huge differences in how my body reacts to exercise. The most noticeable is that I can now get out of breath and my legs can now get tired. I never knew this was not normal because I was never that kind of " normal ". The stenosis in my valve would help shut my legs down before they could get tired before but now, boy do they get worn out!

Once again I am forced to start from scratch as I learn all about my body and how it reacts to exercise, hydration and nutrition. Even my breathing needs some adjustments. I say this like its drudgery but I am actually going at this with a renewed sense of optimism for the future.

My future plans may include an Ironman in 2013 but it is something that I don't dare wish for until I know my body will let me do endurance type exercises again. I don't know that I could stand to have the same dream snatched away from me again. As trite as it may sound, I am taking it one day at a time now and enjoying the journey because you never know for sure if the destination you have in mind is the one you will arrive at so you may as well enjoy the ride there.

Since I chose a tissue valve at the young age of 49, I will likely need to have it replaced again sometime in my life and I am good with that. I've learned a lot from the whole experience and am quite sure that the lesson is not over yet. I found a terrific refuge in the forums on Cardiac Athletes and can only hope that somehow, sharing my experiences will help someone else.

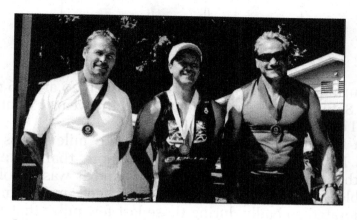

Update ! I wrote the above back in 2011, just 4 months after surgery to replace my defective aortic valve. One month later, I came in 3rd place in my age group in that sprint triathlon ! I still consider that feat as a minor triumph in which I am quite proud. I never did do the Olympic distance triathlon but instead shifted my focus to running and biking. In September of 2012 I entered my very first bike race, a hilly 85 mile lap around a local lake. I earned a bronze medal coming in 15th place overall by completing the trek in 4:47.

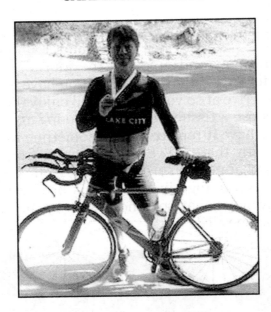

During the winter of 2011 I ran between 20 and 26 miles every Saturday for several months and this year, I wanted to see if I could go farther.

In December I was already at the 20 mile fitness level when I attempted the first run of more than 26.2, the marathon distance. I ran 28 miles and it was absolutely horrible from mile 22 to 28. In fact, my form had deteriorated so badly during those last few miles that I hurt my foot and wasn't able to run for a week.

Despite this setback, over the course of one month I ran a 30, and then 40 mile run ! I am training for a run of 52.4 miles, or two marathons, at the end of this month and if that goes well, I have already mapped out a course and will attempt to run the same 85 mile lap around the lake that I did for my bike race. I expect my time to be considerably greater on foot than bike !

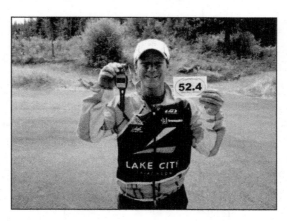

People ask me why I run and I can't honestly say it's for my health because clearly a 5 mile run would be great for one's health. Sometimes I think it's because I still can, even after open heart surgery but maybe that only made me realize that I just love to run and that ability was almost taken away from me due to my heart. Knowing that it could all end the next time I strap on my shoes makes each run all the more enjoyable, and me all the more thankful.

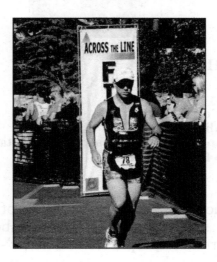

CHAPTER 17

Tony ' CopperTone ' :

" Three strikes ... NOT out !!! "

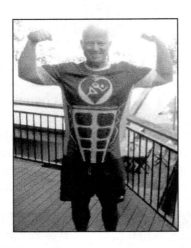

CARDIAC ATHLETE 17

First name: Tony
Forum name: "CopperTone "
Country: Australia
Diagnosis: Coronary Artery Disease; Heart Attack
Treatment: Two Bypass Grafts

The following account is a brief overview of the unfolding and continuing story of three family members of Cardiac Athletes, Coppertone, Intrepid MJ and 'Tiger'-Lilli.

As I write this in February of 2012, I am a 49 year old father of three adult children and grandfather of two. Though not a particularly talented athlete, I have lived my life with a definite focus on physical fitness, enjoyment of sport and outdoor activity, eating sensibly, healthy lifestyle and encouraging my children to do the same.

For most of my adult life I trained regularly and participated in a variety of sports as diverse as surf lifesaving, kayaking, surfing, triathlon, cycling, mountain running, wrestling, various football codes, multisport racing and orienteering. I made a living in a series of careers that put my sporting and fitness skills to good use as a sea kayak guide, river kayak and canoe guide http://www.sunshinecoastkayaking.com.au/ wilderness survival skills instructor, police search and rescue squad member and high angle rope rescue technician. I spent many years coaching and managing junior sporting teams in kayaking, surf lifesaving, cross country running and wrestling.

I guess most people that knew me saw me as either a fitness fanatic or a bit of a try hard athlete, having a go at everything and making the good athletes look even better. Although I was usually in the second half of the field in most triathlons or running events, sometimes at the very back. I could hold my own in a kayak or surf racing ski and had a few little wins here and there. Though I was never going to threaten on a national level, I still enjoyed training like a world champion and got much satisfaction in just taking part in any sport and reaping the fitness rewards.

I spent most of my life in pretty good health and had much confidence in the fact that I was super fit and from a cardiovascular standpoint I felt that I was in top shape. Even at the age of 42 while working in a pretty stressful frontline policing career I found the time and energy to train six days a week for the 2005 Coolangatta Gold Surf Ironman Race. This race is about the equivalent of a half ironman triathlon, taking the elite athletes about four hours to complete and over 40s competitors like myself, a little under 6hrs. Consisting of a 24km racing surf ski (ocean kayak) ocean paddle, a 3.6km ocean swim, a 6km ocean paddleboard section and 14.6km of beach sand running it is a gruelling test of stamina and ocean skills.

Having completed the event in October 2005 I was pretty ecstatic as it was an event I had been dreaming about doing for many years. I guess you could say that I was at the peak of my fitness and confidence.

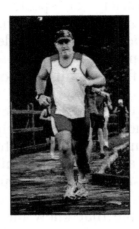

Then in early 2006 my health started to deteriorate, I was physically and mentally well below par. Though I could not put my finger on what was wrong and though it was not all that obvious to others, I just did not feel right. I carried on training and shrugged off my malaise. My blood pressure was a little high and my stress levels were up, though as a Police Officer that was sort of to be expected.

Earlier, I had been for a cardiac treadmill stress test and was told that at 42 I was as fit as a very fit 25 year old and that there was nothing wrong with my heart or cardiovascular system. In mid-June I checked into the Caloundra Private Hospital to have AC joint surgery to my right shoulder. I had injured the shoulder in June 2005 whilst effecting an arrest during a violent domestic violence incident that I was attending.

Whilst being prepped for surgery I was informed by my surgeon that my blood pressure was so high that he could not risk performing the surgery that day. I recall my blood pressure was reading 175/110, an off the chart reading for a man of my health and fitness levels. My surgeon suggested that I may indeed have some cardiovascular issues and that before he would consider further surgery, I should consult my General Practitioner with a view to some cardiac checks.

This news was a complete shock as I was feeling fine

physically, though I knew that I had been having increasing anxiety and stress type problems over the previous months. In fact I had consulted my doctor about some severe symptoms that could best be described as panic attacks. My doctor decided that it must just be work related stress that was causing these symptoms. I was quickly reassured that my blood pressure was just a symptom of my anxiety and that I should seek ways to relax. This reassurance was of some help, though I was starting to feel a sort of foreboding sentiment, cracks were starting to form in my armour.

Then on June 22nd at about 2am, after having run nearly 20km earlier in the evening, I experienced the worst symptoms ever. I woke up feeling nauseas, sweating, with tingling down my right arm and pain in my right thumb and fingers. Although I could hardly believe it, I knew I was having a heart attack so I called for an ambulance.

Arriving at the Nambour General Hospital I was treated as a heart attack victim for a few hours and I was informed that I was to be transferred to Prince Charles Hospital, a specialist cardiac hospital in Brisbane about 100km south, for an angiogram first thing in the morning.

By the change of shift, I had recovered so well that the staff changed their diagnosis and kept me in the General Hospital for three days of observation, during which time I displayed no more symptoms. I was released from hospital with a diagnosis of " pericarditis " (a swelling of the heart sack caused by a virus) and told to take it easy for a few weeks.

I took it easy, stopped training and took some time off work. Over the next six weeks I experienced similar frightening symptoms on at least five occasions and I was rushed to hospital by ambulance on three of those occasions. I underwent a series of cardiac stress tests that were supposed to show whether I had been having heart attacks or whether I had blocked coronary arteries. All the tests bar one were normal. The abnormal test showed that under intense exercise a very small portion of my heart was being deprived of blood/oxygen, possibly indicating a very small blockage. I was told that this test was so marginal and so small that it was nothing at all to worry about. I was assured that anybody who went as far as I did on the stress test (Bruce Protocol on the treadmill) without chest pain or more signs of blockage was perfectly healthy and not at risk. I was assured that I was absolutely fine !

I was advised that I needed to see a psychiatrist rather than a cardiologist. Put it simply, the problem was in my head not my heart. Personally I was now absolutely terrified. The heart attack symptoms were so real, yes I was surviving but the symptoms were getting stronger and the incidence of them was increasing.

Thinking back, I remembered that on my first admission on June 22nd I was told that the only absolutely accurate way of testing for blocked coronary arteries is to do an angiogram procedure. This is where a catheter on the end of a wire is placed into femoral artery at the groin and guided up into the heart where dye is pumped into the arteries and x-ray images are then viewed of how clear the arteries are, highlighting any blockages. However in order to receive an angiogram the patient has to meet certain risk factors, show certain symptoms and in the opinion of the doctor be at risk of a heart attack or cardiac arrest. In my case, the doctors did not believe that I was at risk and as such there was no need to subject me to an angiogram.

Given the symptoms that I was feeling and the fact that the tests showed a very marginal small area of heart muscle that may be subject to some blockage, I really believed that I should get the angiogram done and prove one way or the other as to whether I had a cardiac problem. I then literally begged my GP to refer me for an angiogram. If I was sick, I needed to know so that I could take measures to recover. If I was well, then I needed to know so that I could get on with my life and address the reasons why I may have been having the symptoms.

Night time from end of June through to the end of July had manifested into a real living nightmare for me. Having most of my symptoms between midnight and about 3am, I began to actually fear going to bed, luckily the Tour de France was being televised live throughout the nights of July and I was able to sit in the lounge room and watch the race till the wee small hours each night. I would usually fall to sleep around dawn, having made it through the night. Though I did not know it at the time, cycling was to become a much bigger part of my life in the years to come.

Toward the end of July I received a call from a catheter lab in a Brisbane hospital informing me that I had been offered an angiogram examination on the 31st of the month. I was surprised, relieved, thankful and now even more worried. After all my requests, why were they finally going to do the test ? I was to find out when I presented at the clinic on the morning of the procedure.

As I was being prepped before entering the angiogram lab, the nurses and technicians informed me that I was only being tested so that they could prove to me once and for all that I was healthy. They told me that I was far too young and fit to have a problem and that after reading about the sort of training regimes that I was keeping up, they believed that if I had coronary artery disease, that sort of intense training would have been impossible for me to either do or indeed survive.

So I was wheeled into the lab, the catheter was inserted, dye was pumped through my heart and the procedure was done. I looked up at the doctor and asked how it went, expecting to be told that my heart was fine. The next few moments were probably the most shocking that I had ever experienced in my life to that point, even considering some of the shocking moments I had experienced in a fairly action packed life thus far.

I was told that I had an extremely bad cardiovascular condition. Words aside, the look on the doctor's face was enough to scare the life out of me, I was in trouble and he could not hide that from me. From that moment my day deteriorated into a downward spiral of shock, disbelief, fear and despair.

I was told that my Left Anterior Descending (LAD) coronary artery (which I later learned that cardiologists nickname " the widow maker ") was 95% blocked and stenosed for over 90% of its length. They told me that the amount of damage that the artery had was in their opinion, so much that it was almost impossible that I was actually still alive. Just the strain of walking up a flight of stairs could be fatal. I had one of the worst cases of cardiovascular disease that they had seen and my only hope of survival was to have a double Coronary Arterial Bypass Graft (CABG) as soon as possible.

Within the space of thirty minutes I had gone from being a perfectly healthy, fit and paranoid hypochondriac with perhaps a psychological anxiety problem to an extremely ill cardiac patient in danger of dying at any moment.

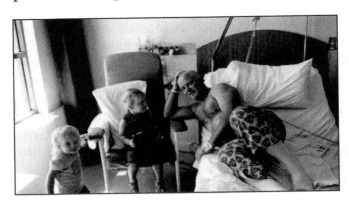

On August 11 I underwent the CABG operation, which I later learned was touch and go as I had so little patent artery wall left on my LAD that it was almost not able to be grafted.

During recovery, I learned that my prognosis was sobering at best. It turned out that my cardiovascular disease was genetic and that my system could not process cholesterol properly causing my arteries to become progressively diseased from a young age. Given the severity of my condition, doctors said that I probably would have died in my early thirties but for one single factor. That factor being that my heart had grown its own natural bypass blood vessels in the form of collateral vessels. The probable cause for this growth was a lifestyle of constant endurance training which put extra demand on my heart so that as my arteries became blocked due to cardiovascular disease, the heart compensated when I was putting it under physical stress by growing the collateral vessels. In short, my fitness based (some say extreme) lifestyle saved me from an almost certain early death.

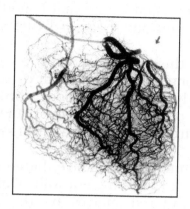

Cardiac angiogram showing collaterals.
Image reproduced from:
http://britscollegebound.files.wordpress.com/2010/08/coll aterals2.jpg

Doctors told me that the genetic process would continue, that my LAD would deteriorate further, my grafts would eventually fail and that I could not expect to live to old age. My best chance, I was told, was to take the array of drugs that they were offering and to engage in only moderate/easy exercise for fear that and intense or endurance based exercise would put too much pressure on my brittle arteries and cause a cholesterol deposit to shift and block an artery or cause the grafts to fail, both scenarios which would most likely prove fatal if they were to happen.

I asked what would happen to my protective collateral arteries if I reduced my exercise and I was informed that the collaterals are a use it or lose phenomena and as such would regress and disappear. Now I was faced with a future quite bleak and depressing.

Over the following weeks I slipped into a frightening depression, the likes of which I had never imagined could exist. Life held no joy nor promise. My family suffered as I became a dependant waste of space. I dearly wanted to get active, but I could find no positive advice anywhere from health, rehabilitation or fitness professionals. All the advice was based on me just accepting that I was now a cardiac patient or " cardiac cripple " and that I should be thankful to be alive and to forget any ideas of living a vigorous active sporting lifestyle.

Yet amidst all this I felt sure that if my endurance based lifestyle had prolonged my life without drugs or surgery and saw me constantly putting my body through events and training that 99% of the people on the planet would never or could never do, surely that could be my answer, my salvation in the future also.

Although I wanted to get active, based on my advice so far I was scared to do anything but walk. Only just being able to walk a few hundred metres by the weekend of the Coolangatta Gold in October 2006, I caught buses and trains from the Sunshine Coast and headed down to the Gold Coast to watch and support my club mates. Taking me twenty minutes to walk from the bottom to the top of the steep Nobbys Hill walkway, a distance of maybe 200 metres, having to stop and rest every few steps, I sat at the top and cried as the competitors ran past me.

The emotion of wanting to get moving and the fear of what might happen if I did overstep my limits was confusing and emotional. Sometime during that day I decided to challenge to medical advice I had received so far, doctors had indeed misdiagnosed me, ill advised me and failed to listen to my input so much in the past, why should now be any different. I needed to forge my own path. Sure I still needed doctors and medications and I am so grateful for the medical technology and skill of the cardiologists and surgeons that gave me my second chance, but I also needed to continue to advocate and think for myself. To that end I then set my first long term goal, I would do the Coolangatta Gold again ! I needed a plan.

Although I thought I had no risk factors for cardiovascular disease, I was wrong. Two uncles, an Aunty and a cousin on my father's side of the family all had heart attacks and/or CABG surgery at young ages. Bluntly put, my father past the condition on to me.   It became apparent to me just how influential genetics are.   I learned that I had Familial Hypercholesterolemia and that even keeping to the strictest of diets, my own body simply produced and failed to dispose of LDL (Bad) cholesterol. Though it was still in my best interests to have a strict and healthy diet, I also needed medication to slow this process down.

Around this time I learned of a cardiac rehabilitation program based in Noosa about 40km from where I live and over the next six weeks I attended the program two afternoons per week. Although the program was a step in the right direction I decided that I needed something more. The physical exercise component of the program, though suited to most cardiac patients, left me craving for more challenge. For the most part I was sitting on an exercise bike surrounded by patients in their 60's, 70's and 80's.

The director of the program, to his credit, noticed that I was acutely depressed and spent quite some time with me discussing my overall picture.   This is quite exceptional given that all the way through my earlier diagnosis and surgical treatment I would spend at most, two or three minutes with a doctor, cardiologist or surgeon. Sitting down and discussing my condition, aspirations or simply having time to ask questions was simply out of the question. This particular doctor, a preventive cardiologist, had a slogan hung on his wall, it read," Treat the patient, not the condition." I liked that, it said a lot about what I thought was missing with medicine in general.

Though my wife and children supported me in every way, my depression deepened and I found that the only way to alleviate this suffocating feeling was to keep active as much as I could. Still in pain from my healing sternotomy and fearful given the warnings about damaging the grafts, I embarked on a walking program that saw me leaving home at about 6am and walking at a slow pace all day until my family got home from work or school.   Sitting at home was not an option, the depressive cloak that enveloped me was too unbearable, I had to keep moving. During these weeks I ended up walking 20 to 40 km in any given day.

As I started to feel a little fitter, I began cycling and taking the same approach, slowly at first just averaging 10 to 14km per hour on flat roads, my rides soon turn into 4 to 6 hour adventures into the Sunshine Coast hinterland and Glasshouse Mountains area.

Though desperately trying to get some advice on getting back into real exercise, I find that advice elusive until one day I hear about a fellow Coolangatta Gold competitor, Alan Coates, who had also undergone a CABG a few years earlier and was now, in his late fifties, competing in the surf again. A very reclusive person, actually getting to talk to him was difficult, however on the day I finally met him on Noosa Beach we immediately had a bond and he shared his own journey from cardiac patient to fearless competitor with me. For the first time in months I felt that I had a positive future, Alan showed me that normal life was a real possibility.

In December 2006 my wife Cathi collapsed, probably due in part to the stress of my own very depressed state. She was hospitalized and found to have a rare genetic heart disorder, Arrhythmogenic Right Ventricular Cardiomyopathy (ARVC). We learned that this is one of those cardiac disorders that is responsible for the sudden death of many teenage athletes and otherwise fit and healthy people (mostly men) in their twenties.

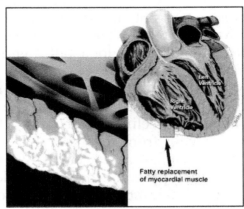

Fatty replacement of myocardial muscle

Image reproduced from:
http://circ.ahajournals.org/content/107/4/e31.figures-only

In 1994 my wife's brother died suddenly from a cardiac arrest aged 32 whilst playing rugby. Suddenly the genetic genie rears its ugly head again. After making some enquiries we were able to ascertain that her brother had died from ARVC, though he had never been diagnosed with the condition as was, right till the day of his death, unaware that he had a cardiac condition.

Cathi was then prescribed medication and we discussed with doctors the ramifications of two genetic cardiac conditions in the family in relation to our three children. Over the next few months all our kids are booked in for various cardiac tests.

During this period I started searching the internet for some sort of support group or other athletic types like me going through cardiac problems. I try for weeks, never having any success and start to think that I am very alone in my attitude and quest. Then one day in April 2007 I type in two words .... **Cardiac** and **Athlete**. From that moment on my world started to change. I was not alone.

That April, still chronically and acutely depressed I travelled to England to meet my relatives and try to get some perspective on my condition. I am also leaving home to give my wife and children a break from my terrible mood. By this point I was jogging and cycling at greater intensities in order to rebuild my fitness. I took with me a folding 20 inch touring bicycle with the intention of doing a few multi day solo cycling tours between meeting and spending time with relatives.

I managed to cycle across Scotland, Yorkshire and Cornwall trying to stand alone and face my fears. By day I ride and soak up life, by night I lay scared and alone in different hostels counting the hours till the sunrise. Since first suffering the panic attacks and/or heart attacks (as both phenomena were indistinguishable to me, and still are), I had noticed that the night time was the worst. I could be active and feeling fine all day and then come crashing down in the wee small hours of the morning. The trip seemed to be working as I forced myself to stand alone, yet also manage to spend time bonding and feeling the love of relatives that I had only actually recently met.

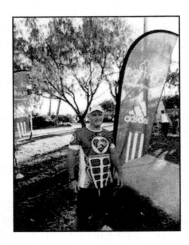

In May 2007 whilst in England I received news that my son Murdoch 22 (a previous surf ironman competitor, Coolangatta Gold team ski paddler, accomplished surfer and professional lifeguard) has just been rescued at Wurtulla Beach after a bout of sustained ventricular tachycardia and blacking out in the surf. During the phone call I learn that he had experienced a couple of dizzy spells and had collapsed at home earlier in the week. Initially told that there is nothing wrong with him (he is too young, too fit and presents a too healthy look) over the week he is hospitalized on three occasions. Eventually he is diagnosed with ARVC, a dilated left ventricle and is suffering acute heart failure. At this point his life hangs in the balance as his body accumulates fluids due to the heart failure.

When I heard this news I was down in Cornwall cycling along the coast. I was completely blown over by this news and every part of my body ached, the depression was taken over by pure fear and helplessness. I was a long way from home, I did not know a single person in that part of the world.

Speaking to Cathi and Murdoch on the phone, they told me to just stay down there and continue my trip and promise to keep me updated with changes in Murdoch's condition. Murdoch also tells me that a mate of his, Adam, a lifeguard that he works with in Caloundra on the Sunshine Coast in Queensland, has just travelled to England to do the summer lifeguard season.

Reluctantly I agreed to stay and I get back on the bike and cycle down the road. I am crying, I feel like vomiting and don't know where I am going nor why. The riding was not helping, I could hardly see the road in front of me and within a few minutes I was feeling very unsafe on the bike so I pulled up at the next beach down the road. It is the first day of the lifeguard season that summer and I gravitated to something familiar.

Call it coincidence, call it serendipity but what happened next is quite amazing. I saw three lifeguards setting up the beach for the day, so I wander on over to have a chat and within a couple of minutes I find myself talking to a bloke that used be in a surf lifesaving team with Murdoch that I coached a few years back in New Zealand. Then he introduces me the other foreign lifeguard, who he himself had only just met that morning and he turns out to be, Adam, Murdoch's mate.

On hearing about Murdoch they invited me to stay with them at a local pub with a bunch of lifeguards from Australia, New Zealand and South Africa and over the next five days I am able to call home morning, noon and night to get progress reports on Murdoch's condition. By the end of the week I learned that he was stable, improving and out of immediate danger.

During this time the support Adam and the other lifeguards I stayed with gave me and all the other locals that we socialized with each night took the edge off the intense fear that I felt. Using the Village of St Merryns as my base for the week, I managed a couple of hundred kilometres of cycle touring during the daytime hours.

On arriving home at the end of May I watched helplessly as Murdoch endures a series of cardiac events over several months. He is told that he needs to be implanted with a pacemaker/defibrillator (ICD) however this cannot be done until his left ventricular dilatation and heart failure symptoms improve (through medication and rest). He is also told that a reading of an episode of ventricular tachycardia needs to be caught on a monitor and printed out. He is constantly tested, however these frequently fatal events are hard to catch unless one is monitored 24 hours per day for months at a time.

From June to October 2007 I am off work diagnosed with severe depression and spend most of my time worrying about my son, my wife and my daughters (the youngest of which is now showing symptoms of ARVC). The only time that my head is straight is when I am training. The physical effort seems to mask the depression and I am able to take a holiday from my worries. During this time I have basically ignored most of my doctors' advice regarding physical exercise and I am training for the Coolangatta Gold six days a week as well as knocking off hundreds of kilometres on my bicycle. However I am taking my medication even though I hate to do so, I recognise that it is necessary.

Two weeks before the Coolangatta Gold Murdoch suffers a long and sustained ventricular tachycardia at Maroochydore Beach. An ambulance is called and his heart rhythm is reverted by paramedics at the scene. A recording of the rhythm is captured on the ECG machine and printed out. This is what cardiologists have been waiting for, proof of the condition and a completion of his diagnosis so that he can have the lifesaving ICD implanted in his chest.

Murdoch is taken to Nambour Hospital where his history is recounted to doctors. Expecting him to be transferred to Prince Charles Hospital where he may finally receive the implant, we are told by the emergency department staff that Murdoch is fine to go home. Whilst in the ED his vitals had returned to normal and he was told that he was fine. We asked for a copy of the ECG print out from the ambulance and we were told that it was not important. Having to demand the printout and after some argument, we were given the printout and were able to fax it to his cardiologist at Prince Charles Hospital via our GP. That printout was the key to a long and frightening puzzle. On receiving the ECG printout Murdoch's electrophysiologist cardiologist arranged for Murdoch to have an appointment within days.

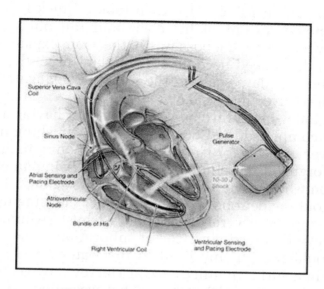

Superior Vena Cava
Coil

Sinus Node

Atrial Sensing and
Pacing Electrode

Atrioventricular
Node

Bundle of His

Right Ventricular Coil

Pulse
Generator

10-30 J
Shock

Ventricular Sensing
and Pacing Electrode

Illustration reproduced from:
http://jama.jamanetwork.com/article.aspx?articleid=204583

I travelled down to Brisbane to support Murdoch and to make sure that there were no more problems. On being called into the doctor's room we were met by one of the junior cardiology registrars and not by the electrophysiologist we were anticipating seeing. This made me a little uneasy, though I remained composed. The registrar asked Murdoch how he was feeling and Murdoch said fine. He shuffled through Murdoch's notes and then said that everything looks fine and that Murdoch should come back in twelve months for a check-up.

I looked at Murdoch and then I looked at the doctor and told him why Murdoch was here. The notes were shuffled again and we were told that there was no such ECG and that everything was fine. I then stood up walked over to his desk and I told him to look again because Murdoch's whole life hinged on this ECG. Tension was mounting and I could see an argument developing here and me being removed from the hospital. Then all of a sudden from somewhere in the notes the ECG copy appeared and the doctor mumbled something about filing. He then took a quick look at the ECG, jumped up out of his chair and ran out the door. Within two minutes the boss was in the room explaining that Murdoch did indeed need an ICD implant urgently. A few days later, 2 days before the 2007 Coolangatta Gold, Murdoch received his implant.

That following Saturday, 14 months after having a double bypass I completed the Coolangatta Gold, finishing midfield in the over 40s category in just under six hours, taking a big step in forging a more hopeful future and being an example to my son who was now having to start life again. This was not without incident however, in the weeks leading up to the event I suffered severe panic attacks whilst swimming. I would have this terrifying fear of suffocation come over me and I could not put my head in the water. I had to be rescued in a surf swimming race at Hervey Bay when I went into a panic in dead flat water. That was about two weeks before the Coolangatta Gold.

Over the next few days I had to literally get club mates to hold my hand and guide me back into the sea at my home beach at Mooloolaba in order for me to put my head in the water. On the morning of the Coolangatta Gold I still had not been able to swim more than twenty strokes without panic. On race day I managed the swim leg purely by spending the whole course repeating a mantra to myself .... "relax, stroke, breathe .... " for 3.6km.

In 2008 I returned to work as a Police Officer, having been advised not to go back to frontline policing, I set about trying to build my career around training and education and joined the district training office on a temporary basis. During that period I completed a Police Operational Skills and Tactics instructors course, qualified as an instructor and began working in that role at my home district.

Work was going fine, I was fit and focused and looked forward to my career. However this was not to be, although my immediate superiors valued my work and encouraged me, those in the upper management level found me to be unsuitable due to my health status. Over a period of months I fought to hold my job however I was forced into a corner, fighting my own illnesses, dealing with my family members' illnesses and having to fight the Police bureaucracy took added toll on my health and I had to concede. Procedures were then implemented to have me medically retired from the service.

In October 2008 I completed my second Coolangatta Gold since my CABG, this time with Murdoch paddling a rescue board for me as my safety support crew during the swim leg. This was such a great feeling to do this together. Incidentally, I improved my time and overall placing in my age category.

In December 2008 the axe finally fell and I was discharged from the Police Service. Although I knew it was going to happen, when it did it really brought out huge feeling of anger and depression. More anger than I thought possible. As I had sort of expected to need some sort of therapy, I planned to spend some time on my bike. As it was, I was ordered by the Police Service to visit a psychiatrist that week and although I had been ordered to see others over the previous couple of years, this consultation left me quite gutted. Up to this point, visiting psychiatrists seemed to have something to do with therapy for my anxiety and depression, this visit left me with the feeling that my former employer was going to grind me down even more.

The very next morning, Saturday the 13th, I packed my touring bicycle and set off southward in an effort to burn off the anger that was boiling inside. I spent the next seven days cycling an average of 162km per day in 30 degree Celsius plus weather to Sydney. On crossing the Sydney Harbour Bridge at ten minutes to midnight the following Friday, I felt that I had proven something to myself. It had been a gut busting and gruelling seven days of self-discipline, endurance, abuse and affirmation that had left me completely and utterly spent, yet satisfied that I could do anything if I tried.

Unfortunately on arriving home by plane three days later I was admitted back into Prince Charles Hospital with a suspected MI. An angiogram was done followed by an MRI and four days of observation in the cardiac ward. As it turned out, although I had pushed myself to extremely high physical stress over the 1134 km (705 mile) ride, my grafts were intact, no MI was detected and I was again diagnosed with pericarditis. I was even told that my riding had not caused the pericarditis and that I had probably picked up a virus during the ride. I had to concede however that pushing myself that hard was probably unwise. I was ordered to take it easy for three months and I did. Though I struggled.

Years later I heard a quote about Andy Irons, former multiple world surfing champion, just after he died. This quote kind of put my behaviour in perspective. " Sometimes one has to go to extremes in order to find one's mediums ". So I have visited my extremes, survived and now I can settle on challenges somewhere below those extremes. By the way, Irons was a super fit athlete and died from exactly the same cardiac condition I have, however he never got to learn that he had it !

On completing my rest period I flew over to Perth, Western Australia to watch my club mates compete in the Australian Surf Lifesaving Championships. When the championships were over I took a 20 inch folding bicycle on a 360km solo tour of the beautiful south west forest areas. Riding conservatively over six days, starting and finishing in Bunbury a port town 172km south of Perth, I managed to regain some confidence in my physical health and ability.

These short multi day bicycle trips have become a general fixture in my life, usually lasting four days and averaging between 100 and 120km per day, every few months I take myself off for a tour. I find that I am able to burn off a few of life's anxieties and shake off the blues when life starts to smother me now and then.

In years gone by I used to do multi day sea or river kayaking trips as my preferred method of escape, however even to this day, I have a fear of getting caught out on the water or on some remote beach and suffering a cardiac event.

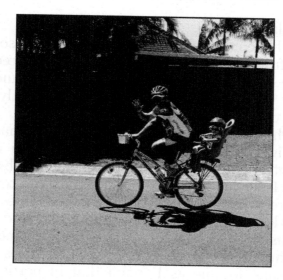

Grandad Tony taking little Lilli for a ride.

I do, however, feel more comfortable on the road cycling as I have this perception that I can get help if I need it. Though this fear is mostly just that, a fear, and I would dearly like to set off onto the water for a decent tour, I still need to work on that goal.

From 2009 and through 2011 life clipped on by and generally seemed to fluctuate between times of optimism, times of minor complications for Murdoch, Cathi and Freyja my youngest daughter, and periods of depression, anxiety and frustration as my own health would take the odd dip now and then.

Murdoch suffered a large DVT and was ill for a time. After months of blood thinning medication the DVT dissolved and he had to have his ICD removed and replaced due to a malfunction with the ICD lead. An adventurous soul, just like his father, Murdoch had to reconcile the limitations his cardiac condition put on his lifestyle. Though the medical advice was that he would not be able to surf again or engage in strenuous exercise, he has found ways to manage his condition and keep his love of surfing alive and active, though with some limitations. He has found a level of exercise that may be okay, though it is an ongoing search for the right balance.

Murdoch's condition has had its benefits also. While restricted from his very physical work and recreational lifestyle, he developed his love of photography and found a talent for academic studies and is currently nearing completion of a bachelor of arts.

Even when I was feeling okay in myself, I had many a sleepless night worrying about Murdoch, Cathi or Freyja. The thought of cardiac events never seemed to be far from our lives. I needed to find some new purpose to focus on, another career path so I set up a personal fitness training business, a kayaking school and a gutter, roof and drive way cleaning business. In reality, I was quite lost and ready to jump into anything. In general these enterprises proved to be problematic for me as I found that in particularly hot weather, I did not have the same ability to cope with hard physical labour that I once took for granted.

I enjoyed the kayaking work, however it has not proved to be a reliable income earner yet. I am not comfortable with the personal training industry for many reasons and I am not medically qualified to help the clients that I would like to work with, those recovering from cardiac conditions or other health problems.

There were highlights of course, taking Cathi and Freyja to France in 2009 and me fulfilling a dream by cycling the Alpe Du Huez climb and then in 2010 completing a cycle ride from Sydney to Brisbane, this time as a member of the 1200kms for Kids Team, a supported group raising money for children's hospital charities.

So heading into the latter part of 2011 I was certainly feeling quite lost and uncertain about my direction in all facets of my life. To be honest I was stagnating and losing my way. I was heading for 49 and did not have the slightest idea about how to approach the next phase of my life.

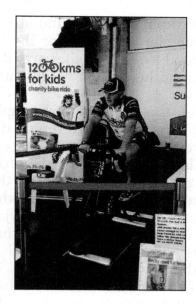

Tony raising thousands
for his children's charities.

All of a sudden as if I had ordered it a restaurant, I was served the biggest dose of " You have focus now ! " that I could have ever imagined. Early in 2011 both my daughters fell pregnant within six weeks of each other. Though at first I was quite shocked and to be honest, I felt that as a family we did not need two babies adding to our stresses, I quickly fell in love with the idea of being a poppa.

Given the recent family history of cardiac complaints both my daughters discussed the issues with their doctors and scans and extra tests were ordered. Freyja already had a question mark over her health given her vague ARVC symptoms. Over the years since my CABG, Freyja had collapsed on a number of occasions and ARVC was suspected, though it is an extremely difficult condition to diagnose.

Though Freyja was assured by her doctor that her baby had very little chance of having any cardiac condition that would affect it as a foetus or infant, he did order specific foetal heart scans to put Freyja's mind at rest. Freyja was only 18 at the time she presented for the first of the echo scans and I am proud to say that she carried herself in a way far more mature than her years. Lightening was to strike again.

During one of the scans a sonographer noticed an anomaly with her baby's heart and reported it to the doctor who then told Freyja it was nothing. Freyja having lived through my misdiagnoses and again the problems Murdoch had in getting diagnosed, decided to follow this up and asked her doctor to arrange another scan at another clinic. This was done and no anomaly was found. Freyja then discussed this with Cathi and I and told us that the original sonographer was absolutely sure and seemed quite concerned that there was a problem. This was again brought up with our family doctor and subsequently Freyja received an appointment to travel to Brisbane for a consultation with one of the two top paediatric heart specialists in the state.

At this appointment it was found that Freyja's baby had two major congenital heart defects and that she would have to be monitored daily for the last four weeks of her pregnancy as the baby would be needing lifesaving surgery. As it happened Freyja moved down to Brisbane to stay at the Ronald MacDonald House near the Mater Children's Hospital four weeks before her due date and within a week complications emerged and she had to have the baby induced three weeks before term.

Lilli was born a beautiful healthy looking good sized baby. Freyja was given a couple of minutes to hold her before she was taken away for echo scans. She was diagnosed with a severe aortic coarctation, a large ventricular septal defect and an undersized aortic valve. Three days after birth she underwent cardiac surgery and although the surgery went well, the trauma saw her whole system start to fail the following day.

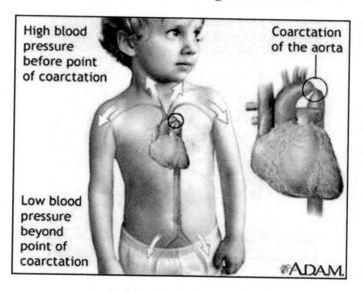

Illustration reproduced from:
http://www.healthcentral.com/high-blood-pressure/18128-146.html

Over the next few days Lilli was literally put on ice as her temperature climbed and she underwent constant " fiddling " as the PICU consultant described it to me, as they adjusted, topped up, took out, put back in and adjusted again fluids, tubes, wires and medicines in a constant battle to stabilise her tiny body.

On about day six her condition began to settle and we all got some relief. At this point it was also confirmed that the surgery to fix the VSD had damaged her ability to pace her heart and that she would need further surgery to implant a pacemaker which in all likelihood would be necessary for the rest of her life. On day nine she had her pacemaker implanted.

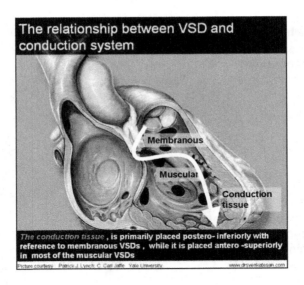

Illustration reproduced from:
http://drsvenkatesan.wordpress.com/2010/06/15/how-does-vsd-affect-the-conduction-system-of-heart-which-is-dangerously-close-to-it/

I can only imagine what dedication, skill and courage it takes to be able to perform surgeries on hearts the size of a fifty cent coin, with the weight of hope and expectation bearing down from the parents of these tiny babies.

By the time Lilli was released from PICU at two weeks old and moved to the close observation ward, she had undergone three cardiac surgeries for four cardiac procedures. When I was diagnosed at 43 with severe cardiovascular disease I felt sorry for myself and angry that I was needing to have cardiac surgery so young and for a condition normally reserved (as I thought) for the older, sedentary, smoking, drinking and overeating section of our society.

Then a year later when my son, another fine healthy clean living young man, went into heart failure at 22 I felt that was just so unjust. Now I was witnessing something so heart wrenching, the agony my daughter was going through with her baby was truly overwhelming. Three days old and undergoing surgery that may have killed her outright, my

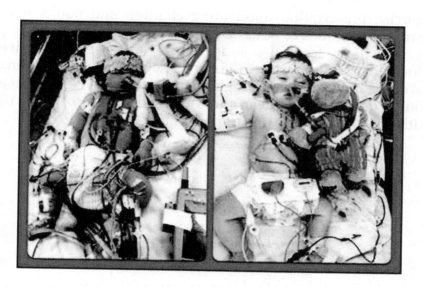

perspective soon changed. By the time Lilli was discharged from hospital after 30 days, I had a mission in life, a direction ... a calling.

As I explained earlier, I had been floundering for some time. Now all I wanted to see, was that Lilli got every opportunity to grow up healthy and as active as she is able and to help her maximise her chances of a full life. After a life time of being a bit of an unqualified fitness expert, years of thinking that maybe I could go to University and get the qualifications I needed to help cardiac patients and others find their way back to health, fitness and a life of activity, I now had all the motivation I needed.

I needed to get the monkey off my back, stand up and be confident in my own health, shrug off anxiety, depression and sickness and move forward again.

In December 2011 I enrolled at the University of the Sunshine Coast summer school and completed a seven week tertiary pathways entrance program which gave me the entry qualification into undergraduate studies. At this moment in time, February 2012, I am now enrolled in the four year Bachelor of Clinical Exercise Science course. My goal is to go on and do post graduate research in the area of exercise for those with cardiac conditions and work in the area of exercise prescription, motivating children and adults with cardiac conditions to be as active and fit as they can be.

Fate in the form of genetics has dealt a series of massive blows to my family in the form of several life threatening cardiac conditions and though the fight to survive has been a source of much pain, fear and anxiety, it has also gifted us with new perspectives and opportunities.

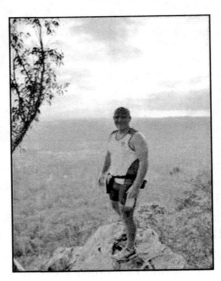

My message

I'll do anything and everything to save my own life and that of my family. I have had to fight and stand my ground on many occasions and I will probably have to in the future. All I want to get across to others is that when all is said and done, you and you alone are the best advocate for yourself and those close to you.

It is more than likely that had we not received the best that modern medical science offers in the form of diagnostic technology, complex surgical procedures and medication, my son, my granddaughter and myself would not have survived. I am eternally grateful for the second chance that we have received at the skilled hands of medical professionals. Yet our journey is also punctuated by a series of occasions when doctors failed to pick up on our conditions, where we were told that there was nothing to worry about.

I do understand that diagnosis is a difficult process, that as patients all three of us were outside the usual norms and that doctors, just like any other people under pressure of workload, make mistakes. This is why I feel that we as patients need to advocate for ourselves and our children.

Certainly listen to doctors, respect their skill and knowledge and process it, however if you believe that they might just be wrong and your life depends on what they are advising, do not stop asking and clarifying until you are truly satisfied. Studies actually show that patients who take responsibility for their own health and are prepared to persist with enquiry, even in the face of criticism and ridicule, have far greater survival rates than those who just accept without question.

The healing process is a partnership between the doctor, allied medical staff and the patient, all have a vital role to play and each have insight and experience unique to their situation.

Equally, the post rehabilitation phase (the rest of a cardiac patients life) can also be challenging, I know this for sure. Support and advice for those seeking a physically active life can be rather thin and hard to come by. The medical profession tends to err dramatically on the side of caution, studies on the benefit of exercise are far outnumbered by studies on the benefits of medication. That is why, as well as forming a good relationship with a cardiologist who will at least understand your need and desire for a level of physical challenge, finding a support network of like-minded souls is so important. Being able to share experiences, training programs, ups and downs with others fighting the same battle provides inspiration and confidence not found anywhere else.

Since the day that I typed the words **Cardiac** and **Athlete** into Google, www.cardiacathletes.com has been an ever-present and vital part of my life, recovery and enjoyment of life.

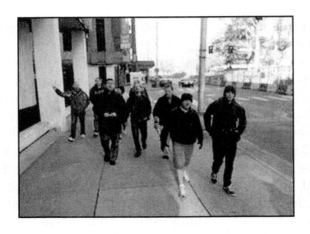

Walking the streets of Harrisburg, PA. 2010, with CA buddies.

The inspiration and friendship that the members share and give each other is incalculable. Had it not been for Cardiac Athletes I most likely would never have achieved as much as I have. Knowing you are not alone is such a comforting feeling.

*(Lars: following on from Tony's last sentence ... as if he and his family hasn't already had more than their fair share of health challenges, in April 2014 as I get this book ready to publish I learn of Tony now having to fight another health war, that of cancer. I admire Tony a great deal. He is truly a CA Superhero. Although repeatedly knocked down by his life challenges, he eventually gets back up, dusts himself down and gets on with business. He is a very modest guy who raises thousands every year for children's hospitals by cycling many thousands of kilometres. If you would like to send Tony Jennings a message so that he knows how much he is appreciated and so that he knows he is not alone, please feel free to do so via his Facebook page here :

https://www.facebook.com/MrCoppertone.1

I am sure he won't mind and will really appreciate your kind and encouraging words. Sometimes even a Superhero needs a lift up or a helping hand.)

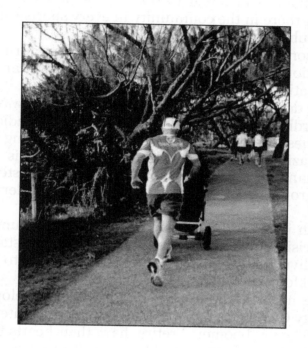

" Knowing you are not alone is such a comforting feeling. "

CONCLUSION

There remains still much to do. There needs to be more AED's out there in the community in every sports centre and athletic club.

I personally believe there should be some form of pre-participation sport heart screening but only if we can address discrimination.

There does seem to be a paradigm shift underway. Many of the cardiac athletes have now appeared on radio, in TV news stories, and had their stories feature in leading journals and magazines. The respect and recognition is coming, slowly, thanks to the media becoming more interested in this special group. Attitudes are shifting as understanding increases.

Health insurance premiums must offer discounts for fit and exercising cardiac athletes and bosses must start to see these individuals as great health ambassadors to have in their workforces.

There needs to be a concerted push to develop Sports Cardiology Centres as demand is about to accelerate as more and more ' baby-boomers ' retire, have their hearts fixed and get back into active sporting lifestyles. There also needs to be experienced and knowledgeable staff fully trained and ready to receive these cardiac athletic ' customer-patients ' and who could also offer cardiac rehabilitation, all under one roof.

Community gym instructors should be able to do a respected Cardiac Rehabilitation Certificate or Diploma course so that any and every sports centre can provide adequate cardiac rehabilitation coverage across great swathes of all countries.

In time, as we all live longer (apparently), there will be more and more people taking part in half marathons, marathons, duathlons, triathlons, Tinman and Ironman competitions, as individuals or in teams, who have cardiac histories, who have fully recovered from their cardiac surgeries and who are now back enjoying challenging their new limitations. They will be the new majority " norm " and the people who do not know their cardiac risks, who have not had a simple ECG, treadmill test, cardiac echo scan, etc., ... these people will become the new minority " abnormal " and " high-risk " competitors.

Stop and ponder that for a moment. There will be **Cardiac Athletes** everywhere, all around us ... and you and I may be one too.

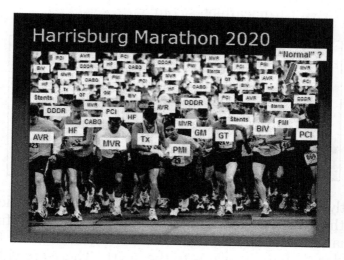

AVR Aortic Valve Replacement; MVR Mitral Valve Repair; Tx Heart Transplant; PCI Percutaneous Coronary Intervention; GT Gene Therapy; PMI post MI; HF Heart Failure; DDDR Dual Chamber Pacemaker; CABG Coronary Artery Bypass Graft.

I hope this humble little book contributes a little more momentum to changing attitudes and policies around the globe and leads to a greater recognition, rethinking and rewarding of this unique group of people ... the proudly defiant **Cardiac Athletes ... A New Breed of Superhero ... Beating Heart Disease Around The World !**

You see, ... Heart Disease made a fatal mistake ... it left some survivors ... who are now seeking their revenge ...

This book is a celebration of the best of the human spirit and of its ability to overcome adversity. Thank you for buying it. You are helping us in our quest to rid planet Earth of all heart disease. I hope you enjoyed the seventeen stories and learned 'heaps'. Lars

THE CA WEBSITES

There are a number of different ways new people can discover us on the internet and all offering entry points into Cardiac Athletes ...

The main CA Website
URL: www.cardiacathletes.com

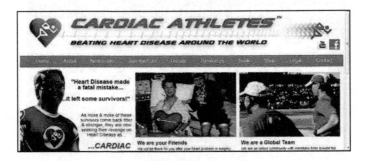

Recently completely revamped to emphasise our mission and goals this website contains a lot of extremely useful free information for anyone interested in health and fitness particularly where it relates to the heart. There are videos to watch, general and specialist FAQ's, heart rate calculators and much more.

The CA Forum
URL: http://www.cardiacathletes.org.uk/forums/

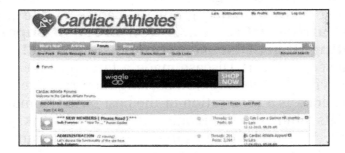

This is a very extensive private forum where Cardiac Athletes from around the world share their tips, advice and success stories. It is arranged almost like a reference book with many sub-forums covering all topics relevant to its members such as training science, nutrition, medication interactions, recovery, psychology, sports cardiology, member sports journals and blogs and much more ... and it is growing and becoming a more and more valuable resource all the time. It is fully searchable so the answers to many of your questions are there to be found. You are able to search for similar cardiac athletes to yourself and ask them directly for the answer to your questions. Members have all embraced the ethos of the forum, the free interchange of information, making free 'info-deposits' and 'info-withdrawals' all for the common good of this unique group of highly spirited individuals who value an active sporting lifestyle regardless of their cardiac histories.

The Facebook Page (Red Superhero banner)
URL:https://www.facebook.com/CardiacAthletes#!/CardiacAthletes

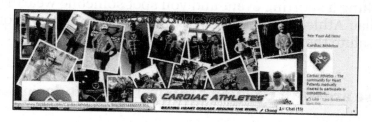

I'm still not sure why Facebook hasn't combined the functionality of their 'Page' and 'Group' community formats. Both have pros and cons, pluses and minuses. So we have both. Many members use these to just dip in and out of real quick in order to keep a finger on the pulse of the group's activities.

The Facebook Group (Blue banner)
URL:https://www.facebook.com/CardiacAthletes#!/groups/478037275561838/

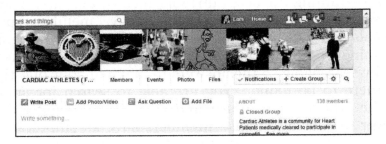

CA Team Kit

You can also support us in our quest and help to spread the word about our heart champions and super heroes by purchasing and wearing our team kit. Just go to the main website and click on the link to the CA Shop or fill in and submit the CA Clothing Range Form. If you happen to be watching a sporting event and you spot someone wearing the Cardiac Athletes Team kit be sure to cheer them on loudly and salute their achievements. Thank you.

These are the 3 Cardiac Athlete Team Kit designs:

1) CA 'Super Hero Fun Event' Team kit
2) CA (Red / Competition) 'Eye of the Tiger' Team kit
3) CA (Grey / Training) 'Eye of the Tiger' Team kit

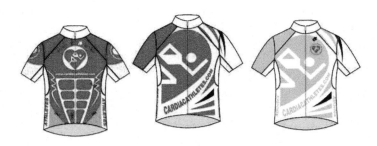

GLOSSARY

Please note, I have compiled this Glossary myself using as much plain English as I could think of so the terms will not be described by way of a concise literary definition and no apologies are offered for this by the editor (me ... Lars).

AED Automated External Defibrillator. This is a small portable electronic device with cables and sticky pads which are placed on the chest. It automatically diagnoses life threatening heart rhythms and delivers a safe and controlled electrical 'de-fibrillation' shock to the heart through the skin. This should stop the chaotic heart rhythm and return it to a normal rhythm. * (*There are not enough of these devices in the community and still too many young sports people are dying of sudden cardiac arrest. If you would like to help Cardiac Athletes reduce these unnecessary deaths then please make a donation to our website. Thank you.*)

Aerobic Physical exercise of relatively low intensity with the energy coming from oxygen in breathed air breaking down fat stores. These are exercises that can be performed non-stop over a long period of time. Jogging, swimming, cycling, walking are all examples of aerobic exercise.

AF Atrial fibrillation, AF or A-Fib is the most common cardiac arrhythmia (heart rhythm disorder). It is due to the chaotic firing of heart cells within the atria (smaller top chambers of the heart) which overrides the normal electrical impulses of the heart pacemaker cells in the Sinoatrial Node or SA Node.

Anaerobic Meaning to 'live without air'/ without oxygen. The opposite of aerobic. It refers to exercise fast, short and intense enough to cause lactic acid build up in the muscles leading to cramping, i.e.; lifting heavy weights or sprinting.

Angina Angina or more correctly angina pectoris is chest pain brought about by ischaemia (oxygen starvation) of the heart muscle usually due to a narrowing of one of the blood vessels supplying oxygen to the heart. Angina can also be caused by coronary artery spasm or heart muscle pinching.

Angiogram An x-ray image made by injecting a special dye into the blood vessels or chambers of the heart so that any defects can be seen more clearly.

Angioplasty A minimally invasive surgical technique for treating diseased heart arteries by temporarily inserting and inflating a tiny balloon on a long thin plastic tube inside a heart artery.

Anticoagulation A medication that keeps blood from clotting. In other words a blood thinner.

Aortic aneurysm The aorta is the largest artery in the body and the first vessel to supply blood to the heart. An aneurysm of the aorta is a sac-like swelling or bulge from this major vessel because of a weakness in its connective tissue wall.

Aortic coarctation The aorta is the major artery coming out of the left heart. It goes up towards the neck and then bends around and down towards the abdomen and legs. Some people are born with a narrowing at the early part of the down section of the aorta. This ' kink in the pipe ' obstructs blood flow and so the left ventricle must pump much harder than normal to push blood through the aorta to the lower body. This can overload and lead to damage of the heart.

Aortic stenosis Stenosis is a term that refers to a narrowing or constriction of an opening, such as a blood vessel or heart valve. In this case the aortic valve is narrowed and constricted. Often this is due to excess fibrosis and or calcification caused by disease.

ARVC   Arrhythmogenic   Right   Ventricular Cardiomyopathy. This is a type of cardiomyopathy (disease of the heart muscle). It appears to be a genetic condition (passed down through a family's genes) which results in the depositing of extra fat between heart muscles cells thereby isolating heart muscle cells from neighbouring ones increasing the likelihood of ventricular arrhythmias (palpitations) happening, fainting or loss of consciousness (syncope) and sometimes sudden cardiac arrest and death.

Ascending aorta The first section of the aorta, emerging from the heart's left ventricle (main pumping chamber).

Asymptomatic Literally means 'the absence of symptoms'. In other words a person is known to have a condition and yet they are showing no outward physical signs such as high temperature, skin rash, etc.

Atherosclerosis A disease process that leads to the build up of a sticky, waxy substance called a ' plaque ' composed of fats and cholesterols inside a blood vessel.

Athlete The Cardiac Athletes definition of an 'athlete' is a person who does regular exercise training in order for them to safely take part in their favourite sports and competitions.

Atrial Fibrillation   AF or A-Fib is the most common cardiac arrhythmia (heart rhythm disorder). It is due to the chaotic firing of heart cells within the atria (smaller top chambers of the heart) which overrides the normal electrical impulses of the heart pacemaker cells in the Sinoatrial Node or SA Node.

Autoimmune A large group of diseases characterised by abnormal functioning of the immune system. The immune system ' gets confused ' and produces antibodies which then attack the normal body tissues.

AVR Aortic Valve Replacement. An abbreviation that

describes an artificial heart valve which has been sewn into the aorta where it leaves the left ventricle (main heart pumping chamber).

Biofeedback The use of electronic gadgets to provide immediate visual and verbal information on otherwise unknown physiological bodily responses such as heart rate. Heart rate monitors worn as wrist watches are an example of this.

Biotech Short for biotechnology. This refers to the use of living systems and organisms (i.e. tissues, bacteria, viruses, etc) to develop or make useful products.

Bypass Surgery that can improve blood flow to the heart (or other organs and tissues) by providing a new route, or "bypass", around a section of clogged or diseased artery.

Bovine Referring to cow, ox, or buffalo.

Bovine pericardial valve An artificial heart valve made from the outer fibrous sac that surrounds the heart. In this case cow pericardium.

Balloon valvotomy Refers to a 'key-hole' surgical procedure where a tiny balloon is inserted on a long flexible plastic tube (catheter) through an artery in the groin or arm and threaded into the heart. When the tube reaches a narrowed heart valve the balloon is inflated. The narrowed or stuck valve leaflets are separated and stretched open as the balloon presses against them. This increases the size of the valve opening and allows more blood flow through.

Bacterial endocarditis A bacterial infection of the heart's inner surface lining involving muscle but more commonly the heart valves.

Bicuspid aortic valve A heart valve in the aortic position which has two flaps (cusps) that open and close instead of a normal aortic valve that has three flaps. It is twice as common in males as in females and is the most common congenital condition of the aortic valve occurring in 1-2% of the general population. Two of the three aortic valvular leaflets stick together during development resulting in a valve that is bicuspid instead of the normal tricuspid configuration.

Bruce protocol A standardized exercise procedure using a treadmill with a 12 lead ECG and 3 minute walking stages of increasing speeds and slopes of the treadmill. This test helps detect if heart muscle becomes starved of oxygen during exercise and higher heart rates due to narrowed heart arteries.

CABG Coronary Artery Bypass Graft. A surgical re-routing of blood around a diseased vessel that supplies blood to the heart. Done by grafting (sewing) either a piece of vein from the leg or an artery from the forearm or from under the breastbone.

Cardiac Referring to the heart.

Cardiac arrest The stopping of the heartbeat, usually because of interference with the heart's normal electrical signal.

Cardiac catheterisation A procedure that involves inserting a fine hollow plastic tube (catheter) into an artery, usually via the groin and passing this tube into the heart. Often used along with angiography and other procedures, cardiac catheterisation has become a primary tool for visualising the heart and blood vessels and diagnosing and treating heart disease.

Cardiac rehab / rehabilitation A program to help people who have had heart attacks, angioplasty, bypass grafts, heart valve replacements, angina, heart failure, pacemakers, ICD's and heart transplants, etc., return to an active life, and to reduce the risk of further heart problems. It is supervised by a specialist team of medical and nurse professionals and includes gradually increasing exercise sessions and education on heart healthy living, and counselling. * (The Cardiac Athlete Trust Fund also provides funding to cardiac rehab programmes around the world. So please, if you wish to, you can make a donation on our website. Thank you).

Cardiology The study of the heart and its function in both health and disease.

Cardiomyopathy A disease of the heart muscle (myo) that leads to generalised deterioration of the muscle and its pumping ability.

Cardiothoracic A term that refers to both the heart (cardio) and the chest (thoracic).

Cardioversion A technique of applying a safe and controlled electrical shock to the chest to convert an abnormal heartbeat back into a normal rhythm. Used to turn atrial fibrillation back into sinus rhythm.

Cardiovascular Referring to the heart and blood vessels that make up the circulatory system.

Cath / Catheter A hollow flexible plastic tube for insertion into a body cavity, duct, or blood vessel to allow the passage of fluids or the insertion of a tiny balloon or pressure monitoring sensor.

Cath lab A specialised operating theatre where cardiac catheterization, a procedure where safe x-ray blocking contrast dyes are injected into the heart chambers and heart arteries creating x-ray images and cine movies which help in the diagnosis of heart disease.

CICU Cardiac Intensive Care Unit. The Cardiothoracic ICU

(C ICU) cares for patients who need heart (cardiac) and chest (thoracic) surgery. Surgical procedures may include operations on the heart, the heart's blood vessels, the chest or the lungs.

Collagen The fibrous protein part of bone, cartilage, tendon, and other connective tissue. It is converted into gelatine by boiling in water.

Collaterals These are small, hidden tributary connecting blood vessels in the heart muscle which open up in response to blockage of a main blood vessel forming natural bypasses.

Conduction defect Special muscle fibres conduct electrical impulses throughout the heart muscle. If faulty they are sometimes referred to as having this.

Congenital Refers to conditions existing at birth.

Congenital Heart Disease Malformations of the heart or of its major blood vessels present at birth.

Coronaries Arteries arising from the wall of the aorta which then arch down over the top outside of the heart and divide into branches. These supply blood to the heart muscle.

Coronary Artery Disease A narrowing of the arteries that supply blood to the heart. The condition results from build-up of plaque and greatly increases the risk of a heart attack.

Coronary Heart Disease Disease of the heart caused by a build-up of atherosclerotic plaque in the coronary arteries that can lead to angina pectoris or heart attack.

CPR CardioPulmonary Resuscitation (CPR) is an emergency procedure to support and maintain breathing and circulation for a person who has stopped breathing (respiratory arrest) and/or whose heart has stopped (cardiac arrest) and to provide oxygen and blood flow to the heart, brain, and other vital organs.   CPR should be performed if a person is unconscious and not breathing.

Cross-training Cross training is defined as training in two or more different sports in a bid to improve your overall fitness and body tone.   It could also mean training in different exercises to improve the fitness and tone of different muscle groups in your body.   It provides variety and reduces the risk of repetitive injuries and postural problems.

CT scan   A CT scanner is a special x-ray machine that rotates around the body and creates extremely fast images of the heart from computer-guided x-ray ' slices ' which are joined together. A CT scan can provide moving images of blood flow within heart chambers and coronary arteries after the injection of a contrast dye. Sometimes referred to as a Computerized Axial Tomography (CAT) scan.

Defibrillator / defibrillation   A portable machine that helps restore a normal heart rhythm by delivering a safe and controlled electric shock to the chest of a patient whose heart is fibrillating and in the final throes of death.

Diastolic   The period of time where the heart is momentarily at rest in between beats. It corresponds to heart blood filling and the lower of the two blood pressures. Systolic is the heart's contracting phase and causes the higher blood pressure reading.

Dilated Cardiomyopathy Abbreviated to DCM this is a heart disease that leads to the main pumping chambers being dilated and too stretched to contract with enough force.

DNF Did Not Finish. In other words did not finish a sports event.

DVT Deep Vein Thrombosis. A blood clot in a deep vein in the calf usually.

ECG / EKG A test in which several electronic sensors are placed on the chest to monitor electrical activity associated with the heart beat just below the surface of the skin.

Echo / echocardiogram A heart test using a high frequency ultrasonic scanner and computerisation to create one, two or three dimensional moving pictures which show how the hearts chambers, valves and blood are functioning to help in the diagnosis of heart disease.

ED Abbreviation for Emergency Department. An area of a hospital specially equipped and staffed for emergency care of patients who arrive with sudden and acute illness or who are the victims of severe trauma . Popularly called the Emergency Room or ER.

Ejection Fraction A measurement of blood that is pumped out of a filled ventricle. Quoted as a percentage number. The normal depth of contraction is 50% wall movement or more.

Electrophysiologist A cardiologist who specialises in the electrical activity of the heart, who is an expert in all heart rhythms and who is able to test and treat these abnormal heart patterns in an EP lab.

Electrophysiology A test that uses cardiac catheterisation to study patients who have arrhythmias (abnormal heartbeats). Controlled bursts of electrical pulses stimulate the heart in an effort to provoke an arrhythmia and the heart is ' mapped ' using special catheters inside the heart with lots of electrical sensors on them. This is displayed on a computer screen as a series of multiple fast moving electrical deflection signals. An EP Study (EPS) is used to decide the risk of sudden cardiac arrest (SCA) of certain patients and whether they need an implantable defibrillator or can be treated with just medicines.

Endocarditis A bacterial infection of the heart's inner lining (endothelium).

Endorphins Hormonal compounds made by the body in response to pain or extreme physical exertion. Endorphins are similar in structure and effect to opiate drugs. They are responsible for the so-called runner's high, and release of these essential compounds permits humans to endure childbirth, accidents, and strenuous everyday activities.

ER Emergency Room (see; Emergency Department above).

Familial hypercholesterolemia A genetic predisposition to dangerously high cholesterol levels.

Femoral artery The main artery of the thigh, found in the groin, supplying oxygenated blood to the leg. Both legs have one.

Fibrosis is the replacement of normal tissue with scar tissue. Scar tissue formation is part of the normal healing process.

Forum An online internet meeting place for the discussion of questions of specialist interest to a group of people.

GERD GastroEsophageal Reflux Disease. Of or relating to or involving the stomach and oesophagus (swallowing tube).

Grafts A portion of living tissue surgically transplanted from one part of an individual to another. In the case of cardiology, graft often refers to a Coronary Artery Bypass Graft but can also refer to replacing part of the aorta with a woven biocompatible material.

Heart attack Death of, or damage to, part of the heart caused by a lack of oxygen-rich blood to the heart muscle cells. Also referred to as an MI or Myocardial Infarction.

Heart failure or more correctly Congestive Heart Failure, is a condition in which the heart cannot pump all the blood returning to it, leading to a backup of blood and pressure in the vessels and an accumulation of fluid in the body's tissues, including the lungs.

Heart murmur Noises superimposed on normal heart sounds. They are caused by congenital birth defects or damaged heart valves that do not close properly and allow blood to leak back into the chamber from which it has come.

HR Heart Rate.

Hypertension High blood pressure.

ICD Implantable Cardioverter Defibrillator. An implantable device that detects life threatening heart rhythms and terminates them by delivering a controlled electrical shock directly to the heart muscle which then blocks and stops this deadly heart rhythm continuing and so normal heart beating can begin again.

ICU Abbreviation for Intensive Care Unit. A specialized center in a hospital where intensive care is provided.

IV or iv. – Intravenous Literally means ' within ' (intra) a vein (venous). IV is also a quick reference to a needle or catheter inserted within a vein.

Ironman A person (male and female) of great physical endurance who competes in endurance contests more commonly involving swimming, cycling, and running. The main Ironman triathlon, is held annually in Hawaii and consists of a continuous 3.8-km (2.4-mi) swim, followed by a 180-km (112-mi) bicycle ride, followed by a 42.2-km (26.2-mi) marathon run performed in succession with ' transition ' periods in-between.

Ischaemia Decreased blood flow to an organ, usually due to constriction or obstruction of an artery.

Key hole surgery Surgery that uses a long thin lit fibre-optic viewing lens attached to a video camera and tiny surgical instruments inserted through small incisions as opposed to the larger incisions of more traditional surgery. This reduces risk of infection and speeds recovery from surgery.

LAD Left Anterior Descending coronary artery. One of the heart's main coronary artery branches coming off the left side of the aorta.

Left ventricle The main pumping chamber of the heart. It is the powerhouse of the ' arterial ' circulatory system and pumps blood out away from the heart to all the vital organs.

Line / iv. / cannula A reference to the administration and monitoring of intravenous (in the vein) infusions of fluids and medications.

Marfan's Syndrome Marfan's syndrome is an inherited (genetic) disorder of the connective tissue which causes abnormalities of the patient's eyes, cardiovascular system, and musculoskeletal system. In the heart this can result in extra stretchy heart valves which then leak or an extra stretchy aorta which then bulges dangerously and could rupture leading to death. Routine follow up tests keep an eye on how quickly changes occur over time.

MI Abbreviation for Myocardial Infarction. Myo (muscle) cardial (heart) infarction (death). Tissue cell death (necrosis) of a region of the myocardium caused by an interruption in the supply of blood to the heart, usually as a result of occlusion of a coronary artery.

Mitral valve The flap-like structures that control blood flow between the heart's left atrium (smaller, upper chamber) and left ventricle (bigger, most powerful, lower chamber).

Mitral Valve Prolapse (MVP) A condition that occurs when the leaflets of the mitral valve between the left atrium (upper chamber) and left ventricle (lower chamber) bulge into the atrium and permit reverse backflow of blood into the atrium. The condition is often associated with mitral regurgitation.

MRI The abbreviated term for Magnetic Resonance Imaging.   MRI uses a large circular doughnut-shaped magnet and radio waves to generate signals from atoms in the body. These signals are used to construct images of internal structures and organs such as the heart.

Murmur Noises superimposed on normal heart sounds. They are caused by congenital birth defects, holes in heart walls or damaged heart valves that do not close properly and allow blood to leak back into the chamber from where it has come.

Myocardial Infarction A heart attack. The damage or death of an area of the heart muscle (myocardium) resulting from a blocked blood supply to that area of the heart wall. The affected tissue dies, injuring the heart. Symptoms include prolonged, intensive chest pain and a decrease in blood pressure that often causes shock.

Myocardium The muscular wall of the heart. It contracts to pump blood out of the heart and then relaxes as the heart refills with returning blood.

NLP Abbreviation for Neuro-Linguistic Programming. This is a sub-branch of psychology which emphasizes that our common behaviours are guided by our regular thoughts and as thought patterns are made up of words we have learned over our life time and our internal conversations, that we can change our behaviour by interrupting these habitual thought patterns by changing just a few words. For instance I created a neural switch from ' Cardiac Cripple ' to 'Cardiac Athlete ' by changing just one word and in the process changed peoples thoughts and behaviour patterns as a result just like the lines of a rail track can be switched sending a ' train of thoughts ' in a totally new direction.

Non-physiologic In other words not the normal changing patterns of bodily functions of an organism. More often this is a reference to heart pacemakers. Some pacemakers mimic the fluctuations of healthy normal hearts and others do not so are referred to as being ' non-physiologic '.

Nuclear imaging Is a method of producing images from the radiation given off by different parts of the body after a radioactive tracer fluid is injected.

Nuclear stress test A safe radioactive dye is injected which targets and is absorbed by heart muscle cells only. When that person is placed under a special imaging machine pictures of the heart can be created which shows any damaged areas or areas not getting enough oxygen.

OHS Open Heart Surgery. An operation in which the chest and or heart are opened surgically while the bloodstream is diverted through a heart-lung (cardiopulmonary bypass) machine.

OR Abbreviation for Operating Room.

Pacemaker A surgically implanted electronic device that helps regulate the heartbeat. It monitors the heart's electrical activity and if it pauses the pacemaker fires an electrical pulse to make the heart muscle contract again.

Paediatric Pediatrics (or paediatrics) is the branch of medicine that deals with the medical care of infants, children, and adolescents and their diseases and the age limit ranges from birth up to 18.

Palpitations An uncomfortable feeling within the chest caused by an irregular heartbeat.

Pericardium The outer fibrous sac or membrane that surrounds the heart.

Pericarditis Inflammation of the outer membrane surrounding the heart. When pericarditis occurs, the amount of fluid between the pericardium and hearts outer wall surface can increase. This increased fluid presses on the heart and restricts its relaxation and filling in a situation referred to as Cardiac Tamponade which is life-threatening unless some action is made to reduce this outside the heart fluid pressure.

PICU Abbreviation for Paediatric Intensive Care Unit. A specialist department dedicated to the acute and emergency care of very sick infants, children and adolescents.

Plaque A deposit of sticky fatty (and other) substances in the inner lining of the artery wall. It is characteristic of atherosclerosis.

Porcine A reference to heart valves that are harvested from pigs, specially treated and sewn onto a support structure for use in humans to replace their diseased valves.

Pressure gradient If the blood pressure is the same on both sides of a structure then there is no pressure gradient. If there is a narrowing in the middle of a blood vessel for instance then there will be a difference in the blood pressure on each side of the narrowing, a pressure difference or pressure gradient. This can be visualised like a gradient slope in the land from highland to lowland. Pressure gradients can be measured across heart valves and across heart walls if there is a hole.

Pump head Originally this was just a locker room term used by heart surgeons for a post-surgery phenomenon that happened to some patients. It is well documented that some people who have open heart surgery using a heart and lung bypass machine can have measurable reductions in their thinking and reasoning abilities which lasts many years. Many theories exist as to why this happens and blood filters have been added to these bypass machines in order to catch and trap any microscopic debris from the bypass machine, tubes or the heart surgery itself that might otherwise shower the brain and cause damage.

Recipient A term used that refers to the person who receives a replacement heart valve or heart transplant.

Regurgitation Abnormal backward reverse flow of blood through a defective heart valve.

Rehab Short for Rehabilitation. This is a treatment or treatments designed to facilitate the process of recovery from injury, illness, or disease to as normal a condition as possible.

Rheumatic fever A disease, usually occurring in childhood, that may follow a streptococcal (bacterial) infection. Symptoms may include fever, sore or swollen joints, skin rash, involuntary muscle twitching, and development of nodules under the skin. If the infection involves the heart, scars may form on heart valves, and the heart's outer lining may be damaged.

Right ventricle The main pumping chamber on the right side of the heart which receives venous blood (depleted of oxygen returning from the body) from the smaller right atrium above and forces it into the pulmonary artery through the pulmonary valve and towards the lungs for refilling of the blood with oxygen.

Sedentary A reference to a lifestyle that is more used to sitting and doing very little in the way of physical exercise.

Spinning Indoor cycling either on a bicycle locked into a special support stand with adjustable resistance on a wheel or performed in a gym on stationary exercise cycles. An alternative to outdoor road cycling for when the weather is too cold or rainy.

ST elevation The ECG / EKG wave has positive and negative deflections labelled P, Q, R, S, and T. The S to T section of the ECG gives clues as to how much oxygen heart muscle is receiving. If the ST segment moves either up or down on the screen or paper it can mean that wall surface of the heart is getting dangerously low in oxygen supply and a heart attack is starting.

Stem cells A stem cell is one of the human body's unspecialised ' master ' cells, which has the quirky ability to grow into any one of the body's more than 200 cell types.

Stenosis The narrowing or constriction of an opening, such as a blood vessel or heart valve.

Stent A device made of expandable, metal mesh that is placed (by using a balloon catheter) at the site of a narrowing artery. This metal scaffold is then expanded on a tiny inflated (then deflated) balloon on a special catheter and left in place to keep the artery open.

Sternum The breastbone in the middle of the chest.

Stress echocardiogram Also known as a 'stress echo', is a test that combines an ultrasound study of the heart with an exercise test. The patient has a set of moving images recorded laying down at rest, exercises up to a fast heart rate and then quickly has a second identical set of moving images taken. This allows the doctor to see how the heart functions when it needs more oxygen and if any wall segments of the heart appear sluggish or non-contracting which would point to narrowed or blocked heart arteries. This test is often used as a screening tool to decide which patients go on to have a more invasive cardiac catheterisation study.

Stress test A test used to ' stress ' the heart in a controlled and safe environment where emergency treatment could be given if it is needed. Used to evaluate heart function, a stress test requires that a patient walks on a treadmill or peddles an exercise bicycle while his or her heart rate, breathing, blood pressure, electrocardiogram (ECG), and feeling of well-being are monitored. When the body is active, it requires more oxygen than when it is at rest, and, therefore, the heart has to pump more blood. Because of the increased stress on the heart, exercise can reveal ECG changes that suggest coronary artery problems not apparent when the body is at rest. The stress test is a screening tool to decide who needs to have further investigation of their heart and coronary arteries using a more invasive cardiac catheter study.

Systolic The period of time where the heart is contracting in between beats. It corresponds to blood ejecting from the heart and the higher of the two blood pressure readings.

Tachycardia Accelerated beating of the heart. A more rapid heart rate than normal.

Tissue valve An artificial cardiac valve made from the pig heart, bovine (cow) pericardium, or other biologic source material.

TransOesophageal Echocardiogram Often shortened to 'TOE' is a diagnostic test that analyses sound waves bounced off the heart. The sound waves are sent through a tube-like device inserted in the mouth and passed down the oesophagus (food pipe), which ends near the heart. This technique is useful in studying patients whose heart and vessels, for various reasons, are difficult to see with standard chest surface echocardiography.

Transhuman A term which means a person has been trans-formed into a being who is more than just a natural human as a result of improvements made by medical science and or having been merged with biotechnology.

Triathlon An endurance event in which competitors perform three sporting activities one after the other with brief ' transitions ' in-between. The most popular involves a swim followed by a cycle race followed by a run. Triathletes compete for the fastest overall course completion time. Triathlon races can vary in distances. However Intermediate or the Standard Olympic distance consists of a 1.5 kilometre (.93 mi) swim, a 40 kilometre (25 mi) bike and 10 kilometre (6.2 mi) run. There are short course ' Sprint ' triathlons, Half Ironman or ' Tinman ' triathlons and also ultra-distance or ' Ironman ' triathlons.

Triple bypass Heart bypass graft operations can be to one, two, three, four or more coronary arteries. A triple bypass is a common operation because it redirects blood to three of the main branches of arteries feeding the heart muscle with oxygen rich blood.

Ultrasound High frequency sound vibrations, which cannot be heard by the human ear. Echocardiography uses ultrasound for the medical imaging and diagnosis of structural-mechanical heart disease.

Ventricular Septal Defect (VSD) Is an opening in the dividing wall (the septum) between the heart's main lower bigger two chambers (the ventricles). A VSD is one of the defects referred to as " a hole in the heart."

Ventricular tachycardia Means the heart's larger main pumping chambers are beating abnormally fast.

REFERENCES

1. http://www.who.int/cardiovascular_diseases/en/

2. Véronique L. Roger, Alan S. Go, Donald M. Lloyd-Jones, et al. Heart Disease and Stroke Statistics—2012 Update. A Report From the American Heart Association. Circulation. 2013; 127: e6-e245

3. Paul A. Heidenreich, Justin G. Trogdon, Olga A. Khavjou, et al. Forecasting the Future of Cardiovascular Disease in the United States. A Policy Statement From the American Heart Association. Circulation. 2011; 123: 933-944 Published online before print January 24, 2011,

4. Coronary heart disease statistics. A compendium of health statistics. 2012 edition. British Heart Foundation Health Promotion Research Group Department of Public Health, University of Oxford.

5. http://www.cadiacresearch.org/topic/asian-indian-heart-disease/cadi-india/premature-heart-disease

6. http://www.heartfoundation.org.au/information-for-professionals/data-and-statistics/Pages/default.aspx

7. Mampuya WM. Cardiac Rehabilitation past, present and future: an overview. Cardiovascular Diagnosis and Therapy. Vol 2, No 1 (March 2012). http://www.thecdt.org/article/view/108/180

8. La Gerche A et al. Exercise induced right ventricular dysfunction and structural remodelling in endurance athletes. European Heart Journal 2011 Dec 6. Epub ahead of print - published with editorial

9. La Gerche A et al. Disproportionate exercise load and remodeling of the athlete's   right ventricle. Med Sci Sports Exerc. 2011 Jun;43(6):974-81.

10. La Gerche A et al. Pulmonary transit of agitated contrast is associated with   enhanced pulmonary vascular reserve and right ventricular function during exercise. J Appl Physiol. 2010 Nov;109(5):1307-17- published with editorial.

11. La Gerche A et al. Lower than expected desmosomal gene mutation prevalence in endurance athletes with complex ventricular arrhythmias of right ventricular origin. Heart 2010; Aug;96(16):1268-74. - published with editorial.

12. La Gerche A et al. Biochemical and functional abnormalities of left and right   ventricular function following ultra-endurance exercise. Heart,2008; 94: 860 – 866.

13. Corrado, D.; Basso, C.; Pavei, A.; Michieli, P.; Schiavon, M.; Thieman, T. J., Trends in Sudden Cardiovascular Death in Young Competitive Athletes After Implementation of a Preparticipation Screening Program. Journal of the American Medical Association 2006, 296 (13), 1593-1601.

BIBLIOGRAPHY

The following are literary sources read in the development of this book but which were not directly referred to within the main body of text. I offer this list to the reader who would like to read further and deeper into the field of Sports Cardiology. I have further sorted these references in ascending chronological order. I have done this because I would like it to be a resource and help you with your own continued reading, researching and developing. Again benefitting us all. It also helps us to really appreciate where our common knowledge today originated from.

2013

1. Drezner, J. A.; Toresdahl, B. G.; Rao, A. L.; Huszti, E.; Harmon, K. G., Outcomes from sudden cardiac arrest in US high schools: a 2-year prospective study from the National Registry for AED Use in Sports. British Journal of Hospital Medicine 2013, 47 (18), 1179-1183.

2. Mahmood, S.; Lim, L.; Akram, Y.; Alford-Morales, S.; Sherin, K., Screening for Sudden Cardiac Death Before Participation in High School and Collegiate Sports. American College of Preventive Medicine Position Statement on Preventive Practice. American Journal of Preventive Medicine 2013, 45 (1), 130-133.

2011

3. Asplund, C. A.; O'Connor, F. G.; Noakes, T. D., Exercise-associated collapse: an evidence-based review and primer for clinicians. British Journal of Sports Medicine 2011,45 (14), 1157-1162.

4. Benito B, Gay-Jordi G, Serrano-Mollar A, Guasch E, Tardif JC, Brugada J et al.Cardiac arrhythmogenic remodeling in a rat model of long-term intensive exercise training. Circulation 2011; 123: 13-22.

5. Evangelos, P., T. Antonio, and B. Montse, Electrocardiographic abnormalities and diagnostic criteria in athletic overtraining. British Journal of Sports Medicine, 2011. 45(2): p. e1.

6. Garber, C.E., B. Blissmer, and M.R. Deschenes, Quantity and Quality of Exercise for Developing and Maintaining Cardiorespiratory, Musculoskeletal, and Neuromotor Fitness in Apparently Healthy Adults: Guidance for Prescribing Exercise. Medicine and Science in Sports and Exercise, 2011. 43(7): p. 1334-59.

7. Kabasakalis, A., et al., Blood Oxidative Stress Markers After Ultramarathon Swimming. Journal of Strength and Conditioning Research, 2011. 25(3): p. 805-811.

8. La Gerche A, Burns AT, Mooney DJ, Inder WJ, Taylor AJ, Bogaert J et al. Exercise-induced right ventricular dysfunction and structural remodelling in endurance athletes. Eur Heart J 2011; 33:998-1006

9. Rowland, T., Is the Athletes Heart Arrhythmogenic?: Implications for Sudden Cardiac Death. Sports Medicine, 2011. 41(5): p. 401-411.

10. Sorokin, A.V., et al., Atrial fibrillation in endurance-trained athletes. British Journal of Sports Medicine, 2011. 45(3): p. 185-188.

11. Wilson M, O'Hanlon R, Prasad S, Deighan A, Macmillan P, Oxborough D,et al. Diverse patterns of myocardial fibrosis in lifelong, veteran endurance athletes. J Appl Physiol 2011; 110:1622-1626.

2010

12. Bhella PS, Kelly JP, Peshock R, Levine BD. Delayed enhancement of the intraventricular septum following an extraordinary endurance exercise. BMJ Case Reports 2010; DOI:10.1136/bcr.06.2010.3096

13. Corrado, D.; Pelliccia, A.; Heidbuchel, H.; Sharma, S.; Link, M.; Basso, C.; Biffi, A.; Buja, G.; Delise, P.; Gussac, I.; Anastasakis, A.; Borjesson, M.; Bjørnstad, H. H.; Carrè, F.; Deligiannis, A.; Dugmore, D.; Fagard, R.; D'Andrea, A., et al., Left atrial volume index in highly trained athletes. American Heart Journal, 2010. 159(6): p. 1155-1161.

14. Hoogsteen, J.; Mellwig, K. P.; Panhuyzen-Goedkoop, N.; Solberg, E.; Vanhees, L.; Drezner, J.; Estes III, N. A. M.; Iliceto, S.; Maron, B. J.; Peidro, R.; Schwartz, P. J.; Stein, R.; Theiene, G.; Zeppilli, P.; McKenna, W. J., Recommendations for intepretation of 12-lead electrocardiogram in the athlete. European Heart Journal 2010, 31 (2), 243-259.

15. Jancin, B., Subclinical Atherosclerosis Seen in Middle-Aged Marathoners, in Family Practice News 2010, International Medical News Group.

16. Jefferies, J.L. and J.A. Towbin, Dilated cardiomyopathy. The Lancet, 2010. 375(9716): p. 752-762.

17. La Gerche A, Robberecht C, Kuiperi C, Nuyens D, Willems R, de Ravel Tet al. Lower than expected desmosomal gene mutation prevalence in endurance athletes with complex ventricular arrhythmias of right ventricular origin. Heart 2010; 96:1268-1274.

18. Link, M.S. and N.A. Mark Estes, Athletes and Arrhythmias. Journal of Cardiovascular Electrophysiology, 2010. 21(10): p. 1184-1189.

19. Pelliccia, A., et al., Long-Term Clinical Consequences of Intense, Uninterrupted Endurance Training in Olympic Athletes. Journal of the American College of Cardiology, 2010. 55(15): p. 1619-1625.

20. Popovic, M.B., et al., The Effects of Endurance and Recreational Exercise on Subclinical Evidence of Atherosclerosis in Young Adults. The American Journal of the Medical Sciences, 2010. 339(9): p. 332-336.

21. Sahlen, A., et al., Effects of Prolonged Exercise on Left Ventricular Mechanical Synchrony in Long-Distance Runners: Importance of Previous Exposure to Endurance Races. Journal of the American Society of Echocardiography, 2010. 23(9): p. 977-984.

22. Scharf, M., et al., Cardiac magnetic resonance assessment of left and right ventricular morphologic and functional adaptations in professional soccer players. American Heart Journal, 2010. 159(5): p. 911-918.

23. Trivax JE, Franklin BA, Goldstein JA, Chinnaiyan KM, Gallagher MJ, deJong ATet al. Acute Cardiac Effects of Marathon Running. J Appl Physiol 2010; 108:1148-53.

24. Wilhelm, M., et al., Early Repolarization, Left Ventricular Diastolic Function, and Left Atrial Size in Professional Soccer Players. The American Journal of Cardiology, 2010. 106(4): p. 569-574.

25. Wilson, M., et al., Cardiovascular function and the veteran athlete. European Journal of Applied Physiology, 2010. 110(3): p. 459-478.

2009

26. Abdulla, J. and J.R. Nielsen, Is the risk of atrial fibrillation higher in athletes than in the general population? A systematic review and meta-analysis. Europace, 2009. 11(9): p. 1156-1159.

27. Boron, W.F. and E.L. Boulpaep, Medical Physiology A Cellular and Molecular Approach Second Edition. Vol. Second. 2009, Philadelphia, PA: Saunders Elsevier.

28. Breuckmann F, Mohlenkamp S, Nassenstein K, Lehmann N, Ladd S, Schmermund Aet al. Myocardial late gadolinium enhancement: prevalence, pattern, and prognostic relevance in marathon runners. Radiology 2009; 251:50-57.

29. de Noronha SV, Sharma S, Papadakis M, Desai S, Whyte G, Sheppard MN.Aetiology of sudden cardiac death in athletes in the United Kingdom: a pathological study. Heart 2009; 95:1409-1414.

30. Maron, B.J., Distinguishing hypertrophic cardiomyopathy from athlete‚Äôs heart physiological remodelling: clinical significance, diagnostic strategies and implications for preparticipation screening. British Journal of Sports Medicine, 2009. 43(9): p. 649-656.

31. Mont L, Elosua R, Brugada J. Endurance sport practice as a risk factor for atrial fibrillation and atrial flutter. Europace 2009; 11:11-17.

32. Reichhold, S., et al., Endurance exercise and DNA stability: Is there a link to duration and intensity? Mutation Research/Reviews in Mutation Research, 2009. 682(1): p. 28-38.

33. Sanchez, L.D., J. Pereira, and D.J. Berkoff, The Evaluation of Cardiac Complaints in Marathon Runners. Journal of Emergency Medicine, 2009. 36(4): p. 369-376.

34. Serrano-Ostáriz, E., et al., Cardiac Biomarkers and Exercise Duration and Intensity During a Cycle-Touring Event. Clinical Journal of Sports Medicine, 2009. 19(4): p. 293-299.

35. Tortora, G.J. and M.T. Nielsen, Principles of Human Anatomy Eleventh Edition. 11 ed, ed. B. Roesch2009: Wiley. 74.

36. van Teeffelen, W.M., et al., Risk factors for exercise-related acute cardiac events. A case,Äìcontrol study. British Journal of Sports Medicine, 2009. 43(9): p. 722-725.

37. Wilson M, O'Hanlon R, Prasad S, Basavarajaiah S, Stephens N, Senior R,et al. Myocardial fibrosis in an veteran endurance athlete. BMJ Case Rep 2009; DOI:10.1136/bcr.12.2008.1345

2008

38. Baldesberger, S., et al., Sinus node disease and arrhythmias in the long-term follow-up of former professional cyclists. European Heart Journal, 2008. 29(1): p. 71-78.

39. Kadoglou, N.P.E., F. Iliadis, and C.D. Liapis, Exercise and Carotid Atherosclerosis. European Journal of Vascular and Endovascular Surgery, 2008. 35(3): p. 264-272.

40. Lakhan S E and Harle L. Cardiac fibrosis in the elderly, normotensive athlete: case report and review of the literature. Diagn Pathol 2008; 3:12.

41. Lawless, C.E. and W. Briner, Palpitations in Athletes. Sports Medicine, 2008. 38(8): p. 687-702.

42. Mohlenkamp, S., et al., Running: the risk of coronary events: Prevalance and prognostic relevence of coronary atherosclerosis in marathon runners. European Heart Journal, 2008. 29(15): p. 1903-1910.

43. Molina, L., et al., Long-term endurance sport practice increases the incidence of lone atrial fibrillation in men: a follow-up study. Europace, 2008. 10(5): p. 618-623.

44. Pelliccia, A., et al., Long-Term Clinical Consequences of Intense, Uninterrupted Endurance Training in Olympic Athletes. Journal of the American College of Cardiology, 2010. 55(15): p. 1619-1625.

45. Rehman, S.U. and J.L. Januzzi Jr, Natriuretic Peptide Testing in Primary Care. Current Cardiology Reviews, 2008. 4(4): p. 300-308.

46. Sachdev, S. and K.J.A. Davies, Production, detection, and adaptive responses to free radicals in exercise. Free Radical Biology and Medicine, 2008. 44(2): p. 215-223.

47. Schmermund, A., T. Voigtlv§nder, and B. Nowak, The risk of marathon runners,Äìlive it up, run fast, die young? European Heart Journal, 2008. 29(15): p. 1800-1802.

48. Tümüklü, M., I. Etikan, and C. Çinar, Left ventricular function in professional football players evaluated by tissue Doppler imaging and strain imaging. The International Journal of Cardiovascular Imaging (formerly Cardiac Imaging), 2008. 24(1): p. 25-35.

49. Vink, A., et al., Histopathological comparison between endofibrosis of the high-performance cyclist and atherosclerosis in the external iliac artery. Journal of Vascular Surgery, 2008. 48(6): p. 1458-1463.

50. Whyte G, Sheppard M, George K, Shave R, Wilson M, Prasad Set al. Post-mortem evidence of idiopathic left ventricular hypertrophy and idiopathic interstitial myocardial fibrosis: is exercise the cause? Br J Sports Med 2008; 42:304-305.

51. Whyte GP. Clinical significance of cardiac damage and changes in function after exercise. Med Sci Sports Exerc 2008; 40: 416-1423.

2007

52. Akerstrom, T.C.A. and B.K. Pedersen, Strategies to Enhance Immune Function for Marathon Runners. Sports Medicine, 2007. 37(4/5): p. 416-419.

53. Andreas, V., Longitudinal analysis of heart rate variability. Journal of Electrocardiology, 2007. 40(1, Supplement): p. S26-S29.

54. Belotserkovskii, Z.B., et al., Structural and functional characteristics of the heart of professional soccer players after retirement from long-term sports activity. Human Physiology, 2007. 33(4): p. 490-495.

55. Ector J,Ganame J, van der Merwe N, Adriaenssens B, Pison L, Willems Ret al. Reduced right ventricular ejection fraction in endurance athletes presenting with ventricular arrhythmias: a quantitative angiographic assessment. Eur Heart J 2007; 28:345-353.

56. Goel, R., et al., Exercise-Induced Hypertension, Endothelial Dysfunction, and Coronary Artery Disease in a Marathon Runner. The American Journal of Cardiology, 2007. 99(5): p. 743-744.

57. Mel'nikov, A., A. Kylosov, and A. Vikulov, Relationships of inflammatory activity with biochemical parameters of the blood and sympathovagal balance of young athletes. Human Physiology, 2007. 33(5): p. 624-631.

58. Nieman, D.C., Marathon Training and Immune Function. Sports Medicine, 2007. 37(4/5): p. 412-415.

59. Pedoe, D.S.T., Marathon Cardiac Deaths: The London Experience. Sports Medicine, 2007. 37(4-5): p. 448-450.

60. Vohringer, M., et al., Significance of Late Gadolinium Enhancement in Cardiovascular Magnetic Resonance Imaging (CMR). S, 2007. 32(2): p. 129-137.

2006

61. Barbier, J., et al., Sports-Specific Features of Athlete's Heart and their Relation to Echocardiographic Parameters. Herz, 2006. 31(6): p. 531-543.

62. Heidbuchel, H., et al., Endurance sports is a risk factor for atrial fibrillation after ablation for atrial flutter. International Journal of Cardiology, 2006. 107(1): p. 67-72.

63. Juerg, S., Myocardial perfusion imaging by cardiac magnetic resonance. Journal of Nuclear Cardiology, 2006. 13(6): p. 841-854.

64. Lim, W., et al., Elevated Cardiac Troponin Measurements in Critically Ill Patients. Arch Intern Med, 2006. 166(22): p. 2446-2454.

65. Maron, B.J. and A. Pelliccia, The Heart of Trained Athletes: Cardiac Remodeling and the Risks of Sports, Including Sudden Death. Circulation, 2006. 114 p. 1633-1644.

66. Möhlenkamp S, Schmermund A, Kroger K, Kerkhoff G, Bröcker-Preuss M,Adams Vet al. Coronary atherosclerosis and cardiovascular risk in masters male marathon runners. Rationale and design of the "marathon study". Herz 2006; 31:575-585.

67. Swanson, D.R., Atrial fibrillation in athletes: Implicit literature-based connections suggest that overtraining and subsequent inflammation may be a contributory mechanism. Medical Hypotheses, 2006. 66(6): p. 1085-1092.

2005

68. Aghajanyan, M., Electrocardiographic Manifestations of Chronic Physical Overexertion in Athletes. Human Physiology, 2005. 31(6): p. 672-676.

69. Babuin, L. and A.S. Jaffe, Troponin: the biomarker of choice for the detection of cardiac injury. Canadian Medical Association Journal, 2005. 173(10): p. 1191-1202.

70. Corrado, D.; Pelliccia, A.; Bjørnstad, H. H.; Vanhees, L.; Biffi, A.; Borjesson, M.; Panhuyzen-Goedkoop, N.; Deligiannis, A.; Solberg, E.; Dugmore, D.; Mellwig, K. P.; Assanelli, D.; Delise, P.; van-Burren, F.; Anastasakis, A.; Heidbuchel, H.; Hoffmann, E.; Fagard, R.; Priori, S. G.; Basso, C.; Arbustini, E.; Blomstrom-Lundqvist, C.; McKenna, W. J.; Theine, G., Cardiovascular pre-participation screening of young competitive athletes for prevention of sudden death: proposal for a common European protocol. European Heart Journal 2005, 26 (516-524).

71. Naylor LH, Arnolda LF, Deague JA, Playford D, Maurogiovanni A, O'Driscoll G et al. Reduced ventricular flow propagation velocity in elite athletes is augmented with the resumption of exercise training. J Physiol 2005; 563:957-963.

2004

72. Greenland, P., et al., Coronary artery calcium score combined with Framingham score for risk prediction in asymptomatic individuals. JAMA, 2004. 291(2): p. 210-215.

73. Mourot, L., et al., Decrease in heart rate variability with overtraining: assessment by the Poincaré plot analysis. Clinical Physiology and Functional Imaging, 2004. 24(1): p. 10-18.

74. Pescatello, L.S., B.A. Franklin, and R. Fagard, Exercise and Hypertension. Medicine and Science in Sports and Exercise, 2004. 36(3): p. 533-553.

75. Salih, C., K.P. McCarthy, and S.Y. Ho, The fibrous matrix of ventricular myocardium in hypoplastic left heart syndrome: a quantitative and qualitative analysis. The Annals of Thoracic Surgery, 2004. 77(1): p. 36-40.

76. Tunstall Pedoe DS. Sudden death risk in older athletes: increasing the denominator. Br J Sports Med 2004; 38:671-672.

77. Whyte, G.P., et al., The upper limit of physiological cardiac hypertrophy in elite male and female athletes: the British experience. European Journal of Applied Physiology, 2004. 92(4): p. 592-597.

2003

78. Banerjee, A.K., et al., Oxidant, antioxidant and physical exercise. Molecular and Cellular Biochemistry, 2003. 253(1): p. 307-312.

79. Conover, Mary Boudreau, Understanding Electrocardiography, Eighth Edition 8th ed 2003: Mosby.

80. Fagard, R., Athletes Heart. Heart, 2003. 89(12): p. 1455-1461.

81. Kujala, U.M., et al., Occurrence of Chronic Disease in Former Top-Level Athletes: Predominance of Benefits, Risks or Selection Effects? Sports Medicine, 2003. 33(8): p. 553-561.

82. Lorvidhaya, P. and S.K. Stephen Huang, Sudden Cardiac Death in Athletes. Cardiology, 2003. 100(4): p. 186-195.

83. Maron, B. J., Sudden Death in Young Athletes. New England Journal of Medicine2003, 349, 1064-1075.

84. Radak, Z., et al., Marathon running alters the DNA base excision repair in human skeletal muscle. Life Sciences, 2003. 72(14): p. 1627-1633.

85.Zipes, D.P., Mechanisms of Clinical Arrhythmias. Journal of Cardiovascular Electrophysiology, 2003. 14(8): p. 902-912.

2002

86. Pelliccia A, Maron BJ, De Luca R, Di Paolo FM, Spataro A, Culasso F. Remodeling of left ventricular hypertrophy in elite athletes after long-term deconditioning. Circulation 2002; 105:944-949.

87. Stein, R., et al., Intrinsic sinus and atrioventricular node electrophysiologic adaptations in endurance athletes. Journal of the American College of Cardiology, 2002. 39(6): p. 1033-1038.

88. Wilson JM, Villareal RP, Hariharan R, Massumi A, Muthupillai R, Flamm SD.Magnetic resonance imaging of myocardial fibrosis in hypertrophic cardiomyopathy. Tex Heart Inst J 2002; 29:176-180.

89. Wong, C.-K. and H.D. White, Recognising "painless" heart attacks. Heart, 2002. 87(1): p. 3-5.

2001

90. Dorsch, M.F., et al., Poor prognosis of patients presenting with symptomatic myocardial infarction but without chest pain. Heart, 2001. 86(5): p. 494-498.

91. Katzel, L.I., J.D. Sorkin, and J.L. Fleg, A Comparison of Longitudinal Changes in Aerobic Fitness in Older Endurance Athletes and Sedentary Men. Journal of the American Geriatrics Society, 2001. 49(12): p. 1657-1664.

92. Portier, H., F. Louisy, and D. Laude, Intense endurance training on heart rate and blood pressure variability in runners. Medicine and science in sports and exercise, 2001. 33(7): p. 1120-5.

93. Thompson, P.D., Exercise and Sports Cardiology. McGraw-Hill Medical Publishing Division. 2001. ISBN 0-07-134773-9.

94. Vikulov, A.D., A.A. Mel'nikov, and I.A. Osetrov, Rheological Properties of Blood in Athletes. Human Physiology, 2001. 27(5): p. 618-625.

2000

95. Estorch, M., et al., Myocardial sympathetic innervation in the athlete's sinus bradycardia: Is there selective inferior myocardial wall denervation? Journal of Nuclear Cardiology, 2000. 7(4): p. 354-358.

96. Mackinnon, L.T., Chronic exercise training effects on immune function. Medicine and Science in Sports and Exercise, 2000. 32(7): p. S369-76.

97. MacKinnon, L.T., Overtraining effects on immunity and performance in athletes. Immunol Cell Biol, 2000. 78(5): p. 502-509.

98. Pelliccia, A., et al., Clinical Significance of Abnormal Electrocardiographic Patterns in Trained Athletes. Circulation, 2000. 102, p. 278-284.

1999

99. Atalay, M. and C.K. Sen, Physical Exercise and Antioxidant Defenses in the Heart. Annals of the New York Academy of Sciences, 1999. 874(1): p. 169-177.

100. Basilico, F.C., Cardiovascular Disease in Athletes. The American Journal of Sports Medicine, 1999. 27(1): p. 108-121.

101. Hood, S. and R.J. Northcote, Cardiac assessment of veteran endurance athletes: a 12 year follow up study. British Journal of Sports Medicine, 1999. 33(4): p. 239-243.

102. Song Y, Yao Q, Zhu J, Luo B, Liang S.Age-related variation in the interstitial tissues of the cardiac conduction system; and autopsy study of 230 Han Chinese. Forensic Sci Int 1999; 104:133-142.

1998

103. Jensen-Urstad, K., et al., High prevalence of arrhythmias in elderly male athletes with a lifelong history of regular strenuous exercise. Heart, 1998. 79(2): p. 161-164.

104. Karjalainen, J., et al., Lone atrial fibrillation in vigorously exercising middle aged men: case-control study. British Medical Journal, 1998. 316(7147): p. 1784-1785.

105. Maron, B. J.; Gohman, T. E.; Aeppli, D., Prevalence of sudden cardiac death during competitive sports activities in Minnesota High School athletes. Journal of the American College of Cardiology 1998,32 (7), 1881-1884.

1997

106. Fuller, C. M.; McNulty, C. M.; Spring, D. A.; Arger, K. M.; Bruce, S. S.; Chryssos, B. E.; Drummer, E. M.; Kelley, F. P.; Newmark, M. J.; Whipple, G. H., Prospective screening of 5,615 high school athletes for risk of sudden cardiac death. Medicine& Science in Sports & Exercise 1997,29 (9), 1131-1138.

107. Uusimaa, P., et al., Collagen Scar Formation After Acute Myocardial Infarction : Relationships to Infarct Size, Left Ventricular Function, and Coronary Artery Patency. Circulation, 1997. 96(8): p. 2565-2572.

1994

108. Miki, T., et al., Echocardiographic findings in 104 professional cyclists with follow-up study. American Heart Journal, 1994. 127(4, Part 1): p. 898-905.

109. Weber, K.T., et al., Collagen Network of the Myocardium: Function, Structural Remodeling and Regulatory Mechanisms. Journal of Molecular and Cellular Cardiology, 1994. 26(3): p. 279-292.

1993

110. Bjørnstad H, Storstein L, Meen HD, Hals O.Electrocardiographic findings of left, right and septal hypertrophy in athletic students and sedentary controls. Cardiology 1993; 82:56-65.

111. Rowe WJ. Endurance exercise and injury to the heart. Sports Med 1993;16:73-79.

1989

112. Northcote, R.J., et al., Is severe bradycardia in veteran athletes an indication for a permanent pacemaker? British Medical Journal, 1989. 298(6668): p. 231-232.

1972

113. Polednak, A.P., Longevity and Cardiovascular Mortality among Former College Athletes. Circulation, 1972. 46(4): p. 649-654.

Lightning Source UK Ltd.
Milton Keynes UK
UKOW05f0825280417

300106UK00013B/150/P

Lady Glenconner's Picnic Papers

and other Feasts with Friends

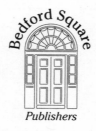

Bedford Square
Publishers

The Picnic Papers first published in 1983, by Hutchinson & Co. Ltd,
an imprint of the Hutchinson Publishing Group

This edition first published in the UK in 2024 by Bedford Square Publishers Ltd,
London, UK

bedfordsquarepublishers.co.uk
@bedsqpublishers

A portion of the royalties from the sale of this book will be donated by the
author and the publisher to Safelives a registered charity in England and Wales
(Registered charity no. 1106864) to support their work to end domestic abuse.

ISBN
978-1-83501-238-3 (Hardback)
978-1-83501-239-0 (Trade paperback)
978-1-83501-240-6 (eBook)

2 4 6 8 10 9 7 5 3

Typeset by Palimpsest Book Production Ltd, Falkirk, Stirlingshire

Printed in Great Britain by CPI Group (UK) Ltd, Croydon CR0 4YY

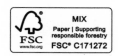

*To my friend Susanna who was
the inspiration for this book.*

Contents

Introduction

I am sadly writing this introduction on my own as Susanna Johnston, with whom I wrote the original *Picnic Papers*, died last year. I have missed her guiding hand on the new edition of this book but I hope she would approve.

Naturally, our undiluted gratitude went to the distinguished contributors who generously shared their picnicking experiences with us. Each and every one gave such encouragement by their enthusiasm and interest that the pleasure of corresponding, planning and talking with them over the venture was intense. Now I have a selection of new contributions to add to the mix and am equally grateful to today's writers for taking the time to share their memories and opinions of eating al fresco.

Susanna and I had both been dedicated picnickers since early youth and consequently find the subject of outdoor eating wholly absorbing. After all, it is a well-established habit. Our Stone Age forbears could be said to have picnicked after a fashion as they applied flint to firewood, culled berries, or sat with mammoth ribs in hand at the mouth of a cave; but whereas for them there was no alternative, for us there is all the excitement of the break away from daily ritual as we set out to find the perfect place to unpack the basket and perhaps even to find on-the-spot food to add to our provisions.

So – what is a picnic? The *Oxford English Dictionary* tells us in a few lines:

> *Picnic* Originally a fashionable and social entertainment in which each person present contributed a share of the provisions; now, a pleasure party including an excursion to some spot in the country where all partake of a repast out of doors... The essential feature was formerly the individual contribution; now it is the al fresco form of the repast.

Picnics, if the *Oxford English Dictionary* is to be trusted, were originally a foreign institution – an institution peculiar to the upper class; the *Annual Register* in 1802 declares that 'the rich have their sport, their balls, their parties of pleasure and their *pic-nics*' – and a year or two later James Beresford, in his popular work *The Miseries of Human Life, or The Last Groans of Timothy Testy and Samuel Sensitive: With a Few Supplementary Sighs from Mrs Testy,* describes one of his female characters as being 'full of Fete and Picnic and Opera'.

During the last hundred years or so picnicking has become such a popular pleasure that the phrase 'this is no picnic' is an accepted idiom to describe an unpleasant or unpopular experience. One of the joys of picnicking is proving how much depends on the setting and, cliché though it is, how much better something very ordinary can taste when eaten out of doors. In a bluebell wood with a campfire blazing, try making a dough of flour and water, add a pinch of salt and nothing else whatsoever. Roll it into a messy ball. Squeeze this lump onto the end of a long pointed stick. Thrust it into the flames and wait for it to turn brown. Here you have a 'damper' the time-honoured picnic delicacy. It is unlikely that it would be equally appreciated if served at a dining-room table by candlelight.

The very suggestion of a picnic tends to produce a strong reaction. Some people loathe them. Sir Steven Runciman, the historian, certainly appeared to disagree with the modern idea of picnicking as an enjoyable pastime. He told us in a letter:

Memories crowd up of depression and discomfort; not quite dispelled by a picnic with Agatha Christie on Dartmoor, at which we drank champagne from silver goblets. Nor have my picnics been really eventful. I remember once picnicking on a Syrian roadside with a local colonel who had been sent to accompany me because I insisted on visiting a crusader castle near the Israeli frontier. Poor portly man, he had to climb to a mountaintop with me. And when we paused on the way back to eat, the Israelis took potshots at us from across the frontier, and the colonel, good Muslim though he was, consoled himself with the wine (local and awful) that I had brought with me. Or a picnic organised in Jericho (in 1931) by Abdul Hamid's retired astrologer, where Susanna's grandmother and I were poisoned. I have picnicked in a snowstorm on the Great Wall of China. In 1931, I picnicked, more happily, with a Rumanian prince on the (then) Bessarabian frontier, looking at suspicious Russian sentries across the river Dniester. That was happier, as was a picnic on a barge on the river Mekong where the royal band played Mozart. But on the whole my experiences have been a trifle *triste*.

However miserable the author of this letter may have been at the time of these ordeals, there can be no denying that his experiences were colourful. Some people feel that picnics are all very well when necessary, provided they are permitted to stick to the smudgy jam sandwich, hard-boiled egg and Bakelite teacup of their youth. We both look back on this type of picnic with nostalgia but never attempt to repeat it.

Some of those who have contributed to this book, Sir Harold Acton, for example, who was the first person to encourage us in this venture, have described unexpected and often nerve-racking adventures that have come about as the result of setting out on a picnic instead of allowing oneself to be securely tethered to a dining room or restaurant table. Some have shown how a day out of doors can be far more entertaining and educative, not to mention beneficial to one's purse, than one in a crowded pub.

Whatever our attitude, it remains a fact that we English, in the main, have an irresistible habit of eating al fresco, in spite of our unreliable climate. We will eat anywhere – in swamps, on haystacks, in sunshine, hail, fog or drizzle – anything to escape the routine of the kitchen table.

Not so for Graham Norton for whom 'planning a picnic is deciding to be disappointed'. For Graham, 'the only recipe anyone needs for a successful picnic is to see a patch of blue in the sky that is, as my father used to say, "big enough for a pair of sailor's trousers" and then pop into the nearest garage shop and stock up on some items packed with fat and salt. Consume these snacks somewhere you can at least see a tree and count yourself one of the luckiest people alive.'

I would like to thank Susanna's lovely daughters Clara, Lily, Rosy and Silvy who allowed me to refresh the original book and produce this new edition. I would also like to thank Johanna Tennant for being unfailingly kind and helpful – nothing is too much trouble, and for her encouragement and eagle eye. My darling daughters May and Amy were also invaluable in helping to bring the book up to date. Thanks to Sarah Harrison and Bedford Square Publishers for having faith in this book and giving me the wonderful opportunity for re-publishing it; thanks also to my agent Gordon Wise for being instrumental in bringing this book back to life. I would also like to thank the Queen who suggested SafeLives Charity which this book is supporting.

Princess Margaret

When we were first compiling this book, Susanna said how marvellous it would be if we could get Princess Margaret to write something for it. I wasn't at all sure she would, as she hadn't done anything like that before, but I broached the subject one evening when Princess Margaret and I were sitting in my Norfolk farmhouse. We'd had one or two whiskies, she liked to drink whisky after dinner, and I said, 'Ma'am there's something I'd like to ask you.' 'Yes, Anne what is it?' 'Well, you know Zanna and I are compiling a book of picnics with some proceeds going to the Glyndebourne Trust?' She said, 'Anne you know I really hate opera.' Because she loved ballet, she knew a lot about it and was always going down to White Lodge, the Royal Ballet School in Richmond Park, and knew all the children there by name, but opera was not her thing. Anyway, she said, 'Well what are you going to ask me?' And I plucked up courage to ask if she could write a piece about a picnic for us and she simply said, 'Yes of course.'

Sometimes she surprised you, and then of course she came back to us with this lovely picnic at Hampton Court. That picnic was what she called one of her 'Treats', which every so often she would lay on for the members of the household, some of her ladies-in-waiting and some friends. Once she flew us to Osborne House on the Isle of Wight and we had a lovely picnic there. Another dinner she arranged for us was at the Tower of London, where they put a table in the midst of the Crown Jewels so we were surrounded by them, that was a great, great treat.

She loved organising these special occasions and being able to control the situation. It was similar when she used to come up to Glen, the house my husband Colin inherited in Scotland. When we were throwing a party, she'd often come the day before and help me with the flowers or check the dining-room table was laid properly. I'd show her the table plan and she'd say, 'Oh I'd love to sit next to so and so' she knew exactly what was going to happen. That was what she liked and it actually made her very easy. What she didn't like was going to someone's house and them not telling her anything, not knowing what the plan was. She hated surprises and that could make things difficult. I wonder if it was because she was going through a difficult time in her marriage, which she couldn't control, so she would want to be very exacting about those areas that she could. An example of this was that she knew precisely where everything was on her dressing table and would notice at once if something had been moved. She also collected shells and once a year one of my least favourite tasks was to wash them with soapsuds in a bath, dry them and put them back in the glass cupboards. I could never remember where they were supposed to go but she knew very precisely. 'Not there, Anne, can't you remember that one always goes there?' She was very particular like that.

Picnic at Hampton Court
HRH The Princess Margaret

Nearly all picnics in Britain end up in a lay-by by the road because, in desperation, no one can decide where to stop. I felt that another sort of treat, slightly different and rather more comfortable, was indicated. In my opinion picnics should always be eaten at table and sitting on a chair. Accordingly my picnic, in May 1981, took the form of an outing to Hampton Court.

This mysterious palace is like nothing else – very complex in structure and design. Built first by Cardinal Wolsey, it continued in construction through many reigns. One can wander through buildings dating from about 1514 to Charles II, William and Mary (with the help of Sir Christopher Wren), and George II. George III, when faced with the choice between it and Windsor Castle, mercifully chose the latter, as Hampton Court is rather like a haphazard village.

The Queen kindly let me take some friends. The best plan, it seemed to me, was to do some sightseeing and have lunch in the middle. So I got in touch with Sir Oliver Millar, Surveyor of the Queen's Pictures, who delighted in taking us round the recently restored Mantegnas, which are housed in their own Orangery. These were saved, happily, from the disastrous sale of Charles I's pictures by Cromwell, simply because Cromwell liked them.

I asked Professor Jack Plumb, Master of Christ's College, Cambridge, who had helped in writing the television series *Royal Heritage*, where we should best have our cold collation. He suggested the little Banqueting House overlooking the Thames. This seemed an excellent place for a number of reasons. It wasn't open to the public then, it was shelter in case of rain and, as far as anyone knew, there hadn't been a jolly there since the time of Frederick, Prince of Wales.

The Banqueting House used to be called the Water Gallery and was a retreat for Mary II. When she died William III pulled it down, because memories were too poignant, and built the Banqueting House on the same site. In the main room the walls and ceiling are by Verrio. The hall and anterooms are tiny, and being quite small it is nice and cosy. As three sides of it are surrounded by a sunken garden smelling warmly of wisteria and wallflowers, with the river flowing beneath its windows on the fourth side, it provided an ideal setting.

I took my butler to ensure that everything would be all right.

We started with smoked salmon mousse, followed by that standby of the English, various cold meats and beautiful and delicious salads. Those with room then had cheeses.

We drank a toast to Frederick, Prince of Wales and departed to inspect the famous old vine which has its own greenhouse and Nanny gardener. After that we wandered among the many visitors from abroad, round the lovely gardens and canals, viewing all the different façades of its many sides. We visited the chapel (redecorated by Wren) and the tennis court where we watched a game of royal or real tennis.

It was altogether a glorious day. The sun was shining on one of its brief appearances that summer, and everyone was happy.

Avocado Soup

> 3–4 avocado pears (depending on size)
> 1 pint (570 ml) chicken consommé
> ½ teaspoonful black pepper, salt and sugar mixed
>   together

pinch of garlic salt
1 teaspoonful Worcestershire sauce
a little dry sherry
double cream

Put all the ingredients except the cream in blender. Leave in refrigerator for an hour or until cold. Serve in consommé cups with a little dab of double cream on each serving.

Roddy Llewellyn

Colin and I introduced Princess Margaret to Roddy Llewellyn, who I invited as an extra to a house party we were having at Glen. Princess Margaret was also a guest, and it was clear from day one that it was love at first sight, so I suppose it wasn't surprising that when I asked him to write about a picnic for our book he said, 'Well the very best picnics I ever had were at Glen.' Roddy became one of our very closest friends and he and Princess Margaret often came to stay at the Norfolk farmhouse I bought from my father when I got married. It became a safe haven for the two of them to escape all the awful press attention. Margaret would say to me, 'Roddy and I think your flower beds need weeding, Anne' and they would go out and weed side by side, kneeling on a weeding mat. It was one of the things she liked to do when she was here, like cleaning my car and insisting on always laying the fire for me. I wasn't allowed to touch the fire. 'I was a girl guide, Anne, you weren't, I know all about fires.' She'd fetch the wood from the basket in my hall and set about getting the fire going. She always sat on the chair next to the fire and when I'm here on my own I often feel that she's still here with me.

When Roddy left to get married, Princess Margaret decided that she was going to make friends with his wife, which we both did. She would load up the car with food and things she thought Roddy and darling Tania, his wife, and their gorgeous girls would like, standing at the boot and supervising what went in.

After her funeral, the Queen held a wake for Princess Margaret at Windsor. I was summoned to see the Queen and she said she wanted to thank me and Colin for giving Princess Margaret such a wonderful time in Mustique, and also for introducing her to Roddy. I thought that was so kind, as she really couldn't say anything like that at the time. I told Roddy about it and he was absolutely thrilled.

Picnic at Glen
Roddy Llewellyn

Style is something sadly lacking these days, but picnics at the Glen have more than their fair share of it. One magic day, several summers ago, the two main ingredients to ensure a successful luncheon picnic were there – sun and water. Delicious home-made pâtés, pies with thick crusts and galantines made possible the coming of *La Grande Bouffe* to Loch Eddy. Gin and tonics tinkling with ice mingled with the conversation, which often exploded into laughter. What seemed like an inexhaustible supply of chilled wine helped to wash down the kipper pâté and galantine of grouse, while huge bowls of salad were accompanied by a collection of stalwart cheeses which would have placated Mighty Mouse in his angriest mood. Lunch ended in a bonfire, a gentle row round Loch Eddy and a snooze on a rug or a walk. Whatever one did, one did it without a care in the world.

Kipper Pâté

> 7 oz (200 g) tin kipper fillets (preferably John West),
>   with most of the oil drained off
> 1 packet aspic, made up as instructions
> juice of half a large lemon
> 300 ml carton cream
> parsley for garnish

Put the kippers, ½ pint (275 ml) aspic (save a little for end), the lemon juice and cream in a liquidiser. When smooth put into an entrée dish and cool in the refrigerator for 45 minutes. Then cover with a little aspic. Decorate with parsley and eat with brown toast.

Galantine of Grouse

> 4 oz (110 g) calves' liver
> 8 oz (225 g) veal or sausage meat
> 1 lb (450 g) fat pork
> 4 rashers bacon
> a small bunch of chopped parsley
> 2 shallots
> 1 clove of garlic
> bay leaf
> breast of three grouse

Preheat the oven to gas mark 5 (375°F, 190°C). Put everything through the mincer except the bay leaf, bacon and grouse. Put the bay leaf at the bottom of the dish, then alternate layers of veal or sausage meat, grouse and bacon. Cook for about an hour then press down with a plate. Eat cold.

Susannah Constantine

I loved the television series Susanah presented with Trinny
Woodall. *What Not to Wear* was a makeover show in the early
2000s which we were all glued to. But I really knew Susannah
from the time when she was going out with Princess Margaret's
son David Linley. They used to come out to Mustique and I
always really liked her. She was devoted to Princess Margaret, it
was something we shared. And Princess Margaret was very fond
of Susannah, almost like a surrogate mother for her. Then, of
course, she and David parted ways and I followed her career, but
I only really reconnected with her recently when she sent me
her memoir to read. She is always so friendly and nice and we
enjoy reminiscing about Princess Margaret when we meet.

Picnic Pandemonium
Susannah Constantine

I was never a fan of picnics and have mostly lied about how much
I enjoy eating in the great outdoors. It's not the unpredictable

17

weather, uninvited insects, dribbled ketchup or accidental mouthfuls of sand that put me off, but the work it takes to pull a picnic together. Usually a drive, walk or sail away, you can't afford to leave anything behind and if you do, the picnic is a failure. You can't have more than one person at the helm for this reason. Too many cooks leave too much room for error.

I have been on picnics where everything has arrived and been beautifully prepared and packed by a silver-fingered cook. Picnics on Macaroni Beach in Mustique with Princess Margaret were always an event to relish, and I have many happy memories of Ma'am presiding at the end of a pop-up plastic table. But this was because I wasn't accountable for not forgetting any number of 'the most important' ingredients.

We have a home on the Helford River in Cornwall. It's been in the family eons and as anyone who has holidayed in the UK knows – it's impossible to avoid picnicking. Resentfully I've *had* to embrace this very British of traditions.

Being extraordinarily greedy and a bit of a foodie I can't bring myself to lighten the workload with bought sandwiches and a packet of crisps. I'm not a nutritional snob. I'll eat anything, but one of the primary ways I like to show my family love is through food. And cooking is one of the few things I'm better at than my husband Sten.

Whatever the season or temperature it's always the same. Chipolata sausages. Home-made garlic mayonnaise and crispy parmesan chicken nuggets. Roasted new potatoes with rosemary. Carrot and cucumber batons, hummus. Tunnock's Teacakes for pudding. Lots of greaseproof paper, tinfoil and Tupperware. The menu doesn't change but the venue does and while you don't expect a picnic to come with danger to life, our best and most memorable involved torrential rain, huge waves and an almost-upturned boat.

★

It was a calm and beautiful morning when we set off. A gentle breeze nudged our Rib from its mooring packed with cold box, portable barbecue, three small children and a dog called Archie. Health and Safety has never been a strong point in our family, and we thought not a lot as the wind picked up. By the time we approached Porthbeor beach near St Mawes in an ever-increasing swell, it became clear we had been caught out in a squall with gusts reaching 60 mph. Approaching the beach we were reduced to a crawl, battling huge, cold waves and crashing white water. If ever our ex-RNLI Rib was going to capsize it was now. With the surf breaking we were all tossed off the rubber sides but managed stay onboard. Archie fell out and between waves my husband screamed. 'Jump now!'

Soaked, scared and in peril of losing our picnic I seized the food, threw as much as I could on to the sand and yelled at the kids to grab on to me. We all survived unhurt. There is nothing like adrenalin to boost an appetite. Our picnic never tasted better, and we have never forgotten the day 'we *nearly* drowned'.

Angela Huth

When Angela was pregnant and bedridden, she writes about how Princess Margaret used to go over to her house with Tony (Armstrong-Jones) on a Saturday evening with a delicious cold supper, including the china and the glasses, and Tony would set up a film in the bedroom which they would all watch together. Angela was a close friend of Princess Margaret, which was how I got to know her, and we often used to go and stay with her and her husband in Oxford where he was a don. She was a novelist who wrote among others a terrific book called *Land Girls*, which was turned into a film starring Rachel Weisz. Her story about Princess Margaret shows how thoughtful she could be. I remember when I was having a very difficult time with my two older boys and then Christopher had his terrible accident, she would constantly phone up to see if I was all right and would send a car to pick me up and bring me to Kensington Palace for lunch. She'd say, 'Anne you've got to eat you know, you've got to keep your strength up – for Christopher's sake.' She was incredibly kind like that, which I don't think is something many people know about her.

The Perfect Picnic
Angela Huth

There are picnics of the mind and picnics in real life. Most people have experienced both and know the difference between them.

In the imagination the *déjeuners sur l'herbe* which we attend seem to be very similar. There is always warmth, but cool shade, iced white wine, grass that doesn't prickle, butterflies – a veritable Impressionist picture, happily out of focus. If the imagination were unkind enough to look closer, the dream would be broken.

In reality the dream is broken, almost inevitably, as soon as the very idea of a picnic is cast abroad, and the hamper packed. (Hamper indeed: where are the hampers of yesteryear, those magnificent wicker baskets, lids slotted with knives and forks, and stacked with their special plates? It is supermarket cool boxes in which we pack our feasts of today, and they are not at all the same.)

But disillusionment is of no matter to the determined picnicker. Once launched on the expedition, he blooms with optimism however black the cloud that billows from nowhere, however large the spots of rain. On, on he drives past those Picnic Areas whose corrugated lavatories and official rustic tables make him sad to think this generation of townsfolk think *they* are proper picnic places. On to a small stretch of balding coast with a misted view over a grim sea. The wind might die down, but until it does where better to eat than the stuffy cosiness of the car, thick with the smells of melons, cheese and wet dogs? Children shriek, there's strawberry jam on the steering wheel and, by heavens, it's almost the fun we had imagined.

For there is probably no hardier race of picnickers than the British. On Bodmin Moor I have watched summer sleet sizzle the flames of the barbecue on which lie dozens of drenched *langoustines*, where in a nearby bowl *fraises du bois* turn to pulp. But the smiles of the crowd gathered under their anoraks wavered not. I have seen members of the edge-of-the-motorway brigade sprayed black with mud by passing cars as they enjoy their sliced-bread sandwiches. I have seen trainspotters relishing Chinese takeaways on a stack of mailbags at Paddington Station on a November afternoon.

But happily, whatever the disappointment of real-life picnics, in retrospect it is the delights that are remembered. And thus our nostalgia for picnics. We continue to persevere with them, for when they work they are occasions of particular pleasure.

My own first memories of picnic life were at the age of twelve: curried egg sandwiches at sunless Overstrand. My sister and I – scoffing at our parents' tweed coats and mackintoshes. Eight years later there were picnic lunches at point-to-points in Hampshire – occasions of supreme sophistication, those. The backs of Land Rovers were let down to reveal the last of the real hampers of delicious food. I don't remember precisely *what* food. I have no recollection of quiches in those mid-fifties days – they were to become fashionable much later. But I do remember sturdy wicker baskets with separate compartments for bottles of drink, and standing round with tiny glasses in fuzzy-gloved hands, sipping cherry brandy and sloe gin against the cold.

The point of those picnics was not, of course, the food (or even the horses) but the chance to brush against the fancied member of the opposite sex and be offered a sausage on a stick with a look of such penetrating desire that the legs would tremble in the gumboots like grass in a wind. How beautiful they were, those sporting young men in their riding macs that clacked like a field of cabbages when they moved – their greenish trilbies cocked saucily over one eye, their incredible eyelashes, and small

23

patches of mysteriously long hair on their cheeks. No wonder the contents of the hampers were of no consequence.

But of all memorable picnics the one nearest to perfection of imaginary picnics took place in Cornwall four years ago. It was the inspiration of those master picnickers, Marika and Robin Hanbury-Tenison. She was one of our finest cooks. He is a renowned explorer. They have feasted off rattlesnakes and spiders in many a foreign jungle in their time, but at home on Bodmin Moor their picnics were incomparable.

It was May, very warm. We were asked to wear Edwardian clothes, and to meet in the bluebell woods. These woods were sprawled about along a valley – crumbling old trees, lichen-covered – their frizz of new leaves a-dazzle with spring sun. Our chosen place was on the mossy banks of a stream: a place where wild thyme grew. Tables were laid with damask cloths and spread with a feast in keeping with the Edwardian era. We lay on cashmere rugs, crushing bluebells. We ate iced strawberry soup, chicken and bacon pie, cherries in wine and pyramids of meringues. Suddenly through the trees came our elegant Ambassador to Japan, Sir Fred Warner. He wore a blazer, straw boater and almond-pink silk tie. Behind him rustled his wife, Simone, in forget-me-not blue, who sang to us in her clear piping voice while her small sons fell in and out of the stream. There will never be another picnic like that middle-aged frolic in the bluebell woods, but there will be others of surprising and enchanting character, and in old age we perennial picnickers will still be there, sharing the present delight beneath umbrella or parasol, remembering all the while the hampers of our youth.

Strawberry Soup

> 2 chicken stock cubes
> 1 pint (570 ml) water
> 2 lb (900 g) fresh or frozen strawberries
> ½ teaspoon mixed herbs
> salt, pepper
> ½ teaspoon ground ginger
> 1 small carton natural yoghurt
> 2 tablespoons finely chopped chives

Combine the chicken stock cubes and water, bring to the boil and stir until the cubes are dissolved. Add the strawberries and herbs, season with salt and pepper, and mix in the ground ginger. Bring to the boil again, simmer for 5 minutes and then rub through a fine sieve to remove the seeds. Stir in the yoghurt, mix until smooth, and serve hot or iced with a garnish of chopped chives.

Milton Gendel

Milton, an American Italian art critic and photographer, lived in what was described as 'The most wholly desirable house in Rome.' The Palazzo Pierloni Caetani was situated on the Isola Tiberina, a little island in the middle of the Tiber river. I do remember it was very damp. He had been introduced to Princess Margaret's best friend Judy Montagu by the British socialite Lady Diana Cooper, and they were married in 1962. Judy was a very old friend of my husband Colin, and we often went to stay with them, as did Princess Margaret. It was one of Princess Margaret's favourite stops in Rome along with La Pietra which was the home of Harold Acton, which we also visited. Milton and Judy had a little girl, Anna, who had a total of twenty-four very well-chosen godparents, one of whom was Princess Margaret. When Judy died very suddenly at the age of forty-nine, Princess Margaret stepped in and invited Milton and Anna to the royal palaces during the summer when Anna was on school holiday. Milton always had a camera on him and was constantly snapping away, I think because he was always around the royal family he got intimate relaxed photographs of them. He took a rather wonderful one of the Queen wearing a headscarf preparing burgers to feed her dogs at Balmoral. When he asked if he could take one more photograph she apparently replied, 'Well, I'll be very surprised if you've got any more film left.'

Picnic in Rome
Milton Gendel

For generations the English have been domesticating the Sublime by choosing its precincts for their picnics. There is no beauty spot in creation, on Alp, lakeside or riverbank, in jungle or desert, that has not served as a setting for a group of English people with picnic baskets, spirit lamps and teapots in cosies. At least this was so before the highway picnic became current, with picnickers on folding chairs and the open boot of the car serving as buffet.

Once, in the spring, a few decades ago, Rome offered a happy conjunction of scenic sublimity and picnicking English to provide appropriate foreground figures. Evelyn Waugh, in the Holy City for his annual Easter devotions, was the star of the occasion. Jenny Crosse, daughter of Robert Graves and correspondent of *Picture Post*, was always the moving spirit on such occasions. She rang up Babs Johnson, the writer known as Georgina Masson.

'Evelyn Waugh is here with Diana Cooper – you know – she's Mrs Stitch in his novels. I thought we might have it at your place.'

The self-educated daughter of an Indian Army officer, Babs brought the competence, pertinacity and inspiration of a Mrs Beeton to her various interests. The two ladies devised the guest list, which contained enough flannel-coated men and hatted or bandanna-ed women to provide the cast for a proper English picnic.

Then Evelyn Waugh announced that he would come to the picnic only if he did not have to sit on the ground. With some regret Babs Johnson gave up the thought of the remoter romantic glades of the villa, where daffodils were springing and cherry trees blossoming, and moved her tables and chairs out in front of the vaulted stable that old Prince Filippo Doria let her have as a grace-and-favour home in his park.

A lovely limpid blue and gold April day framed Babs's stable-yard rock garden. Jenny bustled about serving Frascati, mascarpone and ricotta seasoned with salt and pepper and garnished with a sprinkling of paprika. Next came tufted raw fennel, to be pulled apart and dipped in olive oil with mustard, and eggs stuffed with anchovies. Round loaves of crusty bread, the descendants of those found – baked hard – in the ashes of Pompeii, were set out together with plates of prosciutto, minuscule slices of spicy salami, rounds of lonza and mortadella.

When Evelyn Waugh arrived he was allotted a little table to himself where he sat plump with a commanding air, more lordly than any rank-proud gentleman on the Grand Tour.

The talk turned on the personality and history of Pius XII, the reigning pontiff. Jenny and Babs were censorious. The Pope was austere, autocratic. Sympathetic to German *Kultur*, he had not been outspoken enough against the Nazis. True, the Vatican had contributed to the gold ransom extorted from the Roman Jews during the German occupation, but it hadn't prevented their deportation or the massacre of the hostages at the Fosse Ardeatine. A devout Catholic guest blushed with discomfiture at the protracted and irreverent discussion. Evelyn Waugh, now impatient, banged his fork on the table.

Jenny placatingly held out a bottle of Frascati.

'Some wine, Evelyn?' He fixed her with a cold blue eye. 'Mrs Crosse,' he said, with compelling emphasis, 'has anyone ever remarked on the uncanny resemblance between you and the late unlamented Mrs Roosevelt? Undoubtedly she was one of the most ill-favoured women the world has ever seen.'

A stunned silence followed this pronouncement, as its author returned to spearing rounds of salami. It was broken by Diana Cooper, out of the depths of her bonnet: 'He's just *too* awful.'

Jenny retreated to the stable converted into a sitting-room where Babs was uncorking some wine. 'Are you crying?' Babs asked. Jenny repeated what had just been said to her. Babs, a sturdy woman with iron-grey hair, a determined look and a kind eye, listened with growing indignation. She had been brought up near the Khyber Pass, where respect was paid to the New Testament on Sundays and holidays, but where daily life was ruled more by the Old Testament. She was also uncompromising in her view of women's rights.

'Jenny,' she said, 'you go right out there now and hit him as hard as you can. You're a woman and he won't dare hit you back.' Jenny looked shocked, but obediently turned and went back to the rock garden.

Evelyn Waugh peered up at her with a bland expression as she addressed him: 'Evelyn, I have always admired you as a writer. After your behaviour today I want you to know that I no longer admire you as a man. But, as Christians, perhaps we meet on common ground. So I *forgive* you.'

As a master of dry comedy he must have relished the turning of his elective worm into a monument of moral dignity. The company certainly did: there were shouts of laughter, followed by praise for Jenny and belated reproval for Evelyn Waugh.

'I don't care much for picnics,' said Waugh when it was time to go. 'But I enjoyed this one immensely. And I shall never forget it.'

Anchovy Eggs

eggs
mayonnaise
anchovy fillets
salt
pepper
lemon juice
mustard
cayenne
basil

Hard–boil the eggs. Crack the shells and drop immediately into cold water to minimise the darkening of the yolks. Shell and cut in halves lengthwise. Mash the yolks and moisten with mayonnaise and well–pounded anchovy fillets. Season to taste with salt, pepper, lemon juice, mustard and cayenne. Refill the whites with this mixture and sprinkle with chopped basil.

Harold Acton

Harold Acton might well have been at the picnic described by Milton Gendel, as he was a great friend of Evelyn Waugh. An art historian, novelist and poet, he was said to be the inspiration for the character of Anthony Blanche in *Brideshead Revisited*. Villa la Pietra, just outside Florence where he lived, was Princess Margaret's other favourite place to stay in Italy. I used to go and stay at this exquisitely beautiful villa with her. 'Come on, Anne,' Princess Margaret would say to me, 'we've got to be well behaved here,' and she was. People used to be desperate for an invitation to lunch, they knew Harold loved good caviar, which cost a bomb, so they would phone up and say they had a present for him and could they pop in... there was quite a lot of that going on. But as we arrived he would always be standing on the steps to greet us: 'Ma'am welcome to my humble abode, which is at your disposal.' Princess Margaret used to give me a look and I'd get the giggles and she'd tell me off for laughing. The house really was magical, it was full of wonderful paintings, the sheets were all of the finest linen and he had just the right amount of divine soap and bath essence in the bathrooms, which he had specially made. Harold was a wonderful conversationalist, you really had to be on form when you saw him, but I felt honoured to have known him and of course delighted to have him in the book.

A Picnic at the Ming Tombs
Harold Acton

The Tuscan countryside has been amenable to picnics since the fifteenth century, when Lorenzo the Magnificent invited his cronies to rustic repasts in the bosky Mugello and in cool Camaldoli. Cured ham and pungent cheese stimulated a thirst for the vintages celebrated in Francesco Redi's dithyrambic *Bacchus in Tuscany*, which in turn stimulated a flow of rhyme and melody. Lorenzo's best poems are redolent of picnics.

The more refined cakes and sandwiches of my childhood were consumed with appetites sharpened by climbs up Vincigliata or Monte Morello, and by games of hide-and-seek and blind man's buff, but I remember the delicious cakes better than the company. We lounged on the grass as in Manet's *Déjeuner sur l'herbe*, though none of the girls reclined naked in our midst, for we were strictly supervised by a governess. Since nothing more sensational occurred than a bleeding nose or a bruised knee, my memory of those bygone picnics is hazy.

The neighbourhood of Beijing where I spent seven happy years, was even more amenable to picnics. A novel called *Peking Picnic* was popular at the period, but I forget if the title was justified by the contents. Picnics, however, were traditional in ancient China, whose greatest poets considered wine essential to the enjoyment of nature. Many a Chinese scroll depicts parties of poetical tipplers in a secluded spot among mountains and bamboo groves.

The Western Hills near Beijing were often chosen for al fresco meals, but after the Japanese invasion it was deemed foolhardy to venture far from the city, since roving bandits and marauding soldiery infested the countryside. The Ming Tombs, for instance, twenty miles north-west of Beijing, were officially out of bounds.

A spirited American lady, whom I shall call 'Mrs Schooner', was determined to take the risk before returning to Massachusetts, and she invited me to join her for a picnic at the Tombs, perhaps because she could find no other escort. She told me she had hired a motor car with some difficulty by paying the driver through the nose. 'He's a cutie but he's kinda yaller. He was even scared of taking me to the Summer Palace.'

Unwilling to appear pusillanimous, I agreed to accompany her to the Valley of Thirteen Tombs. She knew no Chinese, whereas I was fairly fluent in the language. Though she was double my age she had twice my energy: her enthusiasm for everything she saw was infectious. The hired car was filled with a rich variety of edibles from the Hôtel de Pékin where she was staying. She told me she was bringing foie gras as well as smoked eel and half a dozen bottles of Pouilly. 'I won't let you starve, dear. You are a good sport to keep me company. All the others I invited made some lame excuse, the darned cissies!'

Mrs Schooner whooped with laughter as we set off from the hotel. 'Wouldn't it be fun if we were kidnapped by bandits?' she said gaily. She was dressed and made up as for a morning's shopping in Bond Street – an invitation to rapine, I thought, in spite of her certain age. The road was so bumpy that she clung to me when we swerved past a file of camels. By fits and starts she related her life history. 'At high school I was a champion wrestler and I've had four husbands to wrestle with. None of them gave me the love a girl expects: they were more interested in my dollars. I had a hunch that I'd find my fifth in China, that's why I'm here. So far nothin' doin'... '

She talked so much that I was distracted from the scenery – a sweeping bare plain dotted with burial mounds and an occasional stele. The October weather was serene, the sky like Venetian glass.

After an hour my hostess said, 'I'm getting thirsty, dear, what about you? Let's stop the car for a nip of dry martini. It's in the big thermos flask.' So the driver stopped near a file of donkeys, loaded with panniers and bundled blue figures on top of them. Nothing if not democratic, she filled a glass for the driver, but he said '*Pu kan*' ('I dare not'), so she offered him some chewing gum and swallowed his portion herself.

Apart from the donkeys the road was deserted. 'How far have we still to go? For twenty miles it seems more like a hundred. I'm glad I brought plenty of nourishment.'

I heartily agreed, for her incessant monologue had become wearisome. The car jogged along almost as slowly as the donkeys and by the time we approached a white marble *p'ai-lou*, or cere-monial gateway, Mrs Schooner announced, 'I'm famished. Let's hop out and eat!' As a magnificent pavilion was visible yonder, I proposed that we should stop there. It contained a huge stone tortoise supporting a memorial tablet. Its massive coral-red walls and yellow-tiled double roof against a background of rippling lapis lazuli hills were as impressive as any in the Forbidden City.

'Okay,' said Mrs Schooner. We spread a rug on a patch of coarse grass and unpacked the baskets of victuals with enough glasses and cutlery for at least half a dozen people. 'The situation is pretty but it sure is lonesome,' Mrs Schooner remarked, peering through her binoculars.

'Well, what did you expect? This is where the Ming emperors of the last truly Chinese dynasty were buried with their wives and concubines.'

'It doesn't look like a cemetery to me. Have we come to the right place?'

Certainly the Valley of Thirteen Tombs had nothing akin to the cluttered cemeteries of Europe and America. It was all too grandiose: its monumental buildings were still brightly coloured though decayed, and the landscape was on too vast a scale. No soul was in sight. One was reminded of the Egyptian pyramids and of Shelley's 'Ozymandias': 'Look on my works, ye Mighty, and despair!'

'I guess I'd have liked to be an imperial concubine,' Mrs Schooner mused aloud. 'They must have had loads of fun without responsibilities.'

'I doubt it, for they had jealous wives to contend with. Many were poisoned or drowned in wells.'

'Don't talk of poison, this pâté's yummy. A pity we can't make toast here. Just spread it on a cracker.'

While I was drawing the cork from a bottle of wine, three ragged men with guns appeared suddenly from nowhere. 'Bandits,' said our terrified driver and scampered off. The men sauntered up and stared at us while we were eating. They stared as if they had never seen 'foreign devils' before. Robust, with high cheekbones and ruddy complexions, they were typical northerners of peasant stock. 'I guess the boys are hungry,' Mrs Schooner remarked. 'Hi there!' she called, offering them some of our chicken and ham and buttered rolls. 'Ask them to sit down and introduce themselves.'

When I spoke to them their faces lit up with broad grins. They sat cross-legged beside us with their battered guns, and once they had sampled our fare they ate like ravenous tigers. Our knives and forks perplexed them; accustomed to chopsticks, they preferred to eat with their fingers. They dangled the layers of fat on the ham above their open mouths and swallowed with a noise of trickling water.

Though they were not very communicative, I gathered that they were disbanded soldiers, irregulars who had been fighting the Japanese, whom they ironically referred to as 'dwarf bandits'. Now they intended to make their way home to villages in the north. Concerning ourselves they were inquisitive. 'How old are you? Are you husband and wife? Where do you come from and what is your honourable country?' – the usual questions. Our wine had less appeal for them than the cocktails, but they soon polished off the food. Not a scrap was left for our driver. 'Serve him darn well right for leaving us in the lurch!' was Mrs Schooner's comment.

'*Tsamen tou shih p'êng-yu*' ('We're all friends'), the men repeated, and they belched appreciatively. One of them, flushed with dry martinis, fired his gun into the air to demonstrate his gratitude.

'Supposing they all start shooting? I guess they're trigger-happy.' Mrs Schooner betrayed slight alarm through her tough veneer. 'Now we've seen a few live bandits, why bother to see the Tombs?'

The men thanked us with formal courtesy, bowing and shaking their own hands. I distributed a few coins for their journey money and we wished each other *I lu p'ing-an*, a safe and peaceful return. Our driver slunk back rather crestfallen as soon as they were out of sight. 'You were in luck. They could have shot you,' he said. 'And I could have shot them,' said Mrs Schooner, producing a pocket pistol from her leather bag.

Having come so far with that definite intention, I was anxious not to miss the Triumphal Way leading to the Tombs, but Mrs Schooner had had enough. 'I'm disappointed in the bandits,' she declared. Already she was bored and grumpy. Her subconscious had yearned for a shindy, a little bloodshed. I left her with the driver to finish the wine and relax while I wandered towards the avenue of statues in the distance. Very strange they looked, standing in couples on that desolate plain. Sculptured lions, horses, camels, griffins, unicorns, elephants, civil and military officials over life-size carved from single blocks of stone, the elephants thirteen-feet high and fourteen-feet long, formed a perpetual guard of honour for the funeral procession of dead emperors.

'You really ought to see the statues,' I urged Mrs Schooner. 'They are quite extraordinary if not unique. Do let me take you there.'

'Nuts to statues. I've a cocktail engagement at the embassy and my thermos flask is empty.'

The actual Tombs were ahead of us and I was sorry not to visit that of Yung Lo, the founder of modern Beijing. But Mrs Schooner was stubbornly deaf to persuasion. On the way back she was silent and comatose, to my intense relief. Perhaps I was not the right companion for such a picnic. Later I heard that she had spread a romantic report of our carousal with wild bandits armed to the teeth. The remaining bottles of Pouilly were sent to my house with a note of farewell on pink writing paper with a silver monogram: 'When you come to Magnolia, I'll give you a proper picnic. Wombs not tombs, and barbecues on the beach. *Aloha*, as they say in Hawaii, Sincerely, Arabella Schooner.'

Dorothy Lygon

The character of Cordelia Flyte in *Brideshead Revisited* was said to have been inspired by Dorothy Lygon. She had been brought up at Maddresfield Court in Worcestershire and was known as one of the 'bright young things' of the 1930s. Evelyn Waugh was a friend and regular visitor to the house who knew Dorothy as 'Poll'. Dorothy ended up briefly marrying the somewhat uncoventional Robert Heber-Percy who had been the lover of the composer Lord Berners. Berners was very eccentric and lived in a house near Susanna, I remember he had lots of doves and dyed them all different colours. Not surprisingly the marriage didn't last very long and they split up after about a year. Heber-Percy had a housekeeper who was in love with him and she saw Dorothy off pretty smartly.

Picnics from the Past
Dorothy Lygon

Picnics played a definite part in our lives when we were young. They fell into two categories – nursery outings, which were ordinary nursery teas taken to the garden, the woods or the beach, or family picnics, which were rarer and more elaborate, often including some of the household. I remember one of the latter sort on a steamer on the River Severn and another by the weir on the Teme. A third was on the Goodwin Sands, off the Kent coast, large areas of which are uncovered during the extreme tides of spring and autumn. The remains of a German submarine wrecked there during the 1914–1918 war were still visible in the 1920s; the sand was quite firm to walk on as long as there was no water on it, otherwise it shifted round one's feet and started to engulf them in a way that was both frightening and exciting.

The food on these grown-up picnics was always the same, but they didn't happen often enough for us to get bored with it. There were bridge rolls filled with Russian salad, small mutton pies known as Buckingham Palace pies, jam puffs and coffee and chocolate éclairs. The mutton pies were particularly good. There was no need for knives, forks or spoons and I can't remember any being provided. I think we drank lemonade; the men would have had beer or whisky or cider – certainly not wine, nor do I remember ice. For a later recipe the following is one which has evolved over the last year or two; it can be used for sandwiches (made with brown bread well buttered), or put in small ramekins or cartons to eat on its own.

Dorothy's Russian Salad

Allow 1½ eggs per person if the eggs are large, or 2 if small. Hard-boil them and, after peeling, chop roughly and tip them into a roomy bowl. Add salt, pepper, a good sprinkle of Worcestershire sauce and enough single cream to moisten the mixture. Next add herbs, some kind of onion (either chives cut with scissors or spring onions or minced shallots), then parsley and/or whatever you have available – dill, chervil, tarragon and fennel are all good. Sometimes I have added chopped shrimps or prawns quite successfully. It can be made in advance and kept under cling film or foil in the refrigerator. I have not tried freezing it, but have found it a good flexible basic recipe.

Buckingham Palace Pies

> short pastry
> 1 ½ lb cooked mutton, beef, chicken or rabbit
> 2 shallots, finely chopped
> butter
> stock
> rich brown gravy
> salt, pepper and Worcestershire sauce
> beef jelly

Preheat the oven to gas mark 7 (425°F, 220°C). Make a number of tartlet cases with the short pastry. Cut out two circles, one smaller than the other, for the tops of the tartlets. Fit the larger circles into a greased mince pie tin, which usually makes 12 cases. Cut a hole in the smaller of the circles. Bake blind until lightly browned.

Cut slices of cooked meat into small squares, rejecting any fat or sinew. Cook two finely chopped shallots in butter and mix with the meat in a pan with enough stock to cover it. It should then be cooked slowly for about an hour until the meat is extremely tender. Remove the meat, cover with a good rich brown gravy seasoned with salt, pepper and a dash of Worcestershire sauce, and fill the cases with this mixture. Put a little meat jelly on the top, cover with the pastry circles, one on top of the other, and fill the hole with beef jelly.

Mamie's Comfort

Fill a large thermos with hot Bovril mixed to required strength and lace generously with port and brandy. A very useful hot drink for a cold picnic.

Clementine Beit

Being tied up and robbed by the IRA is happily not an everyday occurrence but it was something that happened to Clementine Beit. She was a cousin of the famous Mitford sisters and was married to Sir Alfred Beit who had inherited an incredible art collection including works by Goya, Velasquez and Gainsborough. They bought a Palladian house just outside Dublin called Russborough, partly to house all their marvellous paintings. Of course, people knew about it, and one day an IRA gang led by the heiress Rose Dugdale broke into the house when they were all at home. Everyone was tied up and nineteen paintings were stolen. Eventually the police turned up and freed Alfred. Two hours later, as he was telling them which paintings had been taken, they asked him if Lady Beit had been at home. 'Oh god, yes she was!' he said. He'd totally forgotten about her! Eventually they found her in the cellar bound and gagged. I think she'd been mouthy and annoyed them, which is why they'd dumped her in there.

We knew the Beits through parties and the social scene in London and I became one of a group of ladies Alfred used to take out to events and play tennis with. It was after I was married, but Colin was often in Mustique and Clementine was thrilled to have a break, so was delighted when we used to go off with Alfred for an afternoon. Despite being enormously rich he was very careful with his money. If we went to Wimbledon we used to have to cut the order of play out of the newspaper so he didn't have to buy a programme, and bring our own cushions so he didn't have to hire them. We were allowed strawberries, or ice cream or coffee but not all three.

They didn't have any children and Clementine adored her dog so it was totally fitting that she wrote about a dog picnic for us.

Glory's Picnic
Clementine Beit

Our Ridgeback dog, Glory, loved picnics. He always seemed to know when one was being planned and would get into the car when he saw that it was about to be loaded up; everything was then packed around him and we would set off. On arrival at the picnic spot, he would sit and watch the baskets being unpacked, drooling with anticipation. We always took his dinner with us, and when he had wolfed it down he would do the rounds, pleading with everyone that he was still starving. There were never any scraps left to tidy away before leaving if Glory had been on a picnic!

Glory's Picnic Pudding

Spread 3 or 4 slices of bread – preferably brown – with dripping or butter, including the brown jelly from your dripping bowl if possible. Chop up some scraps and leftovers, mince (raw or cooked), and a little chopped or grated cheese (if liked by dog). Chicken skin was much liked. Cut the slices of bread into fairly small squares. Put alternative layers of bread and scraps into the dog's bowl, moisten with warm gravy or Oxo and mix up lightly with a fork – the mixture should not be too soggy. Cover the bowl with foil.

In Africa we always took water for Glory.

Jasper Guinness

Jasper's party trick was to go into an Italian bar and drink the entire top shelf! He did like a drink, and picnics could never be too far from the house as inevitably many of the guests would end up unable to stand and having to crawl back. He was also a Mitford – his grandmother was Diana Mitford, and his mother, Ingrid was one of my closest friends. I adored Jasper, who tragically died at the age of 57. He lived in Italy with his wife Camilla with whom he bought and did up a glorious Tuscan villa, Arniano. Camilla is an interior designer and we used to talk about Indian fabrics as Colin and I always dressed in Indian clothes that we'd brought back from our trips there. I urged her to go to India to buy materials, which she did. In the process of creating the beautiful garden at Arniano, Jasper discovered a real love of plants and became a botanist, teaching himself landscape garden design. He went on to design other gardens for the great and the good in Tuscany. His sense of fun shines through in his Whoopee picnic.

Whoopee Picnic
Jasper Guinness

Nothing I like more than a picnic. Easily planned, but when the day dawns, I find, one does not always feel exactly one's best. But it's 'yoydleoy' and down to the market we go. First stop: the butcher. I've always been fond of spare ribs, unlike the Italians. They don't set much store by them and, as a result, they damn near give them away. The key word is '*rosticciana*'. Then off to the greengrocer for potatoes, lettuce, tomatoes, lemons and, most important, a huge watermelon (*cocomero*).

Now, as Sherlock's friend asked him, 'Where do we buy the ingredients for the sauce?' '*Alimentari*, my dear Watson.' Sherlock's shop has the advantage of selling not only honey, oil, bread, tomato ketchup, butter and cheese, all of which are to be snapped up on the spot, but also rum, vodka and Cointreau, which are vital for the good of the watermelon.

Home immediately. Time to get someone else to make the salad, the dressing, to wrap the potatoes in foil, and to make the sweet and sour sauce. Time for me to make the Bomba and collect some wood. Time for everyone to have a Camp. Sod. Good Lord. Here they come. Where's the wheelbarrow? Pile it all in, escort them to wherever we're going, light the fire, settle them down, give them a drink and have a lovely time.

Spare ribs: on the grill.

Sweet and sour sauce: take tomato ketchup (Heinz is best), squeezed lemons, honey, rosemary, and anything else in the cupboard.

Potatoes: wrap in silver foil and bung on the fire.

Salad and dressing: search me.

Bomba

Slice the very top off a big watermelon. Take out the inside with a spoon and your hands. Squidge the insides through a colander into a pot. For a big melon put one bottle of rum, one of vodka and a little Cointreau into the empty shell of the fruit. Add as much of the juice as will fit in, leaving room for ice. Vary strength as seen fit.

James Lees-Milne

James Lees-Milne came to Holkham once or twice and I was thrilled when one of his diaries was published in which he comments rather nicely on how I looked. He was a friend of Diana Mitford and said to have been a lover of her brother Tom. He was a very well-known architectural historian and expert on country houses. He married Alvide, Viscountess Chaplin, who was a landscape gardener and whilst he is said to have had an affair with Harold Nicholson in the 1930s, she apparently had one with Harold's wife, Vita Sackville-West. James was not a man for typical country estate pursuits, but he and his wife lived in the mid 1970s at Essex House on the Badminton Estate of Master, the Duke of Beaufort who, when Lees-Milne's dog escaped and messed up the hunt, is said to have declared, 'What's the point of the Lees-Milnes? They don't hunt. They don't shoot. What use are they?'

I Loathe Picnics
James Lees-Milne

I loathe picnics.

It may be hereditary. My parents also loathed them as much as they disliked each other, and certainly as much as they disliked us. By some inexplicable mischance it became an established family custom that on the birthday of my sister, my brother and myself, the five of us went in a hired punt and one canoe on the River Avon for a picnic. To make matters worse, we three children were all born in August. So too was my mother, but I think that only one year did we go on four of these ghastly expeditions in this ill-fated month.

We embarked at Evesham and sailed (if that is the right word) in deadly silence either up or downstream. If we started downstream there was the impending horror of having to battle against the current on the way back. If we started upstream there was the weir, which meant dragging or carrying the boats several yards overland and the certainty of one of us losing his or her temper. Now the extraordinary thing was that in those distant days when summers were summers and the sun shone from morn till eve, it always rained on our birthdays, not intermittently, but consistently, heavily and often catastrophically. Of course we knew beforehand that this would be the case. Nonetheless we went because our parents supposed that we children enjoyed the outings, and that they must dutifully subordinate their strong disinclination to our pleasure. It was only when we were grown up that we dared admit how much we had disliked these expeditions. Our parents groaned. 'If only,' my mother said, 'you had told us so when the eldest of you was five.'

In retrospect these countless picnics merge into one because almost invariably they followed the same pattern and the same proceedings repeated themselves. First there was the unloading of basket, rugs, cushions, sunshades, umbrellas, waterproofs and dogs from car to punt and canoe. Next, the embarrassing scene of my father bargaining with the boatman about the charge, which, if I remember rightly, was thirty shillings for the first three hours and five shillings for each subsequent quarter of an hour. This calculation enraged my father who refused to understand why, were we to spend four hours on the river, the last should cost him a whole pound.

'But you might not come back,' the saucy boatman once dared to remonstrate.

'Do you suppose,' my father replied, drawing himself up to his full six foot two and half inches, 'that I would want to go off with your beastly canoe, leaving you with my new Minerva four-seater? Think again, my good man. Besides, don't you know who I am?' Who was he, anyway?

If we started upstream my mother, who insisted upon having the canoe to herself and the dogs, in spite of my father's warnings, invariably got caught in a whirlpool. She would go round and round and round, desperately paddling in one direction, for she could not reverse, until the bull terrier and the Pekineses, made giddy by these gyrations, would jump overboard. This meant that my mother (whose raffia hat had already been knocked off by an overhanging branch) capsized before her madly rotating canoe reached the bank. My father, cursing and swearing 'I told you so', would stretch out the punt pole, exhorting her to grasp it while he towed her ashore. His propulsion of the punt, with the struggling body of his wife at the end of it, was an exceedingly awkward operation for him and an uncomfortable experience for her. At least her immersion settled the vexed question of where to have the picnic. If she hadn't fallen in we would have spent ages looking for the right landing place, the right amount of shade (should a ray of sun come out), and the right amount of protection from the inevitable thunderstorm. As it happened, we were obliged to picnic on the sewage farm, next to the gasometer and just beyond the railway siding.

Before we unloaded the picnic basket and other paraphernalia my mother was obliged to strip to the skin, clean off the stinking mud with tufts of rushes and then be wrapped, shivering, with those rugs on which, had the accident not occurred, we would have sat. Thus she squatted like some Egyptian mummy under an igloo of umbrellas. By now my father was in a filthy temper. He, who was by nature a very practical man, refused to do anything but read the *Morning Post* (always a bad sign) which he was obliged to do standing up. He left us children to unpack the basket and spread the paper plates and food on the soggy ground (every rug and mackintosh enveloping my mother). The smell of sewage, gas and my mother was very unappetising.

Reclining on one elbow with nothing to lean against, even when not eating and drinking with the free hand, has always been torture to me. Besides, the sewage farm did not provide grass, but cinders, if I remember correctly, over which there passed at regular intervals a long, revolving arm which sprayed disinfectant. Memory tells me too that there was seldom enough to eat on our picnics. It never occurred to my mother to tell the cook what food we needed. It was left to the cook to supply chunks of bread and dripping (which children in those days were supposed to like), fids of salty gammon, a few unripe plums and, of course, the birthday cake. On this occasion the bull terrier had sat on the cake, which thereby became a total washout. There would be cider (a great treat) to drink, but not the delicious sweet sort out of a bottle, rather our own home-brewed, bitter sort, unclear and cloudy like some unwholesome liquid from a specimen bottle. There were never enough mugs, and we had to share. I have always had a horror of sharing mugs and would show my disgust. This enraged my father who thought it pathetic. 'Effeminate' was the word he used. Besides, the cider, heady stuff, attracted all the wasps in the Vale of Evesham, as well as little black flies which could not be extracted and had to be swallowed.

After this disgusting and inadequate meal we children had to pack up. We could not take home the remains and my mother – quite rightly – had a horror of litter. We were not allowed to throw the paper in the river, not even the plum stones in case a fish might swallow one and choke. We had to dig a hole with our fingers. Then we had to count the knives, forks and spoons. There was always one missing. From behind the *Morning Post* my father would growl, 'We are not leaving until you have found it.' When it was found my father would put down the paper and yawn. My mother's teeth would chatter. My father would remember an appointment with a man about a horse. He had to get home at once.

We would re-embark. There would be a row among the children about which of us was going to have the canoe because 'shooting the rapids' was the only enjoyable part of the expedition. I, being the most selfish and determined, usually won. Wet, cold, cross and under-nourished, we returned to the boathouse. Looking at his watch, my father would rejoice that we had been on the river for exactly two hours and fifty-five minutes.

How I loathe picnics.

George Christie

A contributor with a similar attitude to picnics as James Lees-Milne was George Christie. I absolutely loved George and his wife Mary, they were great friends. I knew them because George's father John Christie had taught my father at Eton before going on to marry Audrey Mildmay and founding Glyndebourne Opera for her. I used to go and stay with George and Mary at Glyndebourne, first of all in the house and then when their son Gus took over I stayed in a lovely little cottage quite near them. It was all such a pleasure! I've always loved the opera since my grandfather, who was very musical, introduced me to it. I used to dance along to whatever he was playing and frequently went with my father to the operettas, which he adored.

I asked George to write about a picnic because of course Glyndebourne is renowned for the picnics everyone takes to eat in the grounds before the opera, and he agreed. I went to take a photograph of him with my little box brownie and suggested it might be rather fun to take one of him in the ha-ha with the cows behind and picnickers off to the left. Of course he plunged straight into the ha-ha wearing his dinner jacket and I took what

I thought was a rather good photograph! I had imagined he would write about how amazing picnics are at Glyndebourne but, in fact, he writes about how he doesn't like picnics at all and can't understand why people who come to the opera prefer sitting on a rug, which is really very uncomfortable, rather than going into the dining room, which then was quite small but where they could get a very good dinner in comfort.

It's wonderful that George's son Gus Christie has also given us a picnic for this book. Gus inherited Glyndebourne and is married to the brilliant opera singer Danielle de Niese. His picnic gives us a sense of how Glyndebourne has evolved since George's time, and how the passion for picnicking among the audience is undimmed as the provisions and space for it in the gardens have improved.

Glyndebourne: A Critical View of the Picnic
George Christie

Picnics are difficult to stomach. I for one don't have much appetite for them. The human body, it seems to me, is not a suitable shape for eating in comfort at ground level. Eating in this fashion ought to be anti-digestive; so it should follow that the second half of performance at Glyndebourne gets a dyspeptic reception. Less than fifty per cent of the audience can be fed in the restaurant – so something over thirty thousand people picnic in the Glyndebourne gardens each year – a disturbing volume of dyspepsia in my book.

However, the British music critic confounds this theory. He is convinced that the Glyndebourne audience is recklessly receptive to the second part of a performance, having suffered or tolerated the first. Is the Glyndebourne audience a glutton for punishment, as I suspect? Or is the Glyndebourne audience simply a glutton, as the British music critic would like us to believe? Or does the British music critic himself tend to picnic at Glyndebourne and so prove the theory that cynicism is born of dyspepsia? Thirty thousand eating their way through their picnics in the relentless rain of the 1980 summer must surely have tested the audience's resilience. But their frailty remains to be proved. The box office for 1981 was as snowed under as ever. Perhaps the audience comes for the performance rather than the picnic...

In 1976 a device was introduced to make picnics more palatable at Glyndebourne. A large marquee was put up in the grounds, a result of the munificence of W.D. and H.O. Wills. At a ceremony held to celebrate the opening of this marquee, I made a few fatuous remarks about hoping for a wet summer. It turned out to be the hottest, driest summer in recorded history, and the marquee was a wasted asset. Everybody was praying for the rains. The next three summers answered their prayers and swamped the place – so we had to extend the marquee (and, I hope, the receptivity of the audience as well as that of the British music critic).

The picnic ritual at Glyndebourne is relentlessly publicised. Many of the foreign critics devote the first part of their 'appreciation' to a description of the resemblance of the Friesian cattle on one side of the ha-ha to the audience grazing on the other. They invariably devote the next part of their 'appreciation' to a nostalgic, rather than pertinent, walk down Glyndebourne's memory lane; as a token to their profession as critics, they throw in at the end a line or two about the performance which straddles either side of the picnic.

One of the little foibles of Glyndebourne's picnickers is to tie bits of string round the neck of their bottles and moor them to the banks of the ponds to keep the wine cool. One audience member fell in while dragging his bottle out. A resourceful usher showed the luckless man to the wardrobe department, who helped him out with a smart costume from the Bal Blanc scene from the final act of *Eugene Onegin*. The man enjoyed his Blanc de Blanc and turned out to be a critic from California. The enthusiasm of his article was effusive. The temptation to encourage critics to moor their bottles is a strong one, but I suppose it must be resisted!

Gus Christie

My Dad's description of the Glyndebourne picnics is a hard act to follow but I'm delighted to report that our audiences are still as passionate, if not more, about having a picnic in the long interval – thank god, the English are creatures of habit and will often return to their same favoured spot and, I imagine, with the same picnic food each year. When the new theatre was built thirty years ago, there was not much provision for undercover picnickers on wet nights and the foyers around the theatre were crammed with tables and rugs on the brick walkways and it resembled a very glamorous refugee camp. We have now sprouted marquees and stretch tents, so that people can spill out into the gardens on the wet and windy nights as well.

The garden continues to evolve and we have pushed the fence out into the field and created some beautiful new picnicking areas amongst meadows teeming with orchids. One of mine and many people's favourite spots is under the dappled shade of the walnut trees near my mum's abundant rose garden.

You rarely see people spread out on rugs these days and I agree with my dad about the discomfort of ground-level picnicking but nothing beats sitting out on a summer's evening surrounded by others enjoying themselves and our blessed setting.

The local wildlife can be problematic, the canny jackdaws in particular, who now know that the bells summoning the audiences back into the theatre at the end of the interval signals that in about ten minutes the lawns will be clear and it will time to move in for the leftovers. So now we have sporadic crop-scarer bangs and are even imitating the jackdaw alarm calls to keep them at bay, and allow audiences to return, on the balmier nights, for a last drink at dusk.

Josceline Dimbleby

I was so delighted when Josceline said she would write about a picnic for us. She is a wonderful cook, married then to David Dimbleby. I had met her former father-in-law Richard Dimbleby because he was so much a part of the Coronation. He was the pre-eminent voice of the BBC and was doing the commentary for the television broadcast. He either owned or had rented a houseboat which he brought up to be as near to Westminster Abbey as possible and was great fun at the rehearsal. He had a very high vantage point as the abbey was built up on either side of the aisle with rows of seating almost up to the rafters. He teased us maids of honour, saying he was going to be keeping an eye on us all from up there. I remember rather nervously saying to him, 'Well I hope we don't mess it up. I do hope it all goes according to plan!'

Josceline's Devonshire picnic is so evocative and her recipes are of course mouthwatering!

Devonshire Picnic
Josceline Dimbleby

Halfway up to Totnes on the River Dart there is a peninsula of majestic oak and beech trees; it has green sun–dappled banks and we know it as Picnic Point. Almost every day during the school holidays in Devon we picnic. We sail to coves along the coast, or we drive on to Dartmoor for long walks through forests, rewarded by a home-made pasty eaten on the mossy banks of a stream. On wild-weather days we row to the other side of the river by our house, to a disused quarry so sheltered from all winds by its cathedral–like walls that plants grow there of an exotic character quite unexpected in England. But Picnic Point is the most magical place of all. It has a natural fireplace on a promontory looking down into the deep green water, and although there are always signs of others having had a fire there shortly before, we have never, in all our years of Devon life, had to share Picnic Point with anyone.

The boat journey up the Dart is beautiful; most beautiful of all is the calm of early evening in the last yellow sunlight when we often sail up for a picnic supper. One evening we cooked a huge rib of beef – smoky, tender and rare – which we ate by the light of the fire while the children, inspired by the dark woods all round and the river noises, told ghost stories.

Our picnic cooking has been simplified by a large two–sided grill into which the food is clamped and turned over all at once – none of that endless forking of sausages while the smoke chokes and blinds you. We simply put stones on either side of the fire, balance the grill over it, and sit back sipping scrumpy and savouring the smell of the cooking. My children normally profess to dislike sausages, but good butchers' sausages cooked in the smoke of a driftwood fire and stuffed into a fresh bun roll with some mustard and crisp lettuce are always welcome. The other success on the grill is marinaded meat and chicken – the aroma of Indian spices wafting into the English country air has a nice incongruity, and a bold flavour is just what keen outdoor appetites need.

Sometimes when we have set out late we eat on the boat. Tastes are more exciting in the open air, so hot food seems extra special. I often stuff a mixture of grated cheese, onion and herbs, bound with whisked egg, into buttered baps; cook them, wrapped in foil, in a fairly high oven for 15–20 minutes before we leave the house; and wrap the foil up in layers of newspaper. They keep hot for hours, even in the chill of a sea breeze.

Our Devon picnics are an everyday affair. The food is appreciated as much as any I prepare, but the crowded summer days give one no time for elaborate preparation. The special-occasion picnic which I have time to think about, gives me the creative challenge I enjoy best. For Glyndebourne, I once made a game pie decorated musically and inscribed with the words of the opera we were there for, *Così Fan Tutte*. When my children were small we used sometimes to take a large group of their friends for a birthday picnic tea and games in Richmond Park. It gave me great satisfaction to produce an array of brightly coloured cakes, jellies and biscuits set out on the grass on a large white sheet.

Then there are picnics abroad: often uncomfortable, hot, prickly, often not in the perfect spot, but more of a pleasure to shop for. In the East I have had wonderful picnics, prepared in grand, old-fashioned style. I remember one lunch sitting in basket chairs high up above the Ganges at Chunar in central India, eating delicate samosas, spicy meatballs and marinaded chicken out of a basket lined with starched white linen, as we watched and heard a panorama of life on the great river below us.

Having been brought up with all manner of picnics a major part of my life, our nautical Devon feasts have now become most familiar to me, and as a spot which has everything, even its own vegetable crop, the succulent samphire, growing on the mud at low tide, Picnic Point on the River Dart for us reigns supreme.

Grilled Spiced Chicken

(for 6-8)

I find this the most popular picnic food of all. All you have to do is remember to spare a few minutes the night before to prepare the delicious marinade, and in the morning the chicken pieces, tender and aromatic with Indian spices, will be ready to take on your picnic. They will cook well either over charcoal or on a simple grill over a wood fire. If you must, you can cook them in advance on your grill at home – in any case they are excellent cold. You can use any joints of chicken but I find inexpensive chicken wings very successful. Of course, you can vary the spices according to what you have.

1½–2 lb (700–900 g) small chicken joints

For the Marinade

> 1 onion, sliced roughly
> 1-inch (2.5 cm) piece of fresh ginger, peeled and
>   chopped roughly
> 6–8 cloves garlic, peeled
> 3 teaspoons ground coriander
> 2 teaspoons ground cinnamon

2 teaspoons ground cardamom
½ teaspoon chilli powder or cayenne
3 tablespoons red wine vinegar
3 tablespoons sunflower oil
1 tablespoon tomato purée
1 rounded teaspoon salt

Simply put all the marinade ingredients into a liquidiser or food processor and whizz to a smooth paste. Pour the marinade over the chicken joints, stir to coat thoroughly, and leave in a covered bowl in the refrigerator or a cool place overnight.

Grill over a high heat on both sides until almost blackened.

Beef and Onion Flatbreads

(for 5-6)

These are rather like a wholemeal pancake incorporating minced beef and onion. You can wrap them up in foil while they are hot and then in thick newspaper to keep them warm until you reach your picnic place. Alternatively you can eat them cold. Either way, take with you a box of cut lettuce, tomato and fresh mint leaves and wrap the flatbreads round a stuffing of this mixture. They are delicious and nutritious, and children love them too.

1 large onion
4 oz (110 g) minced beef
½–1 teaspoon chilli powder
12 oz (350 g) wholemeal or 85% wholewheat flour
sunflower oil for frying
salt

Peel the onion and chop very finely. Mix with the minced beef in a large bowl. Season with chilli powder and a generous sprinkling of salt. Add the flour and mix in with your hands. Gradually stir in up to 4 pints (150 ml) water – enough to make the mixture stick together. Knead on a well-floured board for 3–4 minutes. Then take egg-sized handfuls of the dough and shape these into round balls. Sprinkle board and rolling pin with flour to prevent sticking, and roll out the dough as thinly as you can. Heat about ¼ inch (5 mm) oil in a large frying pan. Fry the breads one by one at a medium-to-high heat, turning once, until brown on each side. Drain on absorbent paper and pile on a serving dish in a very low oven to keep warm until you are ready to leave.

Arabella Boxer

Another famous cook who contributed a picnic is Arabella Boxer. She was great fun and we all loved being invited to dinner by her and her then husband, the magazine editor and cartoonist Mark Boxer, as you knew you were going to get a very, very good dinner. We all had her cookbooks, *First Slice Your Cookbook* was an absolute bible, we couldn't have a dinner party without using an Arabella Boxer recipe. Not that we were cooking them ourselves, as back then most of us had cooks. (Shamefully I cooked my first meal in my eighties when I found myself living on my own in Norfolk.) The air picnic she wrote for us was brilliant. The food on aeroplanes was always disgusting, and usually rather bad for you, so that years later when my best friend Margaret Vyner and I made our annual trip to India we used to take an Arabella Boxer Air Picnic with us. She was always rather strict about no alcohol, which we found rather harder to stick to, but we did limit ourselves to just one or two glasses of wine and always ended up arriving in fine fettle.

A Picnic for the Air
Arabella Boxer

In the early days of travel, passengers invariably took their food with them. Towards the end of her life, my Scottish grandmother admitted that she had never eaten a meal in public; perhaps she didn't eat when travelling, or perhaps she just didn't travel. For us, living as we did in the north of Scotland, overnight train trips were a part of life; travelling back and forth to school, visits to the dentist and optician – all involved lengthy journeys. One of the nicest things about them was sitting on the top bunk of a third-class sleeper – only our parents travelled first-class – unwrapping the greaseproof paper package of food that was meant to sustain one through the night. Torn between greed and potential travel sickness, I always ended up eating everything, but have felt unable to face the same foods since; sandwiches made with roast beef or chicken still make me feel slightly faint.

On the Trans-Siberian Express, travellers took their own uncooked food with them; the train had a special 'cold' carriage for storing semi-frozen food. Passengers would take with them a large bag of *pelmeni*, a sort of Russian ravioli, and at each station a large pot of water was kept boiling over a brazier, so that the *pelmeni* could be cooked while the train stopped. In England we were not so lucky, and all food had to be prepared in advance and packed.

Few people take packed meals on trains any more, although it would be sensible to do so. There is something slightly daunting about eating alone, surrounded by strangers who are not eating, and trips to the dining car – if there is such a thing – are fun, though expensive and gastronomically disappointing. If, however, one is travelling by air, there is a very strong case for taking one's own food, and one's own drink as well. In the early days of Laker flights this was essential, for food was not provided, and it seemed an eminently sensible economy. From the passenger's point of view, taking one's own food on any regular airline is not of course an economy, since meals are provided free, but rather a sensible form of insurance. This is especially true, paradoxically, when travelling first-class, for the food and drink that are then pressed on us are even less suited to our needs than the ordinary fare. In fact, I have recently discovered that most airlines will provide special vegetarian meals if they are ordered a day or two in advance. Being lower in protein, and more easily digested, they provide a reasonable alternative for occasions when preparing a 'home-cooked' meal is impractical.

When flying, our system is under strain from a number of different factors. The most obvious one is pressure: although the aircraft is pressurised, for technical reasons it cannot be brought down to the pressure that most of us are accustomed to – sea level. Instead, it is kept at the pressure found between six and seven thousand feet – within moments of entering the plane our bodies have to adjust to a significant change in environment. Pressurisation causes the gases in our system to dilate, creating an unpleasant feeling of distention. For this reason it is important not to drink fizzy liquids.

The second main reason for feeling less than well is the dehydration of the air in the cabin. This puts the kidneys under strain since it is their job to regulate the balance of water in the blood. When we are in danger of becoming dehydrated, the pituitary gland produces large amounts of anti-diuretic hormone, causing the kidneys to re-absorb into the bloodstream much of the water which would have been excreted. In order to offset this dehydration, it is vital to drink a great deal; for short journeys, roughly one pint for every hour spent in the air is advisable, while for long trips a quarter of a pint per hour is more realistic. Still mineral water or hot herb teas are ideal.

Alcohol should be avoided at all costs. First it exacerbates dehydration, and secondly it causes extra work for the liver, which is already operating under strain. The liver is responsible for breaking down and getting rid of poisons absorbed into the body, for example those contained in alcohol, caffeine and nicotine. When travelling, the liver is already under pressure and less able than usual to cope with these tasks, so that drinking alcohol and coffee and smoking should be avoided. The liver also controls the degree of acidity in the body, so that very acid foods such as citrus fruits should be kept to a minimum. Champagne is a good example of what to avoid, since it combines three of the worst things: alcohol, acidity and gas.

In addition to the strains caused by pressurisation, dehydration, altitude and speed other stresses are normally connected with travel: fatigue, anxiety and, in many cases, fear of flying itself. All these affect the nervous system, which in turn affects the digestion, therefore foods that put an undue strain on the digestive organs should be avoided. Rich foods, due to their high fat content, come into this category, as do foods that are high in protein. Meat, eggs and cheese should only be eaten in very small quantities, while indigestible foods like hard–boiled eggs and cold potatoes (i.e. potato salad) are also best left out. Highly spiced food like salami is also unsuitable, while garlic is clearly antisocial, to say the least.

A good general rule is to drink as much as possible, remembering to stick to still, non–alcoholic drinks, and to eat as little as possible. The food should be similar to that given to a convalescent: bland, light, easy to digest and appetising. It should be moderate in temperature, neither iced nor boiling hot. Creamy vegetable soups, so long as they are not too rich, salads, small

pieces of chicken or white fish, cooked vegetables (except potatoes), rice, fruit, yoghurt and low-fat cream cheese are all good.
Still mineral water should be carried in generous quantities; it is
no good relying on the stewardess to bring you water, for she
will be too busy, and the glasses are minute. Mineral water, especially a still one, is rarely among the drinks on offer. (A 'bottle'
bag for carrying a large bottle of mineral water can always be
used later to carry off duty-free drink bought on the plane.)
Teabags of herb tea are useful, since these are easily diluted with
hot water when the stewardess does the coffee.

Planning a picnic to take from home is relatively simple, but
finding a suitable meal to bring back, without a base to prepare
it, is another matter. Yet most other countries are better equipped
for this sort of thing than we are, and a brief visit to a delicatessen
just before leaving will usually provide mineral water, vegetable
juice (for a soup substitute), bread, butter, fruit, yoghurt and a
low-fat cheese such as fromage blanc or ricotta.

It is both sensible and fun to shop around to build up a small
picnic kit. A light basket with a lid, or a small cool bag, equipped
with plastic plate and beaker, two plastic containers with lids,
plus knife, fork and spoon, should cover every eventuality. Those
who abhor plastic can find old horn beakers, reminiscent of
shooting parties, in antique shops, while a wooden plate can
replace the plastic one, although it will be heavier. Once the
habit has become established, it takes little time to prepare a
couple of simple dishes before leaving, and the benefit in avoiding,
or at least decreasing, the after-effects of air travel will certainly
repay the extra effort.

Menus for Air Picnics

1. Creamy leek soup
   Potted shrimps
   Brown bread and butter sandwich
   Yoghurt
2. Cold cucumber soup with dill
   Breast of poached chicken wrapped in a lettuce leaf
   Watercress salad
   Crême caramel, baked in an *oeuf en cocotte* dish
3. Prawn and crisp lettuce salad
   Sandwich of brown bread and butter and cress, or
   watercress
   Petits Suisses
4. Beef tea
   Chicken salad
   Matzos or Ryvita
   Grated apple in yoghurt
5. Chicken broth (in thermos)
   Salad of cooked vegetables
   Plums, grapes or cherries
6. Flaked white fish in mayonnaise-type dressing
   Watercress salad
   Brown bread and butter
   Low-fat cream cheese
7. Creamy potato and chervil soup (cold)
   Spinach and mozzarella salad
   Apricots with yoghurt

To drink:
Volvic or other still mineral water
Peppermint, verbena or sage tea

Margaret Vyner

Margaret Vyner is my best friend, I've known her all my life. She was a model who may have walked for the shows but was mainly a photographic model and an artist. I can hardly remember how we met but it was probably at one of the endless weekend parties or dinners we used to go to at that time. Margaret and her husband Henry had a lovely house in Yorkshire, Fountains Hall, near Fountain's Abbey, but we also used to live near them in London. She's my travelling companion, it can be quite hard travelling with people but it was wonderful that we both found someone we could travel with. We want to do the same things and always share a room in hotels; we are very polite around each other, trying not to bang about or turn the light on suddenly in the middle of the night. We've been to India twenty-six times together, travelling all over the country, always chatting away, together with our friend Mitch Crites, the three of us have enjoyed endless picnics together in India.

Dominican Picnic
Margaret Vyner

Dominica, lying between Martinique and Guadeloupe, unloved by many tourists for its black beaches and incessant rain, brought back childhood memories of my grandfather's Victorian conservatory with the smell of damp and warmth and faintly rotting vegetation. The hotel where we stayed was deep in the hilly rain forest. When we arrived it was nearly empty but we were intrigued to find on a noticeboard a mysterious small card advertising 'DOMINICA SAFARIS', which promised a drive round the island followed by a picnic beside a river where we could swim; so, not knowing what to expect, we booked in.

On the appointed morning a brand-new sand-coloured Range Rover appeared, driven by a handsome, bearded West Indian in a matching sand-coloured safari suit and an Ernest Hemingway hat; as we set off we felt that had it been cold he would have tucked a rug round our knees.

The drive itself was breathtaking: in spite of the word safari, we saw nothing but vegetation of such enormity and density that at any moment a Douanier Rousseau tiger might have appeared. We arrived eventually on the site of our picnic: huge rocks, huge ferns and a fast-flowing icy-cold clear river and not a soul in sight. Our driver said that while we swam he would lay out the picnic. When we emerged, starving and half expecting sandwiches and bananas, we were astonished by what we saw. Spread out on a white damask cloth straight from an Edwardian shooting party was the most ravishing and delicious feast imaginable.

First of all, we were given ice-cold rum punches in crystal glasses, and while we sat on the rocks drinking them we gazed greedily at what was to come: stuffed crabs, exotic chicken, avocado mousse, sweet potato bread and mango ice cream. Euphoric after our rum punches (particularly delicious as the Dominican rum and limes are famously good) we set to, and it all tasted as wonderful as it looked, especially as the driver produced a bottle of Clos des Mouches tasting of primroses. Like all good picnics, it seemed to go on for hours, and the experience of enjoying wonderful food and drink in a jungle setting – ferns, plantains, the warm damp air and the only sound (apart from sighs of gluttonous pleasure) that of the running river – was unforgettable.

Two years later we came back to Dominica longing to repeat the experience, but we looked in vain for the card at the hotel, asked in vain about Dominica Safaris, and were met with blank faces – it seemed not so much to have vanished without trace as never to have existed: it had been a *Marie Celeste* of picnics.

Stuffed Crabs

Land crabs are used on the island for this first–course dish.

> 6 small hard-shell crabs
> 3 oz (75 g) freshly made breadcrumbs
> 1 fresh hot pepper, seeded and chopped fine, or hot
>   pepper sauce to taste
> 3 tablespoons chopped chives
> 2 tablespoons chopped parsley
> 2 cloves garlic, crushed
> 1 tablespoon fresh lime juice
> salt and freshly ground pepper
> ¼ teaspoon allspice

3 tablespoons Madeira or dark rum, preferably
    Martinique or Guadeloupe *rhum vieux*
butter

Preheat the oven to gas mark 4 (350°F, 180°C). Plunge the crabs into boiling water and boil for 8–10 minutes. Remove and cool. Take out the meat from the shells and claws and chop it finely. Discard the spongy fibre. Scrub out the empty shells, if small, and reserve. Mash 2 oz (50 g) of breadcrumbs into the crabmeat until the mixture is quite smooth. Add the hot pepper, chives, parsley, lime juice, salt, pepper, allspice, Madeira or rum, mixing thoroughly. Stuff the reserved crab shells with the mixture. If using three or four larger crabs, use the meat to stuff six scallop shells or put in ramekins. Sprinkle with the remaining bread-crumbs and dot with butter. Bake for 30 minutes, or until lightly browned.

If live crabs are not available, buy 1 lb (450 g) of fresh, frozen or tinned crabmeat, or buy plain boiled crabs.

Chicken Calypso

(serves six)

5 tablespoons olive oil
4 lb (1 kg 800 g) chicken, cut into serving pieces
1 lb 2 oz (500 g) rice
1 medium onion, finely chopped
1 clove garlic, chopped
1 green bell pepper, seeded and chopped
1 small hot green pepper, seeded and chopped
8 oz (225 g) mushrooms, sliced

½ teaspoon saffron
piece of lime peel
1 tablespoon lime juice
¼ teaspoon Angostura bitters
2 pints (1 litre 140 ml) chicken stock
salt and freshly ground pepper
3 tablespoons light rum

Heat 3 tablespoons of the oil in a skillet and sauté the chicken pieces until brown all over. Remove to a heavy casserole. Add the rice, onion, garlic, bell pepper and hot pepper to the oil remaining in the skillet and sauté, stirring until the oil is absorbed, being careful not to let the rice scorch. Add to the chicken in the casserole. Add the remaining 2 tablespoons of oil to the skillet, and sauté the mushrooms over a fairly high heat for 5 minutes. Add to the casserole with the saffron, lime peel, lime juice, bitters, stock and salt and pepper to taste. Cover and simmer gently until the rice and chicken are tender and the liquid absorbed – about 30 minutes. Add the rum and cook uncovered for 5 minutes longer.

Hartley Augiste's Rum Punch

(serves one)

2 fl. oz (55 ml) Dominica rum or light rum from
    Martinique or Guadeloupe
½ fl. oz (15 ml) lime juice
3 teaspoons simple syrup (see below)
2–3 dashes Angostura bitters
3–4 ice cubes
maraschino cherry

Combine ingredients in a cocktail shaker and shake hard. Strain over ice cubes.

Simple Syrup

  I lb (450 g) granulated sugar
  ¾ pint (425 ml) cold water

Combine the two in a bowl and stir from time to time until dissolved. Use in drinks instead of sugar. 1 tablespoon of syrup = 1½ teaspoons of sugar

Mango Ice Cream

  4 eggs
  4 oz (110 g) sugar
  ¾ pint (425 ml) milk
  I cup of mango pulp mixed with 2 oz (50 g) sugar
    (extra to above)
  ½ teaspoon vanilla essence

Beat the eggs lightly with the sugar. Scald the milk and stir into the eggs. Cook the egg mixture on top of a double boiler over hot water, stirring constantly until the mixture coats the spoon. Cool and add mango pulp. Freeze to a mush. Remove from the refrigerator and beat well. Freeze again.

Mitch Crites

It was Colin who first met Mitch Crites when he was building houses on Mustique. On the suggestion of Princess Margaret, Colin had asked the theatre designer Oliver Messel to design all the houses on the island. For his own house Colin wanted to create a Taj Mahal–like home and brought in Mitch Crites, an American living in India who dealt in Indian arts and crafts, to advise him and buy Indian furniture and artefacts to furnish the house. Colin invited Mitch to his 60th birthday Peacock Ball on the island, which is when I met him. I'd been to India once on a trip organised by a magazine with a friend – it had been the most extraordinary holiday with elephants, fireworks and spectacular parties, I absolutely loved it, and had gone mad buying all sorts of unsuitable things which we brought back. Mitch said that if we wanted to go back to India he would look after us. I jumped at the offer, and Margaret and I went to stay with him. We accompanied him on his trips around the country, seeing parts of India we would never otherwise have seen and staying in some pretty rough places, but that didn't matter, we had a brilliant time and Mitch made it all such fun. He is a fluent

Hindi speaker, which made all the difference to how we were received and what we could do. The trip became an annual event and we would return with all sorts of lovely things, saris, scarves, different pieces each year and hold an exhibition in his showroom behind Christie's. Princess Margaret used to come and we'd sell our wares, which people would buy for Christmas presents, we got quite a reputation. Mitch is a very dear friend and I do hope that I will manage one more trip to India, to visit him.

Picnics in India
Mitch Crites

Lady Anne, Margaret Vyner and I bonded at the grand 60th birthday party that Colin, Lord Glenconner and Anne's husband, threw for himself and a shipload full of friends, movie stars and exotic guests on the Caribbean island of Mustique in 1986.

I had been based in India since the late sixties and it was only natural to invite 'Les Girls', as I called Anne and Margaret, to visit my wife, Nilou and me in Delhi and Jaipur, and to tour some of the legendary sites. Over the years, we travelled the length and breadth of India in fourteen fascinating excursions. The one rule that they both insisted on was that Colin was not allowed to join us. But, of course, he did come on his own, shopping for his mansions, restaurants and architectural follies that he loved creating on Mustique and St Lucia. Unlike Les Girls, he could be hard to handle.

I remember once Colin told me that he wanted to buy baskets of costume jewellery for a party he was planning. We took a local tuk-tuk deep into the heart of the 17th-century bazaar in Old Delhi and Colin began selecting glittering bangles and baubles, necklaces and earrings from the local street vendors.

He had told me in advance not to call him by his title but the minute we arrived he loudly announced that he was Lord Glenconner and, instantly, it seemed that we had been transported back to the days of the British Raj. After an hour of haggling, Colin asked for the bill and proclaimed that he wanted to pay by credit card and, naturally, the trolley owner replied that he only took cash. Colin went ballistic and threw the bags of jewellery back in his face. Suddenly, a hostile angry crowd surrounded us. I, somehow, managed to hand over a wad of rupees to the guy for his trouble and we leapt into our waiting scooter and sped off. We were lucky to have escaped unharmed. Colin thought it was jolly good fun and I was left exhausted and a bit shaken.

Anne and Margaret loved being on the road with Meva Singh, our loyal Rajput driver. I would map out a two- to three-week tour in some remote part of the country and we would set off. I sat with Meva in the front watching the road while Anne and Margaret were in the back happily chatting away. The highlight of each day was the ritual picnic. We would often drive for kilometres searching for the perfect site, which had to have shade, a stream or pond, a monument, if possible, and, of course, a nearby 'mustard field' as it came to be called, where they could disappear into the vegetables or tall grass for a moment of privacy.

The picnic menu didn't vary much as it suited the warm and humid weather and we all liked it. It included vegetable cutlets, cheese sandwiches on white bread, boiled eggs, sliced tomatoes, red carrots and cucumbers, ketchup packets and seasoning, mango pickle, local sweets and whatever fresh fruit we could find. Also, mineral water and flasks of boiling water for tea.

After lunch, we would relax a while and then continue the journey. Anne and Margaret were wonderful travelling companions. They never complained and were always up for an adventure. As soon as we arrived in the late afternoon at an old palace converted into a hotel or a jungle bungalow, I would ask the maharaja or local guides what's happening in the area. Are there any obscure monuments, local markets or tribal festivals going on? No matter how difficult and bumpy the road was to get to an 'event', they were always ready. We explored village stepwells, palaces and soaring forts and laughed together from morning to evening. These are precious memories that I cherish until today.

Rupert Loewenstein

Rupert was the Rolling Stone's financial manager and he and his wife Josephine were some of our closest friends. They were very brave coming out to Mustique in the early days when there was no running water or electricity but they fell in love with it, eventually buying a house there. Rupert was part of a group, along with Jonathan Guinness, who bought a merchant bank in the 1960s, not long after which he was introduced to Mick Jagger and has been credited with transforming the Stones into a global brand. He was responsible for introducing Mick Jagger to Mustique, who also became a friend after coming to the golden ball Colin threw one year. Bianca Jagger came looking absolutely wonderful in a gold crinoline dress and Mick looked rather weird in a little straw pixie hat sprayed gold. But Mick fell in love with the island and has been the most wonderful asset to Mustique – he helped finance a new school and played cricket with the villagers. I think his children almost think of it as home. We used to have wonderful Christmases there when he was with Jerry Hall, playing games and indulging in amateur theatricals. One year we let it be known that we were putting on a play in which

Mick was playing the doctor and Rupert his assistant and were in need of people to play his patients. There was a queue halfway round the island desperate to be examined by Mick, with my nanny Barbara at the front of it!

Rupert, who was a Bavarian prince, was also responsible for introducing Princess Margaret to some of her German relatives on Prince Philip's side. Initially she was rather reluctant, but Rupert persuaded her to go and they ended up visiting Germany several times to stay with various friends and relations which she loved. Princess Margaret had a coterie of gentlemen, among whom were Rupert and Colin, who at Christmas used to take her somewhere lovely for lunch, preferably near Bond Street. They would suggest they might take a stroll afterwards whereupon they would vie with each other as to who had bought her the most expensive present in Cartier or Tiffany's.

'Caldo e Cremoso'
Rupert Loewenstein

Although, like many spoilt men, I prefer the pleasures of the table in the great indoors, there can be exceptions. The pleasures of the table embrace not only what is to be eaten and drunk, but also the civilised enjoyment of good company in an attractive and comfortable setting. Increasingly I have found that wit flourishes in an atmosphere of good food and drink. Perhaps that is because I have never known (and indeed, do they still exist?) the salons where brilliant conversation is enjoyed, while the guests are only fortified by warm lemonade and, perhaps, a plate of 'fingers'.

In a happier age, in the days of good King Idris, we stayed with Italian friends in Tripoli. The day after we arrived we were taken in a bus to look at the ruins of Sabratha, some sixty or seventy miles away across the desert. Having admired the antique splendours for an hour or two in the scorching sun, our hostess asked us whether we were ready for luncheon. Thereupon we rounded a corner and saw set up in front of the huge pillars looking on to the sea a table covered with gleaming linen and, behind comfortable chairs, two footmen in neat white coats with appropriately armorial buttons.

What did we eat and drink? Cool white wine from Maser, hot cannelloni, *vitello tonnato*, some cheese with North African bread, and grapefruit sorbet. The unexpectedness in the desert of this luxury, which originally we had taken to be a mirage, and the pleasure of the company of great friends in beautiful surroundings, was such as to make it one of the most enjoyable luncheons I have ever had.

When we complimented our hostess on the delights of the day, she said, 'Always remember, for a picnic some of the food must be "caldo e cremoso".'

Bryan Adams

Bryan became a close friend after he bought one of the original houses on Mustique. He was very close to Colin, which is rather strange because they were so different. Bryan is a vegan and very controlled, immensely hard working and Colin was quite the opposite, but Bryan understood him. When Colin died on St Lucia, Bryan went to the trouble of hiring a plane to come to the funeral with one or two friends. He'd written a song, 'You're My Friend', which he sang in the church at the huge funeral we had where hundreds of local people had a picture of Colin stuck to their shirts and were waving black balloons. Bryan's father was in the army and, like me, he is very punctual. I saw him the last time I was on Mustique and he arranged to pick me up for lunch at six minutes to one, assuming I'm sure, I would be late, but there I was ready to go at six minutes to one, and he got out of his car and saluted me. I had to tell him it was thirty-four years of training as lady-in-waiting!

On the Road Houmous
Bryan Adams

The perfect recipe on the road.

This is my recipe for something to munch on when in the car travelling from town to town. I usually have something to snack on whilst sitting for hours in the back of a car, so I'll pack some of this, some crudités or carrot and peppers, and naturally some sort of crispy flatbread to accompany it.

A napkin is always useful when hitting a bump.

I can chickpeas
4 tablespoons tahini
I whole lemon
olive oil
sea salt
I2 cubes of ice

Drain and rinse the chickpeas and put in food processor with a jar of tahini (to taste) plus the juice of 1 lemon and a big glug of olive oil. Blend on full speed for about 3 minutes until it becomes a smooth paste. Once the mixture is smooth, add ice and continue to blend. The houmous will go pale and creamy. Store in airtight Kilner jar in fridge until needed and serve with basket of flatbread and/or sliced carrots and peppers.

Mary Hayley Bell

We met Mary and her husband, the actor John Mills, when we were accompanying Princess Margaret to a film premiere. Mary was a writer and an actor who wrote *Whistle Down the Wind* starring their daughter Hayley Mills. When I was made Lady-in-Waiting I think Colin rather thought he'd be coming along to everything too and I had to tell him that was not how it worked, although he did sometimes come with us to evening events. On this occasion he came with us to the premiere and when chatting to Mary and John, Colin told them all about Mustique and invited them to come and visit. We had a lovely time with them on the island and I vividly remember one picnic that Colin had arranged where we were all transferred by buggy to Pasture Bay, which was at the end of the island near Princess Margaret's house. The West Indian grape trees up there had all been sculpted by the wind and made the most marvellous sight framing the route down to the beach where Colin had set up a table under the trees. We had a lovely long lunch and then all went swimming together. We really got to know them quite well. I wrote to Mary to tell her about the picnic book and ask if she might contribute to it and she immediately said yes and sent hers very quickly. She was born in Shanghai where her father was serving in the Chinese Maritime Customs Service, so it wasn't a surprise that her picnic was one from her childhood enjoyed in China.

Picnic in China
Mary Hayley Bell

The earliest picnics I remember were in China before the Second World War. To us children they were something very special. My grandmother used to tell of picnics in Shanghai, with as many as twelve helpers, and guests riding on ponies to the beautiful canal by their house, Unkaza, where a vast curry was served with chutneys, poppadoms, shrimps and coconuts, not to mention sweets and coffee.

We had wonderful picnics during our childhood in Macao, where my father was Commissioner of Chinese Customs. He had two small armed launches in order to combat smuggling and gunrunning. We used to go aboard preceded by the dining-room and kitchen staff who carried the food in large canisters, and crates of beer and wine. There would probably be about twenty guests. The anchor would be hauled up, and we would set out for Bias Bay, near Hong Kong. The lunch would probably consist of Chinese food: egg flower soup, deep-fried walnut chicken, paper-wrapped beef with shredded cabbage, fresh shrimp and lobster sauce, fried and boiled rice, crabmeat, glazed apples and pancakes. Everyone ate with chopsticks – in fact, my earliest memories of food are of eating with chopsticks.

Before 'Tiffin', as it was called in the East, we would have a swim from the *Pak Tow* or *Lung Tsing* – whichever launch we were in – while the Chinese crew stood by the machine guns watching for pirates – for pirates there were. After half an hour's siesta we would be rowed ashore to the white gleaming beach of Leper Island, with the mountains behind and a distant view of Hong Kong.

Egg Flower Soup

> 2 pints (1 litre 150 ml) bone stock
> 2 eggs
> vegetable oil
> 2 spring onions, chopped
> 1 teaspoon salt
> 2 tablespoons soya sauce
> ½ teaspoon Ve Tsin (optional)
> 1 teaspoon vinegar
> pepper

Bring the stock to the boil and remove from the heat. Beat the eggs, mix with a little oil, and pour slowly into the stock. Add the chopped onions and salt and bring to the boil again. Add soya sauce, Ve Tsin (if using), vinegar and pepper. Stir with a ladle and it is ready to serve. The beaten eggs separate into hundreds of little threads on contact with the hot stock, which gives the soup its name.

Crabmeat in Steamed Eggs

> 1 large crab
> 2 eggs
> 1 teaspoon salt

1 tablespoon soya sauce

2 spring onions, chopped

2 tablespoons sherry

1 tablespoon lard

Wash the crab and steam for 15 minutes. Remove the meat from the shell. Beat the eggs and mix them with the salt, soya sauce and chopped spring onions. Add the crabmeat, sherry and half a cup of water. Mix thoroughly and add lard. Steam for 20 minutes. It should be the consistency of thick cream. Put in a large thermos and serve with plain rice.

Hugo Vickers

Hugo and I spent hours swimming in the sea together in Mustique where we met at the house of a mutual friend. I'd just been approached about writing *Lady in Waiting* and was really thinking it was beyond me; I didn't see how I could do it and Hugo gave me great confidence to carry on. He was so kind and encouraging. I'd always loved his books. *The Kiss*, which he wrote in 1996 is the most charming book about two sisters in Windsor who he knew and the impact on their lives of one kiss by a man called Dick. I absolutely loved it. So I was thrilled to meet him and now consider him to be a dear friend.

Garter Day Picnic
Hugo Vickers

My favourite annual picnic is Garter Day, the Monday of Ascot week, when the Knights and Ladies and members of the Royal Family process from the state apartments in Windsor Castle to the service in St George's Chapel, their blue velvet robes and bonnets of ostrich plumes swaying gently in the summer breeze. I have now attended fifty-seven of these, starting very young in 1965. My enthusiasm for the day remains undiminished. It never loses its magic. I am on duty in the chapel as Captain of the Lay Stewards.

My day invariably begins in London as I prepare the picnic. Given that I and my guest(s) are smartly dressed, it is important to avoid things that will explode in the hands and stain our clothes. I tend to go for smoked salmon sandwiches, which have minimal bread but a huge and luscious mouthful of smoked salmon in the centre, roughly four slices – with, of course, butter on the bread, a certain amount of lemon and just a dash of pepper. These are nourishing, easy to eat, perfect. Wine or fruit juice according to taste and some chocolate to round it off, all very simple – and it travels in the Diamond Jubilee picnic basket from the pop concert in the gardens of Buckingham Palace in 2012. Driving up the Long Walk towards the castle is special. That is where we eat it. Sometimes we go into the castle's private grounds via Shaw Farm Gate and eat the picnic next to the Sports Ground. In both cases the castle is very much in view.

Between 1980 and 1990 I had a good deal with one of my fellow Lay Stewards from St George's Chapel – Captain Andrew Yates, an elderly naval captain who lived in Old Windsor. He was a founder member of Glyndebourne, and after his wife died, made an annual plan with me. He took four tickets for the opera. I did the driving, brought a guest and prepared the picnic. Andrew insisted on eating it from the boot of the car, which was a bit depressing. He did not want the hassle of carrying it to the lawn. But for his 90th birthday, I surprised him by getting someone to come down and set up an elegant table, as for a dinner party. He loved that. It was also his last Glyndebourne.

Picnics can be fun or they can be a nightmare. Finding yourself in a field with cows or worse still, an angry bull, is not to be recommended – so a bit of reconnaissance is essential. I have a phobia of wasps and they sometimes like to join in a picnic, sending me scurrying. The worst scenario – you swallow one. But if all goes well, there is nothing finer than a picnic on a perfect English summer day, a bottle of wine and a siesta afterwards.

Banana Pudding

Not sure how suitable for a picnic – but my aunt's banana pudding has many enthusiastic followers.

Slice up a quantity of bananas as thin as you can be bothered. In a bowl, crumble up a quantity of Cadbury's milk flake chocolate. Put about two pots of double cream into another bowl, feed in the bananas and the chocolate pieces, and stir them well together. You can add a (considerable) dash of rum if you like. Then just put it into the refrigerator for a few hours till it sets solid. Bring it out, sprinkle some more milk flake pieces on the top to cover it. Delicious.

Colin Tennant

Colin was a brilliant organiser of picnics. Once at Glen he arranged a picnic at the Loch and because his eccentric uncle, Stephen Tennant, thought the colour of heather vulgar, he bought and stuck hundreds of blue paper flowers on the hill. Stephen just said, 'So much better darling boy.'

Mustique
Colin Tennant

A picnic is different. In a cupboard, on a hillside, up a gum tree, down among the dead men – anything out of the daily grind. Herein lies our first problem. In Mustique we have a picnic every day. Second problem, always the same people; and third, always the same food. That's not to say we don't enjoy ourselves. It's like laughing at an old joke. It gets better every time. So here goes, everyone, wait for it!

We meet at the beach.

Lagoon or Macaroni (that's the name of the beach, not the

main course)? Macaroni has waves, and no sandflies. For those that can't handle the ocean, Lagoon has sandflies and no waves. For those that can't handle the sandflies, there's 'off'!

Cold cuts, or chicken? The Great General Store in Mustique rarely sells a whole chicken. More usually on offer are what are termed 'chicken parts'. These are fairer than a regular chicken, because each frozen box contains a number of similar parts, i.e. all legs or all wings. There is no question of having to carve or ask guests, 'Which part would you like?' and being left oneself with a bit of brown. NB Avoid at all costs 'chicken backs'.

A guest. Plenty of choice here. However, remember to tell your guests if the picnic is for somebody's birthday, or alternatively in fancy dress.

A glance in the fridge will tell you all you need to know about cold cuts. The chicken parts are more complicated as they need defrosting and should be grilled or devilled.

Mustique Mule

> 1 fresh coconut (or waternut) per person
> vodka
> lime syrup

Cut off the top of the nut with a cutlass. Pour out some of the milk, pour in vodka, lime syrup and ice cubes. Drink through a straw.

Caution: coconut milk will stain your clothes, irremediably.

Seaweed Supper

For an evening picnic on the beach, wrap whatever fresh fish is available in layers of wet seaweed and grill gently over a fire. When cooked, remove the seaweed and sprinkle with fresh lime juice.

Anne's Ginger Whisky Creams or Pudding

> 1 tablespoon whisky
> 2 tablespoons syrup from stem ginger
> ½ teaspoon powdered ginger
> 2 tablespoons caster sugar
> ½ pint (275 ml) double cream
> 2 egg whites
> 3 pieces of stem ginger to decorate

Place the whisky, ginger syrup, powdered ginger, caster sugar and cream in a bowl and whisk with an egg beater until thick. In another bowl whisk the egg whites until stiff. Fold the egg whites into the ginger mixture, spoon into individual dishes and chill. Decorate with small pieces of chopped stem ginger. Cover with foil and pack into an insulated bag ready for the picnic.

Drue Heinz

When Princess Margaret came to Mustique she always refused to fly back overnight, saying she was far too exhausted. She'd say, 'I think I'll go to America and stay with Drue and then fly back from there,' which is what we always did. Drue was married to Jack Heinz who was heir to the Heinz fortune and exceedingly rich. They had a wonderful house on the Upper East Side in New York and we would go and stay there with her. Drue would throw great parties and dinners for Princess Margaret and there would be endless shopping trips. Princess Margaret loved the shop at the Metropolitan Museum which sold jewellery they had copied from paintings in the collection and which everyone loved. There was a pair of earrings, one white and one black pearl earring which many of us had from there, including Princess Diana. Caroline Herrera was a great friend and used to give Princess Margaret lots of her clothes when we were there. I was allowed to choose one outfit from the ready-to-wear collection, which was amazing.

Drue was always such a kind and generous hostess. She also had a house near Ascot and I remember one party there when she imported a complete fairground into the garden so we could all ride on the dodgems and big swings.

Princess Margaret always invited Drue to her annual visit to the Chelsea Flower show. Each member of the royal family used to take a small party of friends on the Monday afternoon, before the crowds were there. It was one of the treats Princess Margaret used to arrange for us and we'd pretty much have the whole place to ourselves. There was a big tent with tea and drinks and lots of different royal households would go, each household having their own table.

Drue was also a great patron of literature and established various literary retreats. She bought Hawthornden Castle outside Edinburgh and if a writer had had at least one book published they could go along and stay. Lunch would be provided in a hamper outside their room and then in the evening she would throw a huge dinner with all these very interesting people to discuss literature and ideas, you might find yourself sitting next to luminaries like Harold Pinter or Lady Antonia Fraser. She also co-founded a literary press, Ecco Press and the Drue Heinz Literary prize. She had a real sense of fun though, which you can tell from her clambake picnic which I think is so well described.

A New England Clambake
Drue Heinz

By far the messiest of all picnics is the famous American institution called the clambake or, before the price of lobster flew too high out of the water, the lobsterbake. In the twenties and thirties it was entirely different, and even grand. The famous

Marshall Field, for instance, would anchor his great yacht off a beautiful stretch of beach in Maine and instruct his crew to go to it. This meant prepare a clambake for the next evening at sundown for his twenty guests.

Nowadays it is every man for himself. However, the menu has not really changed since the Republic was formed, nor has the way settlers learned to cook the corn and shellfish in the ad hoc ovens, or pits, invented by the Indians. The New England or Yankee clambake is as much a national feast as is Thanksgiving. And most people have a last glorious binge on the beach at the end of August before they return to the city from their long summer holidays.

The first clambake I attended was in Martha's Vineyard on a lovely beach of dunes capped with long willowy beachgrass. I was told to bring a sweater, although the temperature at 5 o'clock was about 85 degrees. I was given a basket to carry, surprisingly heavy. I found out later that it was full of vodka and gin. We arrived to find a blazing fire and much consternation. It was supposed to have turned to embers by then, but the wind had risen and whipped up the blaze. And the smoke – Oh Lord – had everyone coughing, rubbing their eyes, retreating frantically from the 'bake' pits and yelling for drinks.

Soon we were consoled with large gins in paper cups, and someone kept running the line of teary-eyed spectators offering ice, ice, anyone? And along came a teenager shaking peanuts out of a large bag. Unfortunately, most of them fell to the sand as we swayed in the wind, which was becoming stronger and colder. Meanwhile the younger, more durable element had managed to damp down the fire and were endeavouring to place the clams around the blistery seaweed whose water would cook them.

Hours passed, the moon came up, and the wind changed. We had to turn our backs to the fire and wrap our much-needed sweaters around us, at the same time trying to keep the sand from getting into every nook and cranny of our weather-whipped bodies.

But then came the cry, 'Clams up!' Several young men appeared with plates piled with clams, sweet potatoes, corn, a small lobster, and a large paper napkin. My nearest companion turned to grab a plateful when a gust of wind caught us and everything fell into the sand. 'Don't touch it yet, it's burning hot,' went down the line. So we all had another restorative drink.

Eventually we found a bit of everything, gratiné with sand. What to do? Obviously stagger to the sea, wash the sand off the food quickly in the water, and eat it with our fingers. I tried, goodness knows, I tried! But I remember only getting wet to the thighs as a big wave struck, knocking the plate from my hand. Thank heavens it was dark. As I trudged back, jeans clinging dankly to my thighs, someone said, 'What wonderful clams. Didn't you think the lobster was great?' I replied, 'Yes, absolutely wonderful, never had anything so good, but it sure makes one thirsty.'

At least I had managed to hold on to my cup and received an immediate fill-up. As I neared the fire, I managed to salvage a baked potato from a friendly helper. I was torn between eating it or stashing it behind my knee as one does at an Irish point-to-point. We now crouched wetly in the moonlight. Someone started to sing, 'By the sea, by the beautiful sea,' and I looked around wildly for anyone who might be leaving in a car. At last I spied a Land Rover driving off, and begged a lift. 'We're full,' they said. 'You'll have to get in the back.' I clambered in, and what did I see but the remains of the clams, buttery corn on the cob, baby lobster, hard rolls and plates of sweet potatoes. Bumping along the potholed road back to the Vineyard I had the best, and possibly the last, clambake I would ever enjoy.

To Arrange a Clambake

The night before the feast make a small pit of sand and line it with rocks and flat stones. Build a fire and tend it through the day. By night-time the ash should be flat on the rocks. The stones and rocks are by now extremely hot. Then bank the fire and leave it. The next day, early in the morning, make a fire again on top of what is left.

The picnic consists of fresh lobsters, clams, corn cobs wrapped in foil (these used to be wrapped in vine leaves) and sweet potatoes baked in their jackets. Cover the whole thing with seaweed and then put a wet tarpaulin over the top and leave roughly from 9 a.m. until 10 p.m., by which time all should be ready and tender. The seaweed supplies the flavour, keeps the moisture in and steams all the seafood. Now we also add half a broiler chicken, again in layers of seaweed, and this is delicious. People lie in the grass around this non-smoking fire and drink draught beer or cider. It's an all-day event.

About Clambakes

Whatever the size of your bake, dig your clams the day before. Scrub them well to remove sand. Put them in a bucket, well covered with seawater. Add cornmeal, allowing ½ cup to 2 quarts (2.28 litres) water. The cereal helps rid the clams of sand and internal waste. Leave the clams in a cool place. Rinse and drain them just before using.

Clambake

(for 20 people)

200 soft-shell clams
50 hard-shell clams (optional)
4 dozen ears of corn
5 broiling chickens
10 sweet potatoes
20 frankfurters (optional)
20 1½ lb (700 g) lobsters or 5 pecks or an equivalent
    weight of soft-shell crabs
butter, melted
beer or cider
watermelon
coffee

Start preparations at least 4 hours before you plan to serve. Dig a sandpit 1 foot deep and 3½ feet across. Line it with smooth round rocks. Be sure the rocks have not been baked before. Have a wet tarpaulin – generous enough to overlap the pit area by 1 foot all round – and a few rocks handy to weight the edges. Build a fire over the rock surface, using hardwood, and keep feeding it for the next 2½ to 3 hours while the rocks are heating. Gather and wash about 4 bushels of wet rock seaweed. In fact, it is wise to soak the seaweed for at least 45 minutes before use. Have a pail of seawater at hand.

Partially husk the ears of corn. Do not pull them quite clean but leave on the last layer or two. Rip these back far enough to remove the silk. Then replace them, so the kernels are fully protected. Reserve the pulled husks.

Quarter the chickens. You may wrap the chicken pieces in

cheesecloth or divide the food into 20 individual cheese-cloth-wrapped servings, so that each person's food can later be removed as one unit.

Scrub the lobsters or crabs.

Now you are ready to arrange for the 'bake'. Rake the embers from the hot stones, remove them from the pit and line it with the wet seaweed, covering the stones. The lining should be about 6 inches deep. Put over it, if you wish, a piece of chicken wire. If you haven't wrapped the individual servings in cheesecloth, pack the pit in layers. For added flavour, put down first a layer of hard-shell clams, then the frankfurters if you use them, then the lobsters or crabs, the chicken and the soft-shell clams, the sweet potatoes and the ears of corn. You may also put seaweed between the layers. Cover the layered food with the reserved corn husks and sprinkle the whole with the bucket of seawater. Quickly cover with the wet tarpaulin. Weight the tarpaulin down well with rocks. The whole should steam covered for about 1 hour. During the steaming, it will puff up, which is a sign of a satisfactory 'bake'. To test, lift the tarpaulin carefully at one corner so as not to get sand into the pit and see if the clams have opened. If so, the whole feast should be cooked just to the right point. Have handy plenty of towels and melted butter.

Serve with beer or cider, with watermelon and coffee to follow.

Tina Brown

Tina came out to Mustique when Colin was selling plots of land there to write a feature on him for *Tatler*. And when Princess Margaret and I went to stay with Drue Heinz in New York, Tina and her husband Harry Evans were frequent visitors. She's been incredibly kind and supportive to me, she interviewed me when *Whatever Next* was published, in a theatre in New York and it was a riot, we had great fun sparking off each other and she kindly threw a wonderful dinner party for me afterwards.

Picnic at Macaroni Beach
Tina Brown

My family was never big on picnics. To create a memorable picnic at least one person in the household has to exhibit an imaginative interest in food. My mother was a huge culinary failure, and my father was only invested in the sangria. All my memories of family picnic attempts at Wimbledon, Henley Royal Regatta and Glyndebourne are sodden with the inevitable British downpour,

113

hunched under umbrellas in collapsible chairs next to our parked car with the boot open to protect the egg salad sandwiches.

But there is one picnic that left its mark on my memory. It was hosted for Princess Margaret at Macaroni Beach on Mustique, the private island in the Caribbean whose founding Prospero was Colin Tennant, later Lord Glenconner. (His wife Lady Anne – who wasn't there – is the curator of this book.)

The other guests – Reinaldo and Carolina Herrera, Brian Alexander, Roddy Llewellyn, and various villa owners – were all a bit bleary-eyed after one of Colin's costume bacchanalias at Basil's Bar the night before. Colin had plunged around the dance floor holding a fuzzy orange wig which he clapped on the head of anyone who didn't seem to be getting into the swing of things. 'There's no one this wig can't improve,' he cried, as Princess Margaret and Roddy hit the floor for a majestic rock and roll.

The next day HRH was worried that her singing performance had not been up to snuff. 'It was the organist who let you down, Ma'am,' said Tennant diplomatically. 'However, I've made enquiries this morning and the general feeling here is that you were much better than you thought.'

Seated at a trestle table covered by a sparkling white linen tablecloth, we all murmured our assent. The picnic was set up in the spiky shade of gently swaying palm trees on Macaroni's white sands, and like everything associated with Colin, was choreographed and catered to perfection. Groaning platters of Scottish salmon finger sandwiches with fragrant dill, mini Melton Mowbray pork pies, creamy devilled eggs, the yellowest of corn salads, the rubiest of small tomatoes, crisp, viridescent lettuce, and most mouthwatering of all, tiny sausages skewered on cocktail sticks just waiting to be devoured before the dessert finale of guava jam tarts. And then a searing cry emanated from Princess Margaret's direction. 'What! No mustard! How am I expected to eat sausages without mustard!' The whole party leapt to its feet in consternation.

To solve the problem, albeit five decades later, I consulted Chef Jason, who prepares exquisite al fresco lunches for the guests of Barry Diller and Diane von Fürstenberg aboard Mr Diller's yacht *EOS*. Jason kindly created this recipe for mustard.

Lavender Honey Mustard à la Mustique

> ¼ cup brown mustard seeds
> ¼ cup yellow mustard seeds
> ½ cup water
> ½ cup apple cider vinegar
> I teaspoon turmeric
> ¼ cup lavender honey
> I tablespoon of the most fresh lavender flowers one can
> find, lightly chopped

Place seeds, water and vinegar in a bowl for two days. Blend with all remaining ingredients after this time.

Bon appetit!

Cecilia McEwan and Jools and Christabel Holland

Parties at the McEwans' were legendary. Terence Stamp, Jean Shrimpton and, of course, Princess Margaret were among the guests they hosted at their house, Bardrochat near Glen in Scotland. They were a very glamorous family, seen as a Scottish version of the Kennedys. Cecilia was the daughter of an Austrian prince, but she married Alexander McEwan who had learnt how to play the Mississippi blues in America in the 1950s. Together with his brother Rory they formed a duo and became quite famous at the time, appearing on television here and on the Ed Sullivan show in the States. Parties often ended up in a singalong, whether at their house or when they came to Glen; it was all tremendous fun. As well as being the consummate hostess, Cecilia was also committed to charity work. In the sixties she'd worked with leprosy sufferers in Thailand and in the 1990s was part of an aid convoy to Bosnia during the war.

Rory McEwan's daughter, Christabel, has become a great friend. She married Jools Holland, who had also been a guest of the McEwans in Scotland. I love Christabel and Jools. I often say to Christabel, 'I go to bed with Jools whenever I can... (watching him on the television of course).' We go on holiday together every year in August, as guests of a Turkish friend who flies us all somewhere hot on a private jet. I'm very lucky to have young friends, as I get into my nineties most of my friends have died, so it's lovely to know a younger generation. When we are on the yacht our host has toys like jet skis to play with and Jools would say, 'Come on, Anne, let's go for a ride, I promise not to go too fast!' So I'd hop on. I'm rather fond of a photograph I have of myself on a jet ski clinging on to Jools for dear life!

I love the fact that I have picnics both from Cecilia and from her niece Christabel in the book.

Marchmont Picnic
Cecilia McEwan

The picnic for me conjures up idyllic scenes under trees, dappled shade, a rippling stream, with girls in muslin and men in panama hats. Baskets of food, French bread and white wine. This illusion has been spitefully dashed by the Scottish Border climate, where many a memorable picnic has been endured, huddled under the walls of Hermitage Castle, the beauty of which has been shrouded in mist, rain mingling with a fried egg sarnie, and a snell wind anaesthetising the fingers.

Picnics now usually take place on the lawn, where a quick dash for cover can be organised at a moment's notice. A table helps to stop any spillages brought on by uneven surfaces or a surfeit of Bloody Marys. Paper everything (no regrets) – cloth, plates, cups and napkins – and burn the lot at the end. A piece of lamb barbecuing, smelling of rosemary, garlic and cognac. Crisp lettuce, cut very thick, to dip in either dressing or fresh mayonnaise; a personal adaptation of a Spanish omelette, which can be cooked and remain in a quiche dish and be eaten with fingers. A terrine to slap on some French bread while waiting for the lamb to cook. Some radishes, some cream cheese with freshly chopped herbs, apples, butter, salt and a large pepper grinder.

Finally, vital to cooks and guests alike, a great deal of drink. Cold white wine, beer, cider and apple juice.

One eccentricity carried on from childhood at Marchmont is the marmalade sandwich – it has to be at every picnic. This may sound unappetising, but can be interesting if made with brown bread, butter and chunky marmalade. There has to be a plentiful supply as addicts will eat them throughout the picnic, beginning as a first course and finishing up what is left as a sort of pudding.

Papillon of Lamb for Barbecue (Mr McEwan's Special)

A small leg of lamb, boned by the butcher so that when opened flat it resembles the shape of a butterfly. Marinate in brandy, olive oil, rosemary, crushed garlic and pepper. Seal on each side on the barbecue and cook for around 20 minutes depending on the thickness of the meat. It should be pink in the centre when cooked. Cut on a bread board in slices like an entrecôte.

Terrine of Game or Veal

6–8 rashers streaky bacon 8 oz (225 g) pig's liver
1 small onion

1 clove garlic
8 oz (225 g) sausagemeat
parsley, marjoram, thyme
8 oz (225 g) pie veal or breasts of pheasant
8 oz (225 g) pork fat
salt and pepper

Preheat the oven to gas mark 4 (350°F, 180°C). Line a baking dish with bacon rashers. Mince the pork, liver, onion and garlic, add the sausage meat and herbs and mix well. Spread half the liver mixture over the bacon in the dish. Arrange strips of veal or pheasant on top. Cover with the remaining liver mixture. Cover the pan with foil.

Place in a larger dish containing water and cook for one hour. Turn out while still warm and drain excess fat.

A Cooling Water Picnic
Christabel and Jools Holland

We are the current custodians of the ruin of 14th century Cooling Castle and have recently dug out the moat. Hoping to unearth suits of armour left over from the siege by Thomas Wyatt in 1554, or carelessly misplaced bejewelled swords, or furiously refused engagement rings, we actually found miles of barbed wire and one remarkably well-preserved, hand-painted sign bearing the ominous warning: *Beware Falling Stones*.

Ignoring the advice, we have now taken to enjoying this newly created water world from a very un-medieval but marvellously practical modern pedalo that can carry a surprising number of adults and/or children with impressive stability.

In challenging times there is no antidote more enjoyable than a water picnic.

The calming effects of being afloat under the dappled shade of chestnut and willow, with frogs camouflaged to perfection causing shrieks of startled merriment as they leap out of our path, and huge silent fish slipping beneath us like submarines, alchemise into an enchanter's spell to soothe the nerves and raise the spirits.

Having experimented with various food styles, some of them, such as sandwiches and boiled eggs, have proved all too easy to collapse or slip out of small hands, and drop moatwards with a heart-stopping plop before the wails of disappointment.

These little savoury mouthfuls are quick to make, easy to handle and satisfyingly filling.

(Makes 24)

1 onion, chopped
4 eggs
250 ml (8 fl oz) milk
60 g (2 oz) flour
½ teaspoon baking powder
60 g (2 oz) grated cheddar cheese or feta
parsley, chopped
pine nuts
125 g (4 oz) butter

Baking tray for 12 muffins.

Oven gas mark 6 (190°C, 375°F) or top Aga oven. Put the onion, eggs, milk, flour, baking powder, cheese and parsley into a mixer.

Whizz it up for about 30 seconds. Melt a little knob of butter into each muffin hole, fill up to about two thirds and bake for 25–30 minutes.

You can add bits of crispy bacon or chopped sausage for carnivores.

Gaia Servadio

Life was always incredibly sociable when we were up at Glen. One of Colin's friends who lived up there was the art historian William Mostyn-Owen who was married to Gaia, an Italian writer, and they lived in one wing of Aberuchill Castle in Perthshire. I have vivid memories of a wonderful lunch there. We arrived as it was snowing, being Scotland it was practically dark by lunchtime, and Gaia had lit the whole house with candles. It was almost a theatrical experience driving up to the house in the snow with candles in all the windows. No one in Scotland would have thought of doing that but Gaia made it all quite magical. We had a wonderful Italian feast and the children were whisked away for lunch, which Colin thought was perfect. Gaia's daughter Allegra was briefly married to Boris Johnson and was a great friend of my ex-daughter-in-law Anastasia. But it was the memory of that fabulous lunch that encouraged me to ask her to write about a picnic for us and I love her idea of cooking the picnic in situ, taken from her Italian roots, and transferred to a Scottish setting.

The Kingdom of Picnics
Gaia Servadio

My idea of picnicking has sprung from eccentric, distant roots.

When my sister and I were very small and when spring had settled on the Euganean hills, my father would assemble a few cooking pans and put them and myself on his bicycle. My sister had her own bicycle, something I didn't envy because it terrified me. The food for the picnic – and that was the excitement – was to be found and cooked in situ. While one of us assembled dry branches, the other would charm the friars of the Abbey of Chiaravalle, a dream of a Romanesque building, into selling us some of their freshly baked bread. The farmers would let us have a few eggs, still warm; in the fields we would gather rucola, that bitter, pungent leaf, and wild mint. And then we would cook.

Now that I have moved to the kingdom of picnics (Britain), my approach remains basically the same: to enjoy a picnic properly one should find the food for it, and cook it, on the spot. Not that I light a fire when I go to Glyndebourne, but I don't see the point of taking a lot of pre-cooked food, a lot of plates and a lot of people transferring it in order to eat.

My recipe for a Scottish picnic – my home is in Scotland, and most of my picnicking is done there – is as follows. A fair number of children and grown-ups, raw potatoes, salt, plenty of butter, bread and a frying pan. Very fresh trout (still alive if possible) in a plastic bag. Cheeses, thyme, pepper, knives, forks, matches and glasses. Despite the occasional tempest, downpour, gale, etc., the burns and the beauty of Scotland make it a superb picnicking land.

So now we select the ideal spot (of course, someone will discover that the next curve of the burn was better). The children gather stones and dry branches; the fire is lit at once, while volunteers look for chanterelles and ceps (*Boletus edulis*) and others clean the trout in the burn.

Stuff the trout with thyme, salt them and cook them directly on the burning wood (turning them after five minutes). The eggs should be fried in the frying pan with the chanterelles or ceps; the bread toasted on the hot stones with the cheese on top. Nothing tastes better than food cooked on wood.

Drink: water, Scottish water, absolute delight!

At the end of this picnic everybody will be dirty and exhausted. Weather permitting, a dip in the burn is recommended.

Rachel Johnson

I first met Rachel, a hugely talented author, broadcaster and television presenter, when she invited me to speak on her podcast, *Difficult Women*. We got along so well, and I thoroughly enjoyed meeting her. It was just before I visited America to promote *Whatever Next* and she offered to come with me on the tour as my 'Lady-in-Waiting' – she would have been perfect!

Picnics and Scones
Rachel Johnson

One summer we were in Scotland staying at my husband's family 'seat', Kelburn Castle, with many children and friends, among them Kate Bingham, the vaccine queen, a woman of relentless dash and drive.

She would make us bicycle up glens and hurl the bikes over barbed-wire fences, and swim in burns and lochs in our pants, play cricket and race on beaches, and one evening, she told the assembled company the plan for the morrow.

We would get up early and catch the eight o'clock ferry to Arran, pick up mountain bikes, then hide them in the brambles somewhere to climb Goat Fell on foot. 'It'll be fun,' she said, 'We'll take a picnic.'

After dinner, late, Kate and I mustered in the kitchen and made the most sumptuous picnic. We cut thick slices of whole-meal bread, buttered them, then layered slices of roast lamb, cheddar, chutney, and tomato. Each one was the size of a small brick, wrapped in cling film. We packed these with boiled eggs and jumbo slabs of Cadbury's Dairy Milk and water into a back-pack that she would carry without complaint.

The only child of mine who would come was my oldest son Ludo, then a sleepy adolescent. As we ascended Goat Fell, having stowed our bikes, it was like climbing Kilimanjaro, only with midges. We trudged and trudged, munching the chocolate to keep us going, while the Bingham clan scampered ahead, declaiming sonnets and singing acapella.

We two were the last to summit and found everyone sitting about, in reverential silence as they rewarded themselves with the excellent lamb sandwiches. Kate handed me and Ludo ours and we settled by a trig point to tuck in. Ludo unwrapped his and sat, stunned for a moment, in contemplation not of the view (clouds of midges) but his sad fate, sandwich in hand.

At that moment a black Labrador ambled up and swiped Ludo's sandwich and wolfed it as easily as Timmy in *The Famous Five* disposing of a dish of strawberry ice cream. Ludo burst into tears. I gave him half of mine, and he has had a horror of picnics (and fell walking) ever since.

As we live on Exmoor, to me a picnic is portable food you can eat out of your hands and needs no embellishment. Pork pies. Sausage rolls. But above all, pasties (not pronounced 'parsties', please). A warm meat pasty or cheese pasty is the food of the gods, eaten halfway through a long walk along the Doone Valley or Valley of the Rocks, before a swim perhaps, knowing that a cream tea awaits you at the finishing post. '"Food always tastes better in the open air",' my father would quote a repeated line in *The Famous Five*, always adding, '"Said George wagging her tail",' and it does. One is hungrier and there's nothing I love more than feeling hungry and knowing I am about to scoff something sustaining and scrumptious, like an egg sandwich, say.

Though I am very lazy, I can knock up scones – which I regard as a vehicle for clotted cream and raspberry jam – in a jiffy. When it's not raining I take the tray out to the garden and we have picnic cream teas on the grass. Once the broadcaster and all-round goddess Emily Maitlis came to our farm for a snoop and stayed for tea and I'll always remember how she wanted her scone: 'Lots of clotted cream, please, and only a little bit of jam.'

I remind her of it sometimes. 'Only a little bit of jam eh, Maitlis?' and she will reply, 'And LOTS of clotted cream.'

Susanna Johnston

Zanna, as I always knew Susanna, was my husband Colin's first cousin; her mother and Colin's mother were sisters. I always said that one of the best things about marrying Colin was getting to know Zanna, we just clicked. We travelled quite a lot together to Thailand and Myanmar – or Burma as it then was. She was so full of ideas and so interested in everything, always fun to be around. She was a writer and wrote a marvellous book about the art historians Hugh Honour and John Fleming with whom she had lived in Italy for a while when she was much younger and completely fell in love with the country. She and her husband bought a beautiful house in Tuscany, near Lucca, and some of the picnics in this book are from friends who either stayed with her there or were invited for one of the wonderful long lunches she used to have. Italy was such a favoured holiday destination for us and our friends. I think it was a continuation of the time when artistocratic young men in the eighteenth century used to travel around Italy discovering its cultural highlights. The Grand Tour was seen as a rite of passage. Zanna used to drive down to their house in Italy for the summer, smoking all the way, with her husband Nicky, whom she adored. She'd been introduced to Nicky, who was an architect, by his great friend, Mark Boxer and they ended up living next to Mark and his then wife Arabella Boxer in London, which is how we asked Arabella to write for the *Picnic Papers*.

Picnic at Bagni du Lucca
Susanna Johnston

We drove along the Valley of the Serchio, which lies between the Apennines and the Appian Alps, towards Bagni di Lucca, a little spa beloved by English poets and writers throughout the centuries for its warm sulphur baths and for being permanently shaded by overhanging mountains and thick chestnut woods. We were making for the small Protestant cemetery where Ouida (the novelist Louise de la Ramée, who took her own childish mispronunciation of her first name as her nom de plume) lies buried. This cemetery is not easy to storm, and bribery and negotiation with the neighbours is needed.

Ouida died of pneumonia in the severe winter of 1909 at the age of sixty-nine and was buried at Bagni di Lucca after years of degradation and near-blindness, deserted by all but her faithful dog. The English consul of the time is said to have been moved by her bleak end and to have paid for her beautiful tomb in the style of the Della Quercia effigy of 1406 in the Duomo at Lucca. By the time we met our friends at the pretty iron gateway to the cemetery, the Tuscan heavens had opened. We pulled our coats over our heads, covered our baskets as best we could, and belted up the path to a small deserted chapel which, to our delight, turned out to be used for storing bales of hay. These we quickly rearranged to provide ourselves with table and benches – using rugs as a tablecloth. In no time we were very snug, looking out at a drenched Ouida and the over-hanging mountains half-hidden in mist and beating rain. Surrounded as we were by chestnut woods, it seemed appropriate to start with this soup, kept hot in a large thermos.

Chestnut Soup or Zuppa di Castagne

> 1 lb (450 g) chestnuts
> 2 oz (50 g) butter
> 2 onions, chopped
> 2 carrots, sliced
> 1 piece celery, sliced
> salt
> pepper
> 1 litre stock

Score the chestnuts on their rounded side and bake in a slow oven for 10 minutes. Peel while still warm. In the butter, brown the chopped onions, carrots and celery. Add the chestnuts, stock and seasoning. Cook for about 40 minutes until the chestnuts are completely tender and have started to break up. Put the soup through a sieve. Reheat and pour into large thermos.

Chocolate Truffles or Tartuffi di Cioccolata

> ½ lb (700 g) bitter chocolate
> 1 teaspoon milk
> 2 oz (50 g) butter
> 1 egg yolk

1 oz (25 g) cocoa

Melt the chocolate and milk in a double boiler. When smooth take it off the heat and work in the butter and egg yolk. Leave the mixture for 4 or 5 hours. Form into walnut shapes and coat with cocoa powder. These must be eaten within 4 hours and kept very cool. One tablespoon coffee powder can be added to vary the flavour when melting the chocolate.

Tessa Baring

Tessa was one of the group who used to gather at Zanna's house in Tuscany. Zanna had an Italian cook who would come in and prepare food for us and we used to head off to the Italian open-air market in the morning to buy what was required that day. I remember being asked to buy the mushrooms but there were hundreds of different kinds on display and I chickened out – there was no way I was going to be responsible for buying them in case everyone died and it was all my fault! But Tessa bravely volunteered to make the selection and we all survived. We always ate lunch outside under umbrellas, everyone had their children there, it was magical.

A Breakfast Picnic
Tessa Baring

The breakfast picnic is a tradition in my husband's family, a strange race of early risers. I recommend it particularly to people with the kind of small children who wake up at five o'clock on summer mornings and are horribly bored for hours before the day is allowed to begin.

Decide on a morning which is likely to be fine, and choose a place that is remote and beautiful but not too far off a road. These picnics are most fun if shared with friends, or with cousins as we used to. Each family should bring some of the food items, and for some reason it is particularly successful if the age range spans three generations. There is a feeling of excitement and exclusiveness at being the only people about so early in the morning, and someone is sure to remark that it is the most beautiful part of the day, and that other people are very stupid to miss it.

When you arrive at your chosen site, the first task is for children to find suitable sticks to light the campfire, and it adds to the sense of adventure if some 'wild' food is found, such as wild raspberries or, later in the year, mushrooms (but only if there is someone in the group who knows what they are looking for!). My mother-in-law has memories of breakfast picnics as a child, where the speciality was an omelette made from blackbirds' eggs stolen from the nest and cooked in a doll's frying pan. (There was more countryside to go round in those days and such a thing would not have been frowned upon as it would today.) Otherwise the ingredients are those of a normal old-fashioned English breakfast: bacon, fried eggs, fried bread (preferably brown and home-made), sausages and fried tomatoes, which are essential as they freshen up the otherwise rather greasy taste. Potato cakes also go down well early in the morning; they can be prepared in advance and brought in aluminium foil ready for frying.

It is important for someone to bring a frying pan, matches, newspaper, some form of cooking fat or oil, thermos flasks of coffee and orange juice for the children, plates, knives and forks and a few rugs, as the grass will be wet with dew. Also an oven

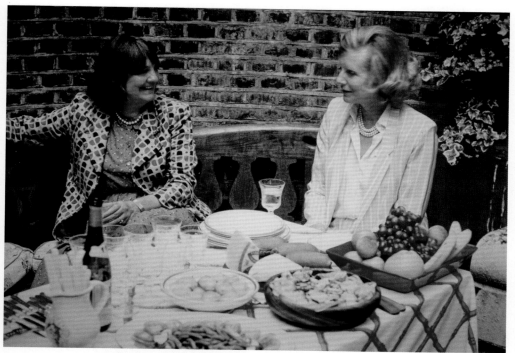

Susanna and me photographed when the original book
came out in 1983

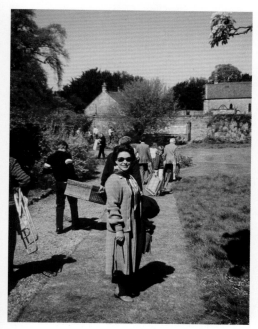
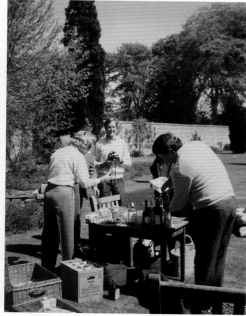

Wicker hampers bearing culinary delights at a picnic with Princess Margaret
and friends in Norfolk

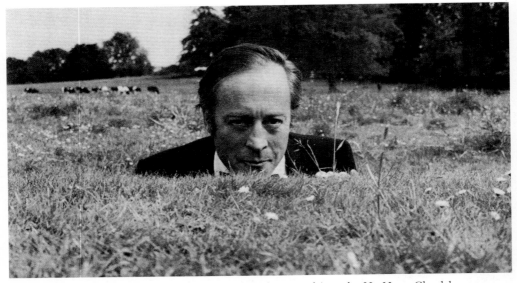

My photograph of George Christie who gamely jumped into the Ha–Ha at Glyndebourne

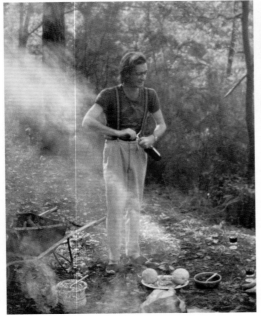

Arabella Boxer with one of
her picnics for the air

Jasper Guinness with his
'Whoopee Picnic'

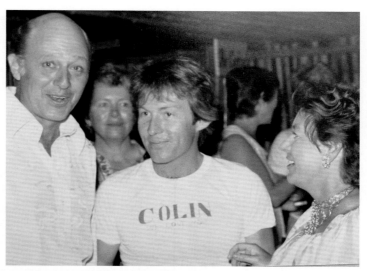

Colin, Roddy and Princess Margaret at one of the many parties on Mustique

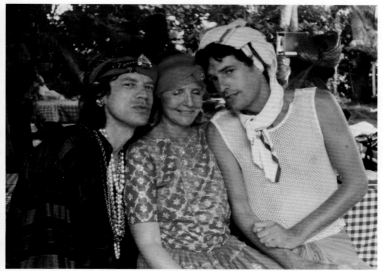

Sandwiched between Mick Jagger and Rupert Everett in the mid 80's

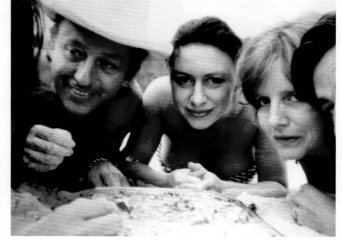

Colin, Princess Margaret and me with friends eating macaroni on Macaroni Beach in Mustique

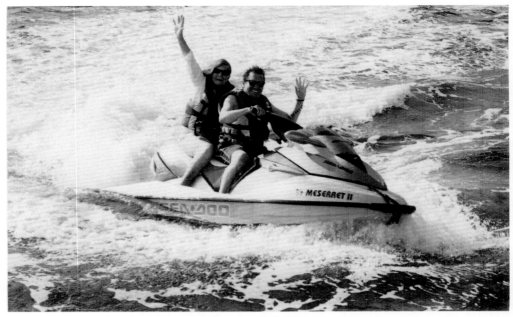

Having a ball on a jet ski with Jools Holland

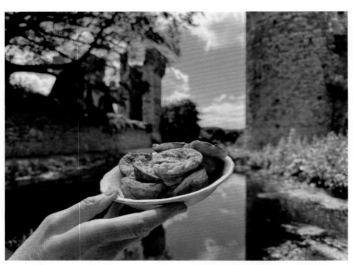

Christabel Holland's cheese muffins at Cooling Castle

With my dear friend Margaret Vyner on one of our trips to India, shopping for fabrics in Jodhpur, taken by our friend and guide Mitch Crites

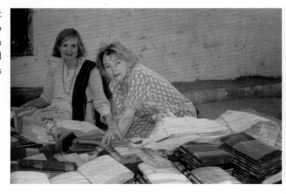

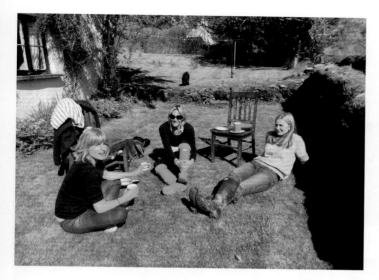

Rachel Johnson with friends Emily Maitlis
and Alice Thomson enjoying homemade
scones and tea in the garden

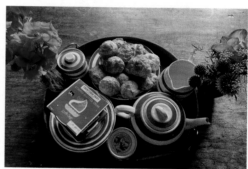

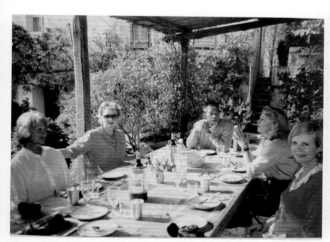

Long lunches with friends at Susanna's house in Italy

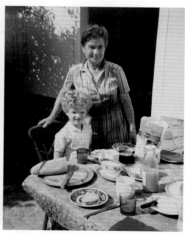

My grandson Euan with Susanna's
wonderful Italian cook Bobbi

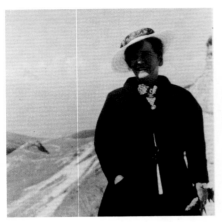

Freya Stark 'Dartmoor Picnic'

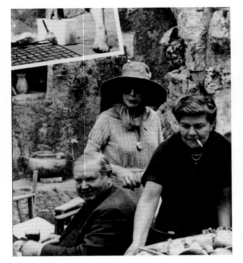

Cliff Parisi as a young boy

Evelyn Waugh, Lady Diana
Cooper and Georgina Masson
at a Picnic in Rome

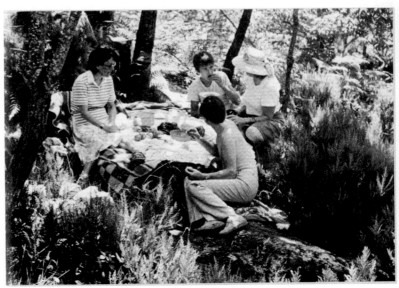

Colette and Sam
Clark picnicking
with friends

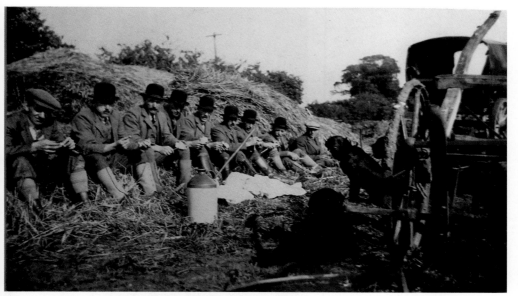

Gamekeepers at Holkham pausing for sandwiches — the bowler hat was produced
to fulfill an order from the Holkham estate for a hat to protect gamekeepers
from low hanging branches, as their top hats kept being knocked off

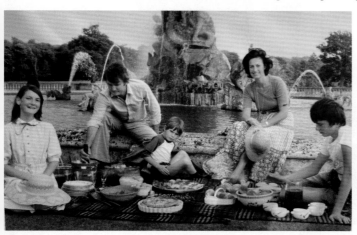

The photograph I took
of Valeria Coke with my
cousin Eddie who became
the 7th Earl of Leicester in
1994 with their children
Thomas, Laura and
Rupert by the Fountain
of Perseus and Andromeda
at Holkham, Norfolk

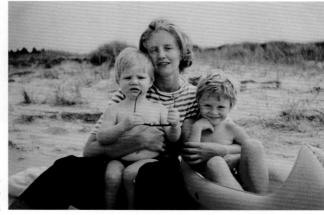

A cold day picnicking with
my boys Henry and Charlie
on the beach at Holkham

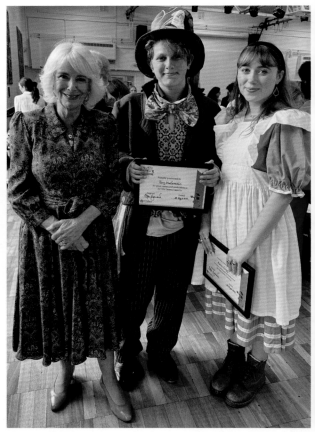

The Queen at a Poetry Together
Mad Hatter's Tea Party with
Gyles Brandreth's grandson,
Rory playing the Mad Hatter
and Hannah Grigg as Alice

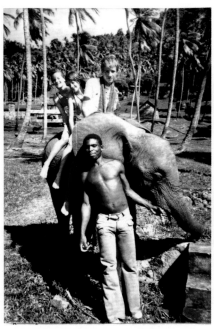

Christopher, Amy and May on Boopa the
elephant being led by Kent, sole beneficiary
of my husband's Will, on St Lucia

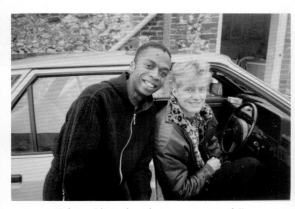

Kelvin O'Mard with Henry in Norfolk

cloth is highly recommended, and something to deal with the inevitable burnt fingers.

When the cooking has been done and you are all sitting round the fire eating the most delicious breakfast you can remember, and feeling that you are the only people in the world, it's a wonderful time for conversation.

A Scottish Recipe for Potato Cakes

2 lb (900 g) potatoes, freshly boiled in their jackets
8 oz (225 g) self-raising flour
salt

Sieve the potatoes on to a floured board, add the salt, and work in the flour by degrees, kneading lightly. Then roll out thinly, cut into rounds the size of a dinner plate, and cut each round into quarters.

Fry.

Michael Grant

Michael lived with his wife in a village near Lucca and was one of Zanna's lunch guests. Sometimes lunch would be at a long table under the fig tree in the garden where lovely ripe figs, if they hadn't been picked in time, would suddenly come plopping down onto the table, which was always laden with carafes of red and white wine and proscuitto and all manner of delicious Italian treats. But sometimes we would take a picnic into the countryside. We would borrow a donkey from the village and load it up with panniers containing the picnic and rugs and wander up into the hills. Obviously deciding where to stop was always a nightmare, 'Let's stop here,' someone would say. 'No, no. I think there's a better spot round the corner, until someone else would put their foot down and say, 'We're having it here, we're not going any further, the donkey is tired!'

Michael was a great classicist and wrote books on ancient Rome.

The Picnics of the Ancient Romans
Michael Grant

Julius Caesar followed up the celebration of his triumphs over his enemies by presiding – sweating profusely, we are told – over an open-air dinner in the public squares of Rome, attended by many tens if not hundreds of thousands of Romans, who drank a good Italian wine (Falernian) and ate, among other things, six thousand eels 'lent' to Caesar by a former political opponent. The dictator liked doing things on a large scale, and this may have been the biggest picnic of all time (picnic? Yes, according to the *Concise Oxford Dictionary*, 'pleasure party including meal out of doors').

Queen Cleopatra did not attend Caesar's party because she was not in Rome, although she arrived shortly afterwards. But if she had been at the dinner she would surely have felt like one of her royal Greek forbears, Queen Arsinoe III of Egypt, who described the picnickers at Alexandria's Feast of Flagons as 'a squalid kind of party – a mixed crowd gorging up stale food'.

Arsinoe would scarcely have been better pleased if she had attended some of the numerous similar festivals in Italy, which gave the opportunity for a good deal of fairly unrestrained eating and drinking. For example, at the annual Festival of Anna Perenna, on 15 March, people camped out with their girlfriends in tents or huts of leafy boughs or reeds, and everyone drank themselves silly. At the Hilaria, the spring festival of the Great Mother, it was the custom to offer the goddess an extraordinarily pungent, garlicky salad ('Its powerful whiff smites the nostrils,' remarked a poet), and no doubt the revellers ate the leftovers. But it was at the various Italian harvest and grape harvest celebrations that the most extensive open-air eating and drinking took place. The emperor Elagabalus once took his court to one of these wine festivals. An outdoor occasion of such a kind did not, perhaps, give him an opportunity for some of his most exquisite alleged touches of banqueting humour, such as letting down a mass of violets and other flowers from the ceiling in such quantities that the guests were smothered to death, but nevertheless we are given a lively account of the coarse talk with which he saw fit to enliven the occasion.

The shepherds in Virgil's *Eclogues* invest the idea of *déjeuner sur l'herbe* with a far more idyllic, romantic glow. However, the *Eclogues* were written not for shepherds but for highly sophisticated Romans: and such Romans, although they were prepared to read about such matters – and had (indoors) adopted the uncomfortable eastern and Greek practice of eating lying down – would mostly have endured almost any torture rather than share the discomforts of what we understand by a picnic. After all, one did not *have* to eat completely out of doors. True, as recent discoveries have shown, it was possible to eat at pleasant little dining places in a Pompeii vineyard, under a pergola. But the architects of the grand houses and villas in the area were adept at distributing a number of indoor dining rooms, suited to the various seasons, at various strategic points of the building, including summer rooms that were *very nearly* out of doors, opening alluringly upon elegant gardens (not upon untutored nature, except for the occasional seascape). A rich, fastidious late Roman, Sidonius Apollinaris, describes such a room, though while gushing about the view he also does not fail to mention a 'glittering sideboard' – and a staircase especially designed to avoid the slightest physical exertion.

However, an earlier Roman, Pliny the Younger, at his country house on the borders of Tuscany and Umbria, actually entertained in his garden, completely al fresco, beside a marble basin filled with water: 'The preliminaries and main dishes for dinner are placed on the edge of the basin, while the lighter ones float about in vessels shaped like birds or little boats.' (Presumably slaves stood around with rakes to pull them in.) For whenever Romans could be lured outside to eat in the open air, they rather liked to have a watery setting. In the reign of Claudius, for example, a lot of people dined out to help the emperor celebrate the opening of a channel between a lake and a river. But the water overflowed, the picnickers got the shock of their lives, and the sponsor of the project ran into trouble.

More successful, in its way, was a rather unusual outdoor party given by Nero's appalling adviser Tigellinus on an artificial lake (or, according to another account, in a theatre specially flooded for the purpose). Tacitus reported it thus:

> The entertainment took place on a raft, towed about by other vessels, with gold and ivory fittings. Their gay oarsmen were assorted according to age and speciality. Tigellinus had also collected birds and animals from remote countries, and even the creatures of the ocean. On the quays were brothels stocked with high-ranking ladies. Opposite them could be seen naked prostitutes, indecently posturing and gesturing. At nightfall, the woods and houses nearby echoed with singing and blazed with lights...

The Romans, if they had to picnic, also liked to use grottoes or caves for the purpose. Some garden dining rooms at Pompeii are artfully designed to look as if that was what they were. But you could also eat in real caves. The Emperor Tiberius did this on one occasion, with results even more disastrous than those which usually attend picnics: a fall of rock occurred that would have killed him, if his friend Sejanus had not interposed his body as a shield – an action that proved beneficial to his future career.

The wine drunk at these out-of-door meals, or indeed at any Roman party, was quite likely to include a tincture not only of resin (as in Greece today) or lime or even ashes (to counteract acidity) but also salt, almonds or goats' milk (to add maturity and flavour); and it was always possible that a red-hot iron had been dipped in it as well, for the same purpose. One also wonders, scanning the pages of Petronius' *Dinner of Trimalchio* and the scarcely less startling *Cookery Book of Apicius*, whether any of the more peculiar dishes described in these works made their appearance at a Roman picnic. Certainly, whatever meat or fish was provided, it would not have been served in any simple form (this elaborateness was no trouble to a Roman cook, who habitually produced his results, however complicated, on mobile, portable, sometimes unroofed charcoal stoves and tripods and gridirons).

Before sewing up your roast dormouse, for example, you ought to stuff it with minced pork and pound it with pepper, pine kernels, asafoetida or 'stinking mastic' (resinous gum smelling of garlic) and *liquamen*. *Liquamen* was the basis of *garum*, one of the very sharp sauces with which the Romans liked to drench every dish, partly because things went bad so quickly. According to one of its recipes, *garum* consisted basically of the chopped, pounded and crushed entrails of sprats and sardines, beaten into a fermented pulp (this is *liquamen*), which was left to evaporate for six weeks and then filtered through a perforated basket into a receptacle. The poet Martial, casting around for words to describe a friend's bad breath, can only remark that it would make even the strongest scent stink like *garum*; here, at least, is one argument in favour of outdoor picnics.

Martial speaks of fans of peacock feathers to keep flies away. But to the Emperor Domitian the flies that are always such a bore at picnics might actually have been an incentive to join in, because he liked having them around, amusing himself by catching them and cutting them to pieces with a specially sharpened metal pen. However, a picnic would not have been a possible milieu for his well-known party joke – serving the petrified senators who were his guests with black dishes and miniature gravestones inscribed with their names – because this inimitably humorous prank required indoor accommodation, with ceiling, walls and floor painted an equally funereal black. However, the insertion of Domitian into a discussion of picnics is probably irrelevant, since that emperor is even less likely than most other prominent Romans ever to have gone on one – and certainly not on a water picnic, since we are told that, although he enjoyed solitary walks, there were certain outdoor noises, notably the splash of oars, that he found intolerably irritating.

Hugh Honour

Zanna met Hugh Honour and his partner John Fleming when she was a teenager living in Italy and, she said, they sort of adopted her, as you might a stray dog. Hugh was a world-renowned art historian who, together with John, wrote the famous *World History of Art*. They lived in a villa called Villa Marchio just outside Lucca, and Zanna ended up buying her house near them. It was always wonderful going there as they were interesting, and excellent conversationalists, but they were pretty eccentric and it wasn't the cleanest house. They had a rather ancient and slow help they called Speedy who knocked us up food, and you tried not to think about the mice you'd seen running around in the kitchen as you ate the pasta she'd prepared. Zanna's husband Nicholas had also been a friend of Hugh's at Cambridge so that helped to cement the friendship further, and she ended up writing a memoir about them. Hugh's picnic is wonderfully literary, based on the novel *Marius the Epicurean* by Walter Pater, and I think conjures up a sense of all the literary figures who travelled through that part of the world.

A White Picnic
Hugh Honour

My ideal of a perfect picnic belongs to the 1950s, not later or earlier. Childhood treats were all very well in a Betjemanesque way. I too 'used to picnic where the thrift/grew deep and tufted to the edge'. But today, driving along the autoroute south of Lyon, I read the signs '*Pique-nique jeux d'enfants*' as a warning rather than an invitation – though the phrase does have a ring of Verlaine about it. Most of my picnics nowadays are eaten on journeys across Europe by road. The company, limited to a maximum of four, is always that of old friends. The food, bought in the town where we spent the previous night, is also well tried – in Italy cold roast suckling pig and the best baked bread to be found anywhere in Europe now (much better than in France where it used to be so delicious), in Spain strongly flavoured ham, in Germany liver sausage, in France a selection of pâtés and galantines and *oeufs en gêlée*. These picnics are no more than brief affairs, however, intervals in a long drive, and never quite match up to my or any other ideal. The *oeufs en gêlée* too often prove to be hard-boiled, not *mollets*. The place where we stop attracts others almost immediately, and seldom seems in retrospect as congenial as the one we had passed only a few minutes earlier or the one we noticed soon afterwards.

For me the perfect picnic must be incidental, just part of a journey through country beautiful in itself and, if possible, with literary or historical associations as well. My ideal picnic began to form twenty-five years or so ago when I lived in Percy Lubbock's villa, Gli Scafari, near Lerici – a house of cool marmorial beauty perched on a rocky promontory above the crystalline blue of the still unpolluted Mediterranean, with a wide view of distant islands and the little fishing village of Porto Venere on the northern arm of the Gulf of La Spezia. The air was drowsy with literary associations. Percy himself had been at Cambridge with E.M. Forster – 'Poor old Morgan,' as he often remarked, 'he never knew quite the "right" people.' Later he had been a disciple of Henry James, whose voice and conversation he could mimic when well-primed after dinner and, for a time, one of Edith Wharton's 'young men' – though he was banished from her little court when he married another wealthy cosmopolitan blue-stocking. Only a few hundred yards away D.H. Lawrence had spent the winter of 1913–14 in a four-room pink cottage on the shore of 'a little tiny bay half shut in by rocks, and smothered by olive woods that slope down swiftly'. Beneath Gli Scafari there was a huge, arching grotto, one of those, we liked to think, that Shelley had explored by boat during the last weeks of his life when he lived at San Terenzo on the other side of Lerici. Byron, on his way from Pisa to Genoa in October 1823, stopped at Lerici for a few nights and made himself ill by swimming far out to sea with Trelawny and eating a large dinner while treading water – one of the most bizarre picnics on record. Next year he was to sail along the same coast on his last voyage, to Missolonghi. But, as we watched from the loggia the passage of shipping out at sea or making for harbour at La Spezia or Porto Venere, there was another figure from the past who haunted our imaginations – Walter Pater.

I had first read *Marius the Epicurean* at school and thought it, as did the young Max Beerbohm, a marvellous 'tale of adventure, quite as fascinating as *Midshipman Easy*, and far less hard to understand because there were no nautical terms in it'. At Lerici I found myself near Marius's country. His villa, White Nights, was among the hills a few miles inland. Pater wrote that 'the traveller, descending from the slopes of Luna even as he got his first view of the "Port-of-Venus" would pause by the way, to read the face, as it were, of so beautiful a dwelling place, lying away from the white road, at the point where it began to descend somewhat steeply to the marshland below'. Each of the windows of Marius's tower chamber framed a landscape, 'the pallid crags of Carrara, like wildly twisted snowdrifts above the purple heath; the distant harbour with its freight of white marble going to sea; the lighthouse temple of "Venus Speciosa" on its dark head-land, amid the long-drawn curves of white breakers'. The description is circumstantial enough to suggest that Pater, who could have passed this way when he went to Pisa, had a particular spot in mind. To find it became the object of many excursions and picnics.

Near the little village of Fosdinovo there are several places which almost match Pater's description. From there one can see the Carrara mountains, uncannily like those in the background to the *Mona Lisa*, which inspired one of Pater's over-familiar purple passages. Glimpses may be caught of an ancient amphi-theatre among vineyards, all that remains above ground of the city of Luni from which Carrara marble was exported throughout the Roman Empire. But to find a point from which Porto Venere can also be seen is difficult. I never succeeded in locating it. If found, this would be the place for the perfect, the truly Epicurean picnic.

Special food would, of course, be eaten, food of a preciosity to suit the occasion and predominantly white. We should begin with fish, cold fillets of sole or shelled scampi and a very pale mayon-naise. Then there might be chicken breasts or quails, stuffed with white truffles and wrapped in the most delicately streaked bacon, lightly fried, accompanied by a white salad such as is sometimes served in Italy in early spring – raw fennel cut into little strips, celery, chicory and paper-thin flakes of turnip sprinkled over with violet flowers to delight both eye and palate. To end we should have a cheese mousse of the type the cook at Gli Scafari used to prepare, firm yet crumbly to the fork and wonderfully light, composed mainly of ricotta (ewe's milk cheese) but according to a recipe I have never been able to trace. We should drink a dry white wine, Verdicchio from the Marche. And afterwards, until the sun sinks into the sea, we would read Pater's 'oft-read tale' again, from the edition printed on handmade paper with title page designed by Herbert Horne, the biographer of Botticelli and one of the last Anglo-Italians of whom Pater might have wholly approved. But the place has not been, and may never be, found. So my perfect picnic remains an untarnished ideal – forever cold and still to be enjoyed.

William Weaver

William was a friend of Zanna's. He was an English translator of modern Italian literature and part of the Italian clan who also had a house in Tuscany, as he describes in this picnic.

A Spontini Picnic
William Weaver

I love music and I love food. Normally I do not enjoy them together. I have walked out of restaurants in protest (ineffectual, I fear) against their muzak or their pianist; I have asked hostesses to turn off the radio or the gramophone; and it is years since I have picnicked on a beach, because the invasion of transistors has succeeded in spoiling that pleasure. So naturally, on a picnic, I would ban any kind of music, reproduced or live (the sight of a guitar immediately suggests the drawl of folk songs and, just as immediately, provokes anticipatory indigestion).

Still, I must admit that one of the most enjoyable al frescos I have had was, in fact, a musical evening on my own terrace. It was several years ago, and Italian Radio was broadcasting *Agnes von Hohenstausen*, a rarely performed opera by Spontini, starring Monserrat Caballe. I learned about the broadcast only after I had invited a few friends to supper.

Fortunately the guests were all music lovers and, in fact, as eager to hear the opera as I was. The radio, however, and the taping equipment were in my cluttered study, which was not the ideal room for dining in. But just outside the study window there is a terrace, with a pergola of grapevines, a table and some chairs. The loudspeakers in the study could be shifted to the window, so that they could be heard by listeners on the terrace. The food, which was cold, had been prepared in the afternoon. It was placed on the table so that guests could help themselves, and they were asked to be on hand a good half hour before the opera was to begin. So we had time for a glass of wine. After the music started, the only noise was an occasional gurgle of more wine being poured and perhaps one or two clanks of dropped cutlery. There were long intervals between the acts, so we could enjoy more talk. And then, when it was over, we had a final glass and exchanged impressions.

We ate one of the many Italian kinds of cold pasta (which I know sounds revolting to the Anglo-Saxon, but is actually delicious), a cold *frittata* – by cold I mean room temperature – and a salad and cheeses and fruit (perhaps grapes from above our heads). And, to be sure, Spontini. Just the right composer for a Tuscan picnic. Verdi would have demanded our total attention, distracting us from the food; and perhaps another composer – I'll name no names – would not have prevented us from talking.

Cold Chitarrucci

>2 lb (900 g) tomatoes
>I cup of basil and marjoram, finely chopped
>salt, pepper
>olive oil
>I lb (450 g) pasta (if possible chitarrucci – the
>   squared-off fine spaghetti)

Prepare the sauce one day before. Peel, seed and chop the tomatoes. Put in a bowl and add the chopped marjoram, basil, plenty of salt and pepper. Leave it to sweat. Drain. Add the oil.

Next day, cook the pasta in the ordinary way. Cool by tossing well in the sauce.

Frittata

>small onion
>I tablespoon olive oil
>2 large tomatoes, peeled and chopped
>I lb (450 g) courgettes, chopped
>8 eggs
>I tablespoon grated Parmesan
>I tablespoon flour
>salt, pepper
>6–7 leaves basil, chopped
>6–7 leaves celery, chopped

Chop the onion and fry gently in the oil. Add the tomatoes and courgettes. Cook on a medium heat for about 20 minutes in a frying pan. Mix the eggs with the cheese, flour, salt and pepper.

When the courgettes and tomatoes are cooked, take them off the heat and add to the egg mixture. Stir quickly. Add the basil and celery leaves. Put back on a medium heat and cook on both sides, turning with the help of a plate. Cool. If the frittata breaks, beat another egg and use for repair work.

John Chancellor

Zanna's brother, John Chancellor, wrote about a country church-yard picnic for us. His daughter Anna Chancellor is an actress who is perhaps best known for playing Duckface in *Four Weddings and a Funeral*.

A Country Churchyard Picnic
John Chancellor

It might be thought that a churchyard is a macabre venue for a picnic. Picnics are, after all, supposed to be cheerful occasions, when you are not expected to entertain thoughts of death. The most fearless and unimaginative of us might hesitate before spreading the contents of a picnic basket upon a tombstone. Who knows how its ghostly occupant would take it?

Some churchyards are more inviting than others. An example of a friendly churchyard is that in the village of Selborne in Hampshire, the home of the immortal Gilbert White. It is

155

universally agreed that Gilbert White has given delight to generations; but who he was and the exact nature of this 'delight' is
known to very few. Nevertheless the book, upon which rests
his unshakeable yet elusive fame, has been reprinted almost every
year since it was published in 1789, with the title *The Natural
History and Antiquities of Selborne.*

The opportunity offered itself one Sunday in September to
make an expedition to Selborne. My son was at school at
Winchester, where once or twice a term I took him out. These
occasions were pleasant enough, but shockingly expensive. I
learned there that it was not only in London that the price of
a meal in a restaurant was scandalous. Admittedly, he did not
make a point of going for the cheaper items, and I was amazed
at the number of gin and tonics that he managed to drink. It
was my sister who, horrified at seeing me pay over a vast sum
for one of these Winchester meals (two of her daughters were
there also), insisted that the next time we took the boy out, it
would be a picnic or nothing.

So we found ourselves on that Sunday in September making
our way from Winchester to Selborne. All the members of the
party were united by the haziness of their knowledge as to who
or what Gilbert White was. My son, furthermore, had the temerity
to doubt the extent of the delight that White had given later
generations. These doubts were, alas, to intensify as the day went
on.

We passed through many a charming village before reaching
our destination. This was the moment to prepare my captive
companions for the great experience ahead of them, to acquaint
them with the 'genius' of Gilbert White. On that very week, two
hundred years earlier, he had made these observations in his
journal:

Black snails lie out, and copulate. Vast swagging clouds...
red-breasts feed on elderberries, enter rooms, and spoil the
furniture... women make poor wages in their hop-picking.
Housed all my potatoes, and tied up my endives... swallows
hawking about very briskly in all the moderate rain... then
we called loudly thro' the speaking trumpet to Timothy
(his tortoise), he does not seem to regard the noise.

There were few swagging clouds on that particular Sunday, and
we lacked the acuteness of observation to notice how many black
snails were copulating.

The entries in his journal explain perhaps why Gilbert White
occupies so firm a place in the heart of the normal, wholesome
Englishman. The English like their heroes to be simple and un-
affected, to be stay-at-home and unambitious, and to be disinterested
in the activities they pursue, thinking of neither gain nor fame.
Gilbert White was all these things. He spent his whole life in the
same house at Selborne; he never aspired to be more than a curate,
and he recorded meticulously, day after day, what he saw happening
in the countryside around him. All this he had put down in *Selborne*,
that little-read classic of English literature, a copy of which I had
not forgotten to bring on this expedition. It was my plan to read
aloud during our picnic one or two of its imperishable passages.

We entered the village, at the end of which we came to
Selborne church and churchyard, described by White as 'very
scanty... such a mass of mortality that no person can be interred
there without disturbing or displacing the bones of his ancestors'.
We squeezed ourselves between several tombstones, very near
the splendid yew tree with an enormous girth which White
measured every year in his meticulous and disinterested way. He
also observed that it was a male tree.

Whilst the others tucked in, I expatiated on the greatness and modesty of Gilbert White and began to read aloud from the famous book. Maybe I chose one of the less stimulating passages – it was about the diversity of soils in the district – or maybe the solemnity of the occasion overcame them, or maybe it was my sister's delicious food, but when I looked up my companions were, one and all, dozing among the tombstones.

Cauliflower Salad

> 1–2 cauliflowers
> salt
> pepper
> cayenne
> 2 eggs
> 1 teaspoon mixed mustard
> 1 oz (25 g) sugar
> 1 oz (25 g) butter
> 4 tablespoons milk
> 3 tablespoons vinegar

Cook the cauliflowers in boiling salted water. Don't overcook – let them retain a little 'bite'. Then leave them in a colander to drain. Divide into small florets and place in a salad bowl. Season well with pepper, salt and cayenne and make the following sauce.

Beat the eggs in a double boiler. Add a level teaspoon of salt, the mustard, sugar, butter, milk and vinegar. Stir over boiling water till it thickens. Then pour over the salad, or bottle and pour over before it is served.

Mint Lemonade

> 4 large lemons
> 8 oz (225 g) sugar
> 1 handful fresh mint
> ice cubes
> 4 bottles ginger ale

Squeeze the lemons and strain the juice. Add the sugar and stir until dissolved. Put into a chilled thermos with mint and some ice cubes. Pack the chilled ginger ale separately in an insulated bag and add just before serving.

Clara Johnston

Clara and I share a love of India. She is Zanna's daughter, who I've known forever. Like lots of young people she travelled in India and knew Bubbles who was the Maharaja of Jaipur. I knew Bubbles too. He gained that nickname apparently from all the champagne that was drunk to celebrate his birth as he was the first male heir to be born to the Maharaja of Jaipur for generations.

A Maharaja's Picnic Tea
Clara Johnston

One afternoon when nothing much was happening in the City Palace, Bubbles, the Maharaja of Jaipur, decided to take us to see his father's old shooting lodge about fifteen miles outside Jaipur. A picnic was prepared and put into the back of the American jeep along with Clare Steel, the uniformed bodyguard, and myself.

In Jaipur, Bubbles is still thought of as the king and those who recognised the T-shirted driver clasped their hands together and bowed as we drove by.

Across a plain, along a thin, straight road, we passed ox-drawn carts brimming with hay and people and stopped for a moment at a lake which stretched for miles without so much as a ripple on its polished surface.

Later the land became hillier and the vegetation more dense. Just before we reached a great dam, Bubbles turned down a driveway lined with rambling shrubs. At the gate two octogenarian servants tumbled down the steps to greet us, as if our arrival had awoken them from a deep sleep.

The house had not been visited for some time and smelled of dust and mothballs. Built in the thirties, it looked like an Italian villa with pastel yellow stuccoed walls, balconies, shuttered windows and a loggia. The house had been used as a shooting lodge for the surrounding area and the hall was lined with stuffed tigers, bears and lions.

Below the front of the house was a stone hideout with square peepholes. Years ago the sport was to tie a bull to the hideout and wait for a tiger to approach. Those who were brave enough watched the event from within, while the rest watched safely from the house.

We sat, unthreatened by tigers, in the garden and the aged servants spread a white linen tablecloth over a round wooden table in the centre of the lawn. The picnic, a mixture of traditional English sandwiches and Indian spices, was spread out on the table by the bodyguard: cucumber sandwiches, spiced chicken, poppadoms, curd raitas and sweets. We drank tea out of a thermos – a picnic item inherited from the English – and watched the sun set over the lake.

Curd (Yoghurt) Raitas

> 1 pint (450 ml) plain yoghurt
> juice of half a lemon
> 2 cloves of garlic (crushed)
> chopped mint leaves
> finely chopped fresh green chilli

Pour the yoghurt into a bowl and beat in the rest of the ingredients. For variations you can add to taste: 1 teaspoon paprika, a pinch of cayenne, a pinch of coriander, coriander leaves or a pinch of cumin. Other ingredients such as raisins, sultanas, sliced bananas, grated carrots, chopped nuts or diced boiled new potatoes can be added. You can make it into a salad by adding raw vegetables.

Poppadoms

Some of the ingredients for poppadoms are not available in England so I have adapted it slightly.

> 3–4 tablespoons flour
> salt
> caraway seeds
> a little mild paprika
> cream or milk

Season the flour with salt and add caraway seeds and red pepper. Mix with cream or milk to a stiff paste. Knead well, roll out a little, cut into cubes of 1–1½ inches (2½–3¾ cm) diameter. Take each cube, roll it and fold it and roll it again, finally beating it with a rolling pin until it is paper thin and the size of a side plate. Prick each slice all over with a fork, lay on a greased and floured baking sheet and bake for three minutes or so in a very hot oven. The poppadoms should blister and be very thin and crisp.

Patrick Leigh Fermor

Patrick Leigh Fermor was terribly good looking, rather a Byronesque character, and I think we were all secretly a bit in love with him. In addition to cutting an extremely glamorous figure as a writer and explorer he was also very charming. He had been in the Special Operations Executive in Crete during the second world war and my father-in-law, who was in charge of the SOE, told me how incredibly brave Patrick was. He organised resistance to the occupation on the island and oversaw the capturing and expulsion of the German commander there. He also wrote about the islands of the West Indies and came to Mustique during the very early days when there was no electricity or running water, but of course he was used to all of that and didn't mind a bit.

The Dales of Moldavia
Patrick Leigh Fermor

It may be rash to intrude this Rumanian feast where so many literary cornucopias are pouring their bounty; for it is the day and the occasion that single out this one, and shadow steals over substance here and veils every memory of what there actually was to eat. (We had set out to pick mushrooms, but they were for dinner.)

The picnic baskets may have contained all sorts of Moldowalkechian wonders – *sarmali* wrapped in vine leaves, fragrant *mititei*, chicken croquettes as light as feathers, a *sterlet* from the Pruth, perhaps, or even, and by the ladleful, wonderful Black Sea caviar from Vâlcov in the Danube delta, on the fringes of Bessarabia; turkey in aspic, almost certainly. Apart from fine indigenous cooking this country seemed to be the meeting place of all that was most delicious in old Russia, Poland, Hungary, Mitteleuropa, France, the Balkans and the Levant. The picnic would have been more likely to start with fierce Moldavian *raki* than with a milder southern *tzuica* of distilled plums; excellent white and red wines, stored in tortuous catacombs, would have accompanied it throughout.

The point of departure was an old and many-legended Cantacuzene country house with inhabitants of indescribable charm. It lay at the heart of a once large but now much reduced estate in High Moldavia, and the time was September 1939. Apart from the two sisters who were our hostesses and their family, there was also, for the summer, Prince Matila Ghyka and three other young English people. (I had become a sort of fixture.) Matila Ghyka, traveller, diplomat, well-known writer on aesthetics – *Le Nombre d'Or, Sortilèges du Verbe*, etc. – and a gastronome famous for his encyclopaedic approach to life, would certainly have had a hand in the planning.

It was a summer of unparalleled beauty and remoteness, but the months passed too fast; the crops were in and the storks were gathering before heading south; and suddenly, not unannounced, the evil omens had begun to multiply quickly, until all seemed black. To forget and exorcise for a day the growing assembly of trouble we set off, on 2 September, to pick those mushrooms in a wood about ten miles away, some of us in an old open carriage, some on horseback; through the vineyards where the grapes were almost ready to be harvested and pressed, and out into the open country. The clearings in the wood, when we arrived, were studded with our quarry. Alighting and dismounting, we scattered in a competitive frenzy, reassembling soon with our baskets full to the brim. In the glade of this mysterious wood, with the tethered horses grazing and swishing their tails under the oak branches, the picnic spun itself out. Soon it was late afternoon and all the bottles were empty and the old Polish coachman was fidgeting the horses back into the shafts and fastening the traces. The ones on horseback set off by a different way. We raced each other across the mown slopes of the vast hayfields and galloped in noisy and wine-sprung zigzags through the ricks and down a wide valley and up again through another oak spinney to the road where the carriage, trailing a long plume of dust, was trotting more sedately home, and reined in alongside.

The track followed the crest of a high ridge with the dales of Moldavia flowing away on the either hand. We were moving through illimitable sweeps of still air. Touched with pink on their undersides by the declining sun, which also combed the tall stubble with gold, one or two shoals of mackerel cloud hung motionless in the enormous sky. Whale-shaped shadows expanded along the valleys below, and the spinneys were sending long loops of shade downhill.

The air was so still that the smoke from Matila Ghyka's cigar hung in a riband in the wake of our cavalcade; and how clearly the bells of the flocks, which were streaming down in haloes of golden dust to the wells and the brushwood folds a few ravines away, floated to our ears. Homing peasants waved their hats in greeting, and someone out of sight was singing one of those beautiful and rather forlorn country songs they call a *doina*. A blurred line along the sky a league away marked the itinerary of the deserting storks. Those in the carriage below were snowed under by picnic things and mushroom baskets and bunches of anemones picked in the wood. It was a moment of peace and tranquillity and we rode on in silence towards the still far-off samovar and the oil lamps and heaven knew what bad news. The silence was suddenly broken by an eager exclamation from Matila.

'Oh look!' he cried. One hand steadied the basket of mushrooms on his lap, the other pointed at the sky into which he was peering. High overhead some waterbirds, astray from the delta, perhaps, or from some nearby fen, were flying in a phalanx. (I shall have to improvise names and details here, for precise memory and ornithological knowledge both fail me. But the gist and the spirit are exact.)

'Yes,' he said, 'it's rather rare; the *Xiphorhyncus paludinensis minor*, the *glaivionette*, or Lesser Swamp Swordbill – *Wendischer Schwertvogel* in German, *glodnic* in Moldavian dialect; I believe the Wallachians call it *spadună de baltă*. Varieties are dotted about all over the world but always in very small numbers. They live in floating nests and have a very shrill ascending note in the mating season.' He whistled softly once or twice. 'Their eggs are a ravishing colour, a lovely lapis lazuli with little primrose speckles. They have been identified with the Stymphalian birds that Hercules killed, and there's a mention of them in Lucian's *Dialogues* and in Pliny the Elder, and I think in Oppian... The ancient Nubians revered them as minor gods and there's supposed to be one on a bas-relief at Cyrene; there's certainly a flight of them in the background of a *Journey of the Magi* by Sassetta – he probably saw them in the reeds of Lake Trasimene, where they still breed; and the chiefs of two tribes on the Zambezi wear robes of their tail feathers for the new moon ceremonies. Some people,' he continued, with a slight change of key, 'find them too fishy. It's not true, as I learnt years ago near Bordeaux. On a spit, over a very slow fire – of hornbeam twigs, if possible – with frequent basting and plenty of saffron, *glaivionette à la landaise* can be delicious... Alas: I've only eaten it once...'

His dark eyes, a-kindle with memory, watched the birds out of sight across the dying sky, and we all burst out laughing. The cosmic approach... It had been a happy day, as we had hoped, and it had to last us for a long time, for the next day's news scattered this little society for ever.

Penelope Chetwode

Penelope and my aunt Sylvia used to head off to Italy and Spain on adventures with ponies. Penelope was a travel writer and my aunt's best friend who used to come up to Norfolk to stay. I remember Sylvia telling me that on the first of their trips, before the ponies, they headed off to Rome in a Mini Minor. My aunt asked Penelope where she had booked for them to stay — certain that there was some lovely little hotel or guest house to look forward to — whereupon Penelope told her she must be quite mad, that she never stayed in hotels and had a tent in the back of the car. They spent ages putting up this awful wonky tent and Penelope got out a little stove to boil something up to eat; it was not what my aunt had in mind, she liked a comfortable bed. After two or three days my aunt said she was taking herself off to an hotel whether Penelope wanted to go with her or not! Despite this unpromising start, Sylvia carried on travelling with her and they loved exploring together. Penelope was married to the poet John Betjeman but after a while they separated and he lived with Lady Elizabeth Cavendish in London, who was responsible for introducing

Princess Margaret to Tony Armstrong-Jones, whilst Penelope lived near Hay-on-Wye.

Suprême de Volaille with St George in Cappadocia
Penelope Chetwode

After an interval of thirty years, I returned to India in 1963 by the overland route. A young doctor friend bought a second-hand Volkswagen Dormobile from a farmer near Wantage and proceeded to make a green roll-up tent on his mother's sewing machine – which has never worked since. The tent, fixed to the roof of the vehicle, could be unrolled and set up as a roomy lean-to shelter within five minutes of arriving at any campsite. The cooking was done in it on two primus stoves, and there was room for three people to sleep on the ground while two of us slept in the Dormobile.

In those far-off days petrol cost the equivalent of 20p a gallon, and by the time we reached Delhi the captain (as we called the doctor) calculated he had spent about £100 on it after driving some five to six thousand miles. We took two months to complete the journey since we wanted to do as much sightseeing as possible in Turkey and Iran, and foodwise our life was one great picnic as we had all our meals *al fresco* except when we spent a few nights in great cities like Istanbul, Ankara and Teheran.

The cooking was done on the primus stoves because the captain had been informed that gas cylinders were unobtainable in many places on our route, and that wood was virtually non-existent throughout Turkey and Iran. I well remember meeting two Swiss boys who were travelling to India on a Vespa and had planned to buy food on their way and cook it on bonfires. Since there was no wood lying about in the treeless wilds of Anatolia they were almost starving – they had to fill themselves up in restaurants in the towns they came through and had hardly any money left.

Primus stoves are so fierce that the ideal pot to use on them is a pressure cooker. I used to cook our supper in one every night, so that we could usually eat within an hour of setting up camp. We eventually got rather bored with the mutton we bought in the Turkish bazaars and thought that chicken would be a welcome change. Accordingly when we came to a small town called Nevsehir, crowned by an Ottoman fortress, we tried to make some men understand that we wanted to buy poultry, but they took us to the police station! There we began to flap our arms up and down and cluck loudly, and everyone laughed and understood perfectly what we wanted. We were taken to a large farmyard on the outskirts of the town where a number of scrawny little cockerels and hens were scratching around. With the permission of the farmer (using the language of gesticulation) we caught two. Now having had a poultry farm, I had learnt the quickest and most humane way to kill chickens. I dispatched the pair by dislocating their heads from the necks, handed one to the captain and advised him to pluck it at once while I did the other, as they are so much easier to feather when they are still warm. Disgruntled murmurs immediately arose from the many onlookers who had accompanied us out of the town, and I suddenly realised the reason. I had let no blood, and Muslims as well as Jews insist on this being done, so we quickly paid for the birds, beat a hasty retreat into the Dormobile, and drove off to Urgup, some twelve miles further on, plucking as we went.

We now found ourselves in the most extraordinary landscape in the middle of Cappadocia: for about twenty miles through a valley erosion has left huge cones about a hundred feet high, some of which look like decaying teeth, others like towers, needles and pyramids formed of ashes and rock. These are collectively known as the Rock-cut Monasteries of Cappadocia because, during the seventh and eighth centuries, whole communities of Christians settled in the area and cut out of the rock churches and monasteries which they decorated with wall paintings in the provincial Byzantine style. It was very rewarding to come across many renderings of St George killing his dragon, as he is traditionally believed to have come from this part of Turkey.

We found a wonderful campsite at the head of the valley in a small sandy field with superb views and a large rock wall to one side over which we hung our bedding to dry during the day. We became so enthralled exploring the churches and monasteries and anchorites' cells that we ended up spending three nights there.

But to return to the supper picnic on the evening of our arrival. I decided to prepare a *suprême de volaille* by cooking the elderly, tough little chickens in the pressure cooker, and the rice in an open saucepan on the other stove. After half an hour I wanted to let the pressure down quickly so that I could get on with making the sauce out of the stock. In the centre of a pressure cooker is a weight; when you lift it off it makes a violent hissing sound which always terrifies me, so I asked the captain if he dared do it. He immediately removed not just the weight but the whole lid, whereupon the cooked birds leaped high into the air and disappeared in the inky blackness of a moonless night!

We were all mad with disappointment at being thus deprived of what had promised to be one of the most gastronomically exciting picnics of our journey, but we did not give up hope. For the next twenty minutes we all crawled about on our hands and knees and, with the aid of two very feeble torches, we finally ran them to earth – literally, for they were covered with the dusty grey soil of the region. Undaunted, we plunged them into a bucket of water and, while the girls washed and jointed them, I made a delicious *sauce suprême* with fat, flour, the stock, a little dried milk powder, and the juice of half a small lemon. I did not add the extra refinement of egg yolks as our egg supply was low and we needed them for breakfast.

We finally sat down in a circle round our old hurricane lamp to a scrumptious meal of chicken and rice and sauce and green beans that we had bought in the market at Nevsehir, followed by delicious little white grapes, and all washed down by unadulterated spring water. Water in Turkey is famous for its excellence and the Turks, who are forbidden wine by their religion, talk rapturously of the water of various regions as others would of the wines in France or Italy.

I think our Cappadocian chicken picnic was the best we had on the whole trip, all the more for being so hard won. I was also very proud of the jam roly-poly I made when we were allowed to camp in the harem of Xerxes in Persepolis but that, as Kipling would say, is another story.

Freya Stark

There is quite a streak of adventure running through some of the contributors to this book. I first met the explorer Freya Stark when we were both staying with the Astors at Clivedon. I told her how much she reminded me of one of my ancestors, Jane Digby, whereupon Freya told me that she knew all about Jane whom she saw as a role model. Jane Digby had been born at Holkham at the beginning of the nineteenth century to Admiral Sir Henry Digby and Lady Jane Elizabeth Coke. She had an extraordinary life and was married four times, in relationships which took her to Germany and Greece where for a while she had an affair with the Thessalian general during the Greek War of Independence. She died in Damascus in 1881 after a long and happy marriage to Sheik Medjuel el Mezrab who was twenty years her junior. I think Jane provided a connection between Freya and I, whom I got to know quite well. I visited her once for lunch at her house in Asola in northern Italy. She was quite small and had had a terrible accident when she was young in a factory in Italy when her hair had been caught in a machine, tearing her scalp and ripping her right ear off. As a result she often wore hats to cover her scars or wore her hair draped over to one side. She was wonderful and such an interesting person to have known.

Dartmoor Picnic
Freya Stark

The best picnics I have known were taken during solitary rides about Dartmoor, on the back of one or other of two home-bred, intelligent animals who would stand still in the heather while I got on or off. When we felt hungry, we would find a flat granite stone and I would sit and undo the sandwiches that Cook had prepared, while the black or the bay nuzzled over my shoulder for the lump of sugar that was coming. The moor spread every-where around, dipping to its rivers, and a quiet happiness blossomed, not only across its brown and healthy spaces, but also from a familiar and beloved atmosphere of countless generations who had felt the same happiness that I was feeling now.

Desmond Doig

Continuing the adventurous profile of some of the contributors was Desmond Doig. A friend of Zanna's, he was something of a Renaissance man: a journalist, artist, photographer and writer, he was the *Statesman*'s roving reporter in Calcutta and is said to have been the first person to write about Mother Theresa. He was also great friends with Edmund Hillary and in 1963 they went together to the Himalayas on an expedition funded by the National Geographic Society to find the abominable snowman. So his wonderful picnic 'When Abominable Snowmen Went Picnicking' was clearly drawn from his own experience!

When Abominable Snowmen Went Picnicking
Desmond Doig

My favourite picnic story comes from Sherpa country below Mount Everest and is about 250 years old. That was the time when the area fairly crawled with yetis – or abominable snowmen.

They became a nuisance, particularly as one of their pastimes was carrying off beautiful young women. In a village called Khumjung, from which some of the most famous Sherpas come, yetis became so thick on the ground that they got in the way. They preyed on precious yaks, dug up valuable potato fields and made the nights alarming with their high-pitched screaming and whistling. Besides, they smelled and were bad-tempered.

The most wise and wily Sherpa elders got together in a series of drunken conferences. How could they rid themselves of the yetis, remembering that they themselves were good Buddhists and couldn't slay the beasts, and that there were some, particularly the lamas, who considered the abominable creatures to be more holy than undesirable.

Unfortunately the person who thought up the prizewinning idea has long since been forgotten. It was, remember, a boozy gathering. The Sherpas of Khumjung, it was decided, would go on one of their popular picnics. Great bowls of potato beer were made by the village ladies, and even more potent bowls of doped *rakshi*, or potato spirit. There were also enough meat dumplings, called *momos*, to build a large house. The curious yetis watched as the villagers, dressed in their brocaded and woolly best, took off to a clearing on a hill nearby and there set to feasting and drinking. Obviously they thought nothing about the fact that every man carried two swords, one made of wood, the other the real thing.

When the Sherpas had had their fill of food and drink, they began to gamble, and then fell to fighting. Wooden swords were drawn and almost every man was 'killed'. Death had never been so noisy and dramatic. Some victims threshed about so much that they almost landed in the river thousands of feet below. Women joined in, torn between lamentation and chopping each other up. The yetis looked on in amazement until it was almost dark. By then the few Sherpas left 'alive' had been dragged by the 'survivors' to their huts. The great pots of doped spirits and hundreds of genuine sharpened swords were left behind. Now it was time for the yetis to have their picnic and, being powerful mimics, it was not long before they feasted and drank, then made a pretence at playing and finally fell upon each other with the swords abandoned by the 'dead' Sherpas.

Great was the slaughter as each side whistled up reinforcements from the dark surrounding mountains, and yetis of all sizes and sexes hurled themselves into the fray. Just a few remained to clear up the battlefield as the Sherpas had done. But when morning came three yeti corpses still remained to be cleared away, and it was on these that the Sherpas descended and removed their scalps as relics to be kept in the village monasteries.

The scalps are still there, in the Sherpa monasteries of Khumjung, Pangboche and Namc Bazar, where they are looked upon with a certain awe and reverence. For years they baffled mountaineers and scientists to whom a few hairs filched from the scalps were sent. The Khumjung scalp became one of the most important clues in the hunt for the elusive snowmen.

In 1960 the mountaineer Sir Edmund Hillary, an eminent American zoologist named Marlin Perkins, and I borrowed the scalp on pain of several very horrid deaths and took it to Chicago, New York, London and Paris. Quite a picnic! It was declared a fake, made from the hide of a wild goat.

Does this mean the epic Sherpa and yeti picnic didn't really happen? It's almost like declaring the Tower of London non-existent if the Crown Jewels turn out to be fakes.

Momos (Tibetan Meat Dumplings)

 1 oz (25 g) yeast
 1 cup (250 ml) warm water
 1 teaspoon sugar
 1½ lb (700 g) plain flour
 8 oz (225 g) minced beef
 1 onion, chopped
 salt
 pepper
 1 tablespoon olive oil

Dissolve the yeast in a cup of warm water with the sugar. Mix with the flour and knead into a dough. Put in a warm place until the dough rises (about 3–4 hours).

Divide the dough into a dozen portions and, using flour to prevent it sticking, roll each portion into a flat round shape about 3 inches (7.5 cm) in diameter.

Meanwhile mix the minced beef with the chopped onion, seasoning and oil and work it into a stuffing. Take a piece of dough and place a piece of this stuffing in the centre. Turn up the sides of the dough to wrap around the stuffing until only a small opening is left at the top; pinch this opening together. Place all the uncooked dumplings in a hot steamer and steam for about 20 minutes.

Lady Diana Cooper and John Julius Norwich

Lady Diana Cooper had a reputation for being the most beautiful woman in England and was also very clever, all the men were keen on her. She was a distant relative of Colin's, and we thought it was a great coup that she agreed to write about a picnic for us. Like Harold Acton and Dorothy Lygon, she also inspired a character in Evelyn Waugh's work. 'Mrs Stitch' who featured in *Scoop* was a well-connected British socialite who could 'fix' things for people. Diana was at the centre of a group of intellectuals in London and acted in films and on stage before her marriage. When her husband Duff Cooper was made Ambassador to France just after the second world war, the soirées she hosted at the British Embassy turned it into a central hub for post-war French literary culture. She wrote as she talked, which I think you can tell from her picnic, and was an extremely charismatic person. I remember going to see her not long before she died in her lovely house in Little Venice. We were taken up to her bedroom where chairs had been put round her bed, and we all had drinks – she was very keen on drinks – while she reclined in bed wearing a lace nightdress and little cape. We were all paying court and utterly in thrall to her.

I've always known her son John Julius through Diana. He became an historian and made several television and radio programmes. He was very good but I always felt he'd been dealt a very strong hand by being the only son of Diana. His Saharan picnics more than live up to the picnics of the other adventurers in this collection!

Memories of Chantilly
Diana Cooper

I have loved picnics for more than eighty years, ever since a feeder embroidered 'Don't be dainty' in cross-stitch was tied around my baby neck. I still do when I am supported by strong hands to the site, and watch the baskets opened and the unexpected unwrapped. Where once it was hard-boiled egg, dry, curly meat sandwiches and perhaps a banana, eaten anywhere, it is now deliberately a surprise of rareness – iced phantasies, cups of fresh fruits, nameless delicacies, gobbled or sipped in selected venues of sunlight or speckled shade and shine... by the water, on the hilltop, darkly in a tropic wood, or warmed on a rug with mulled wine and ginger against the dangerous beauty of blanketing snow.

In arranging picnics I regard the element of surprise almost as an essential. Classical busts of emperors, in a very wide circle – in the heart of a forest in France, where I once lived – all had to be dressed and elaborately hatted, for instance, and I must be the most astonished of the guests. Surprise forbids attendants, anticipation and talk to announce the diversion. On, towards the middle of a summer's evening, with the customary seven or eight friends munching their chicken, that particular picnic's perpetrator said, 'Listen, you've got to be good about this! No, no, you *must* – my neighbour, Madame de X, a sad widow with a very sick son, begged me to cheer her up by bringing you round for coffee and dessert. I knew you'd all be odious about it but it's ten minutes away and we'll be back within the hour. Please help! No, I can't go alone.'

They followed in fury and found themselves in the early night on an eighteenth-century stone terrace with ice creams, liqueurs – no widow – a couple of young lovers and a half moon. Their relief brought the picnic its high spirits – so there we laughed and sang, out of tune, for two hours.

I think my highwater mark of surprise picnics was one that took place countless years ago, when I was living at Chantilly. Cruising around, I discovered a lake surrounded with statues and a sensible, beautiful boathouse. The nobleman who owned it – unknown to me on solicitation – allowed me a picnic on a Sunday. A few guests were staying at my little château in the Chantilly Park. My four or five weekenders and one millionaire from Paris, all expecting a none-too-good lunch at 1.30, were told that we must see this lovely lake at 12.30 – well worth a slight delay. Sudden panic! A message from an 'agent' told me that M. le Comte would be shooting that morning, but should be shot out by 12.30.

So off we all went at 12.40 through a forest where stood some kind of post round which were laid aperitifs (strong) and usual and unusual scraps. 'Good god!' I cried. 'Look what the Count has left us! What courtesy!' Beneath the speckling sun we quaffed and nibbled and blessed nobility.

This little delight was not two hundred yards from the marvellous lake, and one impatient guest sneaked off for a preview. She returned, panting, having recognised my china and pictures, to tell us with a wink from me that she had seen a lunch for eight in the boathouse, with flowers and fruit and bottles – a surprise indeed! And there we feasted, before my total exhaustion.

I have witnessed and delighted in official picnics – and one especially I can never forget, though it was the opposite of surprise. It was with Winston Churchill, no less, in Marrakesh in 1944. The site was chosen with meticulous care, on the brink of a baby canyon chosen at African dawn after two hours' search by Lady Churchill and a daughter and me – a dramatic scenario with a steep footpath through rocks and hazards of all kinds.

The 'start' was at midday and consisted of quite a procession – a food waggon, two or three chairs, linen, rugs, and implements of all sorts in another van, which included a sprinkling of police and detectives. These were followed by four or five picnickers' cars, including (to enliven my heart) Lord Beaverbrook – beloved assistant of the Prime Minister's court – and quite a few young people like flowers, gathered from I knew not where. On arrival at one o'clock the tables were laid, the rugs spread and chairs arranged – I think for the PM, Lord Beaverbrook, and Lord Moran, the great doctor, always in devoted yet mute attendance.

During this planning the young and middle-aged (myself included) took a spirited rash dash down the craggy path to look nearer the rapid, foaming little river and its huge boulders. The young men were soon half-nude and splashing hardily and scrambling none too nimbly over massive rocks. Proudly we swarmed up that fearful path again to a welcome of drinks and appreciation of our description of the dangers we had passed.

The meal, as always, because of its rarity and difference, passed hilariously, with plenty of elderly wit and youthful zest, ending with coffee, dates and brandy galore. 'Lord Moran thinks I should have another glass of brandy.' Several times Lord Moran's unspoken orders were obeyed and I realised suddenly what was inevitable

– namely Winston's resolve to go down the canyon's perilous path. No word of protest either from Lord Moran or from the great man's wife! The young were not perturbed. I was properly alarmed and stood breathless with the elders halfway down to watch, thank god, his safe descent, supported by police and detectives.

At the bottom, where the young and tipsy started trying to scale again with greater enthusiasm these smooth boulders, Winston Churchill must try too and, what's more, with the dragging and pushing of strong detectives, he succeeded in sprawling successfully to the top of them. Watching, I could think only of his steep return, of his fatigue, of his dear heart. I thought of his being dragged up by his arms so soon after lunch. 'A rope, a rope!' If only I could get one round the Prime Minister's middle so he could be pulled up smoothly. No good, no rope. All I could find was a very long and narrow white tablecloth. It would have to do. I seized it and tore down the perilous path. Anxiety shod my feet with sureness, and success crowned the effort. The dear man revelled in the relief of laying his weight upon the offered support, and reached the top daisy-fresh.

I think I have said enough about picnics, delectable as they always must be, unless sodden with rain and wind on a birdless grouse moor. The *change* is the magic. The hungry nomad surely gets no thrill – poor nomad!

Sahara Picnics
John Julius Norwich

I love picnics; indeed, I once had 147 of them running. That was in 1966, when I spent seven weeks crossing and recrossing the Sahara. As far as I remember I enjoyed them all – all, at least, except two, because they had to be eaten during a sandstorm, and the sand always managed to get into one's mouth before anything else did.

There were seven of us, in the capable hands of a first-class *Saharien* guide, Jean Sudriez, who knew better than anyone the secrets of successful desert catering. These include one great fundamental truth: that the food provided for expeditions like ours should be not only nourishing but, within the limits imposed by the circumstances, good. The Sahara demands austerities enough, and there is no point in adding to them unnecessarily. He had accordingly scoured the épiceries of Algiers, and loaded one of our three Land Rovers to overflowing with as wide a variety of tinned delicacies as they were able to produce – to be supplemented, of course, by bread, dates and occasional supplies of other fruit and vegetables from the oases along our way.

The breakfast menu was determined by the need to get the blood circulating again after the almost indescribable cold of the desert night – for the air has no moisture in it to retain the heat, and the thermometer plummets after sunset. We would wake up frozen to the marrow, to be revived (as soon as we had got the fire going) by bowls of steaming porridge, washed down by Nescafé or, more often, a delicious Ovaltine-like drink called Banania, which I vaguely remembered having seen advertised, but had never drunk before and have never tasted since. Bread was a rarity; but we had *biscottes*, Ryvita, tinned butter and industrial quantities of jam.

That would be at about six in the morning; lunch, however, was a more moveable feast, for by nine the sun was literally searing off every inch of skin left unprotected and we would simply stop wherever some unusual feature of the landscape offered the chance of a bit of shade. At high noon, such blessings are rare. The sun blazes down from immediately above one's head and, in the absence of any trees outside an oasis, the best that can usually be hoped for is some little outcrop of rock with a few overhangs beneath which to huddle.

Sometimes we would stretch an awning between two Land Rovers; but the Sahara is a windy place and the operation was seldom as easy as it sounds. Once settled, we would dig into the usual picnic fare – pilchards and pâté, liverwurst and cheese; but the real pleasure came afterwards, with the cool and sloshy – the tinned asparagus, the peperoni and fruit salad that slip down parched throats like a benediction, caressing and refreshing as they go. No wine at lunchtime; in such heat it would have destroyed us, and we didn't even want it. But the water was wonderful because, thanks to our *guerbas*, it was always cold.

The *guerba* is a wonderful thing. A swollen, still furry and all too recognisable carcass of a goat may not be the most attractive of containers for one's drinking water, but its porousness permits just the right degree of evaporation to keep the contents cool, and its position on the outside of the car gives it the full benefit of the breeze. It hangs upside down, by what used to be the legs; a small plug, inevitably if somewhat indelicately placed at one end, serves as a tap. Cold running water in the Sahara noonday, whatever its taste, colour or provenance, is a commodity not to be despised. We each drank well over a gallon a day.

By nightfall it would be cold again, and there would be a new edge to the wind. The fire would be lit – we never missed the occasional opportunity to stock up with firewood or dried bracken, any more than we did with water – and a few more of our precious tins would be emptied into the pot: spaghetti perhaps, or lentils, or chilli con carne as the *pièce de résistance*, with the usual concomitants of sausage, tuna fish and cheese, rounded off with a few succulent spoonfuls of condensed milk flavoured with caramel or Grand Marnier and washed down with *vin rosé*. Those dinners were for me one of the high spots of the day. We would go on sitting round the fire for as long as it lasted, then put on every available sweater, zip ourselves into first our woollen track-suits and then our sleeping bags, and sleep under the stars till it was time for breakfast again.

Such was the basic regime on which we covered some eight hundred miles of desert; and even when we found ourselves in the Tibesti Mountains and had to abandon our Land Rovers for camels it did not change appreciably; the only difference was that camel milk suddenly became available as an optional extra. For two or three days after stopping in an oasis we might supplement it with fresh bread, lettuce and tomatoes, and once we were able to buy a whole *guerba* stuffed full of date paste – which, scooped out with the fingers and carried straight to the mouth, was one of the memorable gastronomic pleasures of my life. But these were bonuses. Tins were the staple, and it is hard to see how we could possibly have improved on them. There was only one serious misfortune that we were called upon to suffer: the *vin rosé* ran out after five and a half weeks. But by then, hardened *Sahariens* that we were, we had learned to take disaster in our stride.

Washing up was never a problem. Though water was naturally far too precious to waste on such a purpose, the desert did every bit as well. One dug the plate or fork or mug into the sand, scoured it round for a moment, and the job was done as well as in any kitchen sink. The sand also solved the problem of what to do with the rubbish. We buried it carefully about a foot deep, then carefully smoothed over the place until there was no sign left of where it had been. This sort of habit is every bit as impor-tant in the deep Sahara as anywhere else – perhaps even more so, since in that dryness nothing ever decays. Once outside the oases, the desert is the cleanest place in the world; and it is also, to me at least, one of the most beautiful. It has a sparkling purity about it unlike anywhere else I have been; one longs for it to remain like that for ever.

Nicky Haslam

I've known Nicky for most of my life. We have a lovely holiday once a year with this great friend of ours who is Turkish and has a huge yacht. Nicky and I are much the oldest of the group and what we like to do is cruise until we get to a lovely beach with sunloungers and hopefully an ice-cream kiosk. Everyone else goes off being desperately active, diving and whizzing about on jet skis whilst Nicky and I like sitting with our ice creams and watching the world go by. He was also a friend of Diana Cooper's and was always at all the parties. He knew lots of film stars and was always throwing wonderful parties for them whenever they were in London. I particularly remember a very glamorous evening he organised for the French actress Leslie Caron – he always ensured that every little detail was perfect.

The party he describes, a birthday picnic he organised for Diana Cooper is typical of the gorgeous evenings he would create for his friends, and fits Diana's own essential picnic criteria by including an element of surprise.

Some Enchanted Evening
Nicky Haslam

Summer, many years ago, in Venice. A light zephyr cooled the
tiles and terraces; the roses and jasmine trembled, the gondolas
nuzzled each other's prows on the narrow canal, the water on
the lagoon beyond stood still as mirror glass. It was cocktail hour,
and it was Diana Cooper's birthday.

'Let's,' I said, 'take the boats and drinks and drift gently among
those deserted little islands for an hour or so.'

'Oh, yes, do let's,' said one of the many guests, Minnie Astor,
maybe, or Dick Avedon, 'there's masses of time before dinner.'

Within minutes we were settled on cushions, the *remi* silently
moving us across the sunset-splashed surface. Dusk came fast, sky
and water became one. The two boats echoed with laughter;
glasses were refilled; our cigarettes' glow reflected in ripples around
us, gradually augmented by first stars and then, in golden fragments, the tiara of lights along the distant Adriatic shoreline.

Now night fell.

'Shouldn't we turn back soon?'

'Suppose so, but maybe just a few minutes more... '

Then: 'What's that sound? Music?' asked Simon Fleet.

'Yes, over there.'

'No, *there,* from *that* island.'

'Surely there's only a ruined lighthouse on it?'

'But I think there are lights as well. Perhaps it's a party,' said
Diana. 'Let's look.'

The boats turned; we drew nearer, the music louder now, the
light flickering on tumbled arches hung with garlands of zinnias.
Diana was the first ashore. She called to us, amazed. 'Quick!
Come!'

We scrambled from the boats. And saw the table swagged with green, the candles amid branches, ice-cold wine and pitchers of Diana's favourite – vodka and grapefruit. We heard the musicians playing a soft bacarolle, while our two houseboys produced baskets of toasted ham and cheese sandwiches, figs with proscuitto, peaches and other Venetian delights that young Arrigo Cipriani had secretly sent across from Harry's Bar a few hours earlier.

With the help of the boys I'd found the island, and we'd spent the day creating this bucolic mise en scène; its ambiance became more enchanting each midnight moment. In fact, until the stars faded. And it being Diana's birthday we sang. And danced.

Colette Clark

A friend who had a famous father and went on to have a famous son was Colette Clark. She was the daughter of the art historian and broadcaster Kenneth Clark, presenter of the series *Civilisation* on the BBC in the 1960s. She was very direct, called a spade a spade and used to have fantastic dinner parties. She brought up her son Sam on her own and he was at school with my son Christopher. He went on to open the successful Moro restaurants with his wife who is also called Sam. I've read that he remembered his mother's glamorous dinner parties and realised what joy and fun food could bring to people. It's rather nice to think that I might have been at one of the dinner parties that inspired such a talented and successful chef.

A Picnic in Portugal
Colette Clark

The best food I have eaten on a picnic was cooked by a farmer's wife in a tiny village in northern Portugal. My brother had asked her for something to take with us on a walk up the foot-hills of the Minho mountains in search of a series of waterfalls, and this is what she provided: two freshly cooked marinated chickens from her own farmyard; slices of cold veal coated in a spicy glacé sauce; meat and egg croquettes (*croquetas*) which were still warm but of such perfect consistency – firm but light – that they could be eaten with the fingers. To this were added home-made bread rolls, tomatoes and fruit from her garden and, to crown it all, little cold pancakes filled with cherry jam and dusted with cinnamon. But it is the croquettes I will remember.

Egg Croquettes

> 1½ oz (40 g) butter
> 1½ oz (40 g) flour
> 8 fl. oz (200 ml) milk flavoured with salt, pepper and
>   bayleaf
> 4 hard-boiled eggs
> 2 raw egg yolks
> parsley, chopped
> pinch of nutmeg
> salt
> fresh white breadcrumbs
> oil and butter for frying

Make a sauce by melting the butter, adding the flour, and cooking to make the roux. Add the milk gradually, stirring all the time. Cook for 5 minutes, then leave to cool a little. Add the chopped eggs, one egg yolk, parsley and nutmeg. Leave on a plate to get cold (it is best to prepare up to this point the night before, or several hours in advance if that is not possible).

Roll into fat sausage shapes on a board covered in seasoned flour, then dip into the beaten yolk of an egg to which you have also added salt. Then roll in a large quantity of fresh white bread-crumbs and fry in a mixture of very hot oil and butter until golden brown (a basket which can be lowered into the fat makes this easier). Drain on kitchen paper one by one, and leave to cool for the picnic.

Meat Croquettes

> 12 oz (350 g) cooked veal or beef
> 1 onion
> ½ oz (10 g) butter
> a small bunch of parsley, chopped
> ½ pint (250 ml) good gravy
> salt and pepper
> 1 beaten egg
> breadcrumbs

Mince the meat in a food processor for just a second or two. Chop the onion and soften in the butter in a frying pan. Add the meat, parsley, gravy, salt and pepper. The consistency should be moist, but firm enough to shape into croquettes once it has cooled down. Then proceed as for egg croquettes.

Christopher Thynne

Christopher was the second son of the 6th Marquess of Bath, the owner of Longleat. He was the Comptroller of Longleat up until his older brother, Alexander, inherited the title in 1993, at which point he was sacked and thrown off the estate. His relationship with Alexander, who was known for having lots of mistresses he called 'Wifelets' wasn't easy, I think having to find cottages on the estate for all these wifelets could be tricky. At one point Christopher thought he was going to have to have one of them living with him but then an alternative was found. When we went to visit Christopher he wasn't getting on with his brother so we only saw the safari park, we didn't go into the house. It was a shame as I was dying to see the famous murals of the Karma Sutra which had been painted inside! Christopher was great fun and loved writing limericks so I wasn't surprised when he wrote us a poem for his picnic.

Anne Glenconner

The Longleat Picnic
Christopher Thynne

Sun is sinking, cars are loaded
Children, food and frying pans,
A basket full of drink and tumblers,
Lemonade and Cola cans.

Dogs are barking, parents shouting,
Dressed in jeans and tweedy suits,
'Have we got a bottle opener?
Sophie, you've forgot your boots.'

The cavalcade of cars starts rolling,
Someone shouts, 'Who's got the pugs?'
Silvy runs back from the Mill House
Loaded with a pile of rugs.

Start again, out through the driveway,
Swirling dust clouds in our wake,
Down the lane and through the woodland,
Heading for the Island Lake.

I love the sound and smell of cooking,
Everybody's had a drink,
One or two are on their second,
Ed is on his third, I think.

Alexander's acting strangely,
Think he's getting rather tight.
Now he's dancing like a dervish,
Someone's set his beard alight.

Tony's chatting up the Duchess.
I think he sometimes goes too far.
The fire's burning rather well now,
Think I'll strum on my guitar.

I'm sure I put it here beside me.
Now it's vanished from my sight.
Oh my god – some stupid bugger,
So that's why the fire's so bright.

Christ! It's getting rather cold now,
Wish that I was in my car,
Put my coat on, pick up litter,
Throw some wood on my guitar.

Time to go now – what a pity,
Just as things were going well,
Life's a picnic – earth's a heaven,
Both to me just now are hell.

Grope our way back through the darkness,
Tree Trunk Bridge I see, I think.
What's that splash? Dad's in the water –
That's goodbye to all the drink.

Matches flare and fade like fireflies,
Someone's fallen in the stream,
Voices calling all around me,
Havoc's reigning quite supreme.

What the hell? – I think I'll stay here,
Wrap up warm – I'll be all right,
I'd only fall into the water –
We're coming back tomorrow night.

Derek Hill

Visiting Derek Hill at his cottage in Ireland was a somewhat terrifying experience. He had bought us plane tickets to Belfast rather than Dublin and, on the way, the taxi ran into a confrontation on the Shankhill Road. The driver made us all lie down in the back of the car to avoid the shooting. We were petrified. But Derek was totally unsympathetic when we eventually arrived at his house. I suppose it was a pretty run-of-the-mill experience for him. He was a painter, Director of Fine Arts at the British School in Rome and a great friend of King Charles. He used to accompany the King on some of his trips abroad to be on hand to advise him as he painted. The King is an excellent artist; he paints beautiful watercolours. Derek did the portraits of various members of the Royal Family, but he also painted a portrait of me which I love.

A Painter's Picnic
Derek Hill

Thinking back over picnics is, I find, no strain to my memory: the landscape, to a painter, is as important as the meal itself. I remember picnics in all sorts of places: in pinewoods in Bavaria, dashing down to a nearby lake to bathe with my cousins while my mother and Aunt Lucy watched, trying to photograph our splashings with trembling hands and shaky results. Then, a few years later when I was a student, picnics in France during painting excursions under those exquisite Ile de France skies of floating clouds and Impressionist river scenes; rarely attended by French friends, who, when they did overcome their dislike of informality and the deep countryside, insisted on correct placement and table linen.

In post-war years there was a vividly remembered picnic in Turkey at a Hittite site – an ambassadorial picnic with the chief archaeological experts in the country as our guides. A liveried chauffeur helped with the 'furniture' and the 'site' – custodians stood at a respectful distance watching the unusual scene. We had a delectable cold Turkish soup called *Leyla* that I was greedy enough to get the recipe for.

Sandwiches, in spite of my grandmother having made a dictionary of them in her handwritten book of recipes, are the one thing that I can do without at any meal, unless they are of the delicious and thinly cut cucumber variety that used to be offered at tennis-party teas. Nowadays they are never thin enough, and the cucumber is seldom peeled. But back to my grandmother: she listed sandwiches of chopped figs and lemon cream, dates, bananas, herring with mustard sauce, olives chopped with ham and cheese, sardines and watercress – an infinite and mouth-watering variety. Today the bread always seems too heavy for the filling, and after one mouthful one feels 'full up to dollies' wax', as Nanny used to call one's bloated state.

If you live, as I do, in one of the wettest climates in the British Isles (Donegal) something warm is needed, and something that can be eaten in a shelter or a neighbour's porch, should the wind and rain be too extreme. It is a rule here never to cancel a picnic because of the weather, which can change completely within a matter of hours. A large thermos filled with risotto or kedgeree is popular, and then a salad packed into a big apple-shaped ice bucket that keeps it cool and fresh; cheese and a tin of Bath Oliver biscuits and slices of almond cake in foil. I am fortunate enough to own a Sardinian wicker basket, which kind Italian friends bought me as a house present; it is 'upholstered' inside with all possible picnic requirements and large enough to hold a banquet.

This picnic essay started about landscape as an ingredient essential to a painter's pleasure, but a more culinary and basic interest has inevitably intervened. Perhaps Bernard Berenson was right when he used to say, 'The trouble with Derek is that he never paints between meals.' I know that even on a perfect day in the most beautiful surroundings, I often regret that my Sardinian basket isn't stocked with paints and brushes rather than the splendid provisions packed by Gracie, my housekeeper.

Leyla Soup (for four)

    1 tablespoon butter
    1 heaped dessertspoon flour
    2 pints (1 litre 150 ml) chicken stock
    2 eggs

1 ½ lemons
freshly chopped mint
2 tablespoons tomato juice
salt and pepper
1 pint (570 ml) yoghurt

Melt the butter and slightly cook the flour in it. Add the stock slowly. Bring to the boil, stirring all the time. Beat the eggs till they froth, add the strained juice of the lemons, and stir into the stock (having first added a few tablespoons of the stock to the egg and lemon) very slowly. Add some chopped mint and the tomato juice. Season with salt and pepper. Bring to the boil again. Add the yoghurt but do not reboil.

Ian Graham

When I came out as a debutante in London in 1950 Ian Graham was a dancing partner of mine. He was keen on vintage cars and used to come and pick me up wearing goggles and a flying jacket. I was quite shy and felt terribly embarrassed to be seen in these cars, which ruined your hairdo. In those days we all had rather neat hairstyles which got blown to smithereens, despite the scarf you would be handed rather crossly when you got in. He fell out of my life and disappeared from the London scene. In fact, he drove a vintage Rolls Royce across America and down to Mexico where he first came across Mayan sculpture, which became his passion and job. He became an eminent Mayanist, involved with preserving and cataloguing ruins. He spent so much time working in Central America it's entirely appropriate his picnic recalls al fresco eating in Guatemala.

Picnic in Guatemala
Ian Graham

On hearing that I take all my meals out of doors during several months of the year, and that I generally eat them sitting on the ground in a forest, you might suppose me to be either mad, or a keen and expert picnicker. Alas, as a picnicker I am neither keen nor expert. My apparent mania for al fresco dining is no more than a consequence of the kind of archaeological work I undertake in Guatemala, and the meals that I provide are decidedly not good picnic fare. Far from being fresh and appetising in appearance, or made up with a due proportion of vegetables and fruit into unusual, perhaps even surprising dishes, mine are nearly always stodgy affairs in which rice, black beans and tortillas routinely play the leading roles, and they are mostly devoured in a perfunctory way during respites from work. Unfortunately, fruit and vegetables soon rot in the tropical heat, and before an expedition is two weeks old they have disappeared from the menu.

Even a French explorer seems to have despaired of the available materials. In describing a journey through these same regions a century ago, Désiré Charnay gives a menu: it starts with *Soupe d'haricots noirs* and goes on predictably to *Haricots noirs rissolés*, but his *vin de Bordeaux* must have made the meal more bearable. Evidently his mule train clanked along to the music of wine bottles, one of which I even found, still unbroken, near a waterhole by which he must have camped. I imagine that in spite of the poor provender, strict etiquette was observed, even in that sweltering jungle; a photograph shows his secretary properly dressed in a frock coat.

Still, I *have* sometimes tried to provide a picnic worthy of the name for a visitor, particularly one who has brought in fresh supplies. And in the absence of such supplies there is always a chance of finding crunch, one of the most delicious being heart of palm. But to obtain something growing in the forest that will contribute freshness, one has to find a tree at just the right stage of growth, and fell it with an axe.

Of these more ambitious picnics, some may be counted successful. At least none has been more unsuccessful as the one mentioned so laconically in *Lolita*. Humbert Humbert, you may remember, tells us that his 'very photogenic mother died in a freak accident (picnic, lightning)'. Nor have any of us yet been struck down by ptomaine poisoning. In this connection, though, I do offer a word of caution that is as relevant to picnics on hot days in temperate climates as it is to the tropics: avoid making up sandwiches or other food with mayonnaise or soft cheese, both of which suit the taste of bacteria all too well. On the other hand, dressings made acid with vinegar or lemon juice put them off.

One picnic I remember, which was nearly ruined by a small mishap, was held in a ruined city of the ancient Maya called La Pasadita, a very small settlement consisting of only a few public buildings perched on a steep hill with vertical rock faces on two sides. Only one building remains standing, and even this seemed doomed to collapse at any moment. Until some fifteen years ago the doorways were spanned by beautifully carved stone lintels, then these were wrenched out by looters. Inside, the walls show the remains of fresco painting, with portraits of rulers and scenes of ceremony. The main elements of our not very sumptuous picnic were: black bean and chorizo salad, empanadas, flour tortillas, mangoes and lemonade.

Black Bean and Chorizo Salad

> 8 oz (225 g) black beans or (much better) lentils
> 1¾ pints (1 litre) water
> chorizo or other spicy sausage
> 1 large onion
> black olives
> 1 teaspoon salt
> olive oil
> wine vinegar
> French mustard

Wash the beans or lentils, add them to the water and bring to the boil and cook, but do not allow them to become mushy. Drain. Cut the sausage into cubes, add chopped onion, chopped black olives and salt and blend with the lentils. Before serving, pour over a dressing of olive oil, vinegar and French mustard.

Empanadas

> *(Makes about 15)*

Pastry

> 12 oz (350 g) self-raising flour
> ½ teaspoon salt
> 4 oz (110 g) butter
> 1 egg yolk
> 2 tablespoons milk for glaze

Filling

    1 lb (450 g) minced beef, or pork and beef (wild boar
       when I made them at La Pasadita)
    1 tablespoon olive oil
    1 small onion, chopped
    1 clove garlic, crushed
    1 tomato, peeled and chopped
    2 tablespoons chopped blanched almonds
    ½ teaspoon chilli powder
    6 dessertspoons raisins
    6 green olives, pitted and sliced
    2 teaspoons capers

Put the flour and salt in a bowl. Cut in the butter until thoroughly mixed. Gradually add enough iced water to form a dough. Wrap the dough in plastic film and keep in the refrigerator while you make the filling.

Heat the oil in frying pan and cook the meat until no longer pink, stirring the while. Add onion, garlic, tomato, almonds, chilli powder, raisins (previously soaked in hot water if hard), olives and capers. Cook over reduced heat for 6–8 minutes, stirring frequently. Add salt to taste. If the mixture is still wet, cook longer. Cool.

Preheat the oven to gas mark 5 (375°F, 190°C). Roll out the dough on a floured surface to rather less than 3 mm thick. Cut in squares of about 4 inches (10 cm). Place a tablespoon of the filling in each square, then fold over on the diagonal, and crimp the edges together with your fingertips. Place the empanadas on greased baking tins and brush with a glaze prepared by beating the egg yolk with the milk. Bake for 15–20 minutes until golden. Place on a rack to cool.

Lemonade

A subtly different flavour can be imparted to lemonade by boiling up the lemon peel in it.

Postscript

As it turned out we were not to enjoy the empanadas, so laboriously baked in an improvised oven in our camp near La Pasadita. I left them during the morning hung in a plastic bag on a tree, out of reach of ants; but some animal, probably a large member of the stoat family, enjoyed them instead. So we had to make do with sardines.

Patrick Lindsay

Another friend who had a passion for vintage cars was Patrick Lindsay. He married my cousin Annabel Yorke and I remember Colin and I went to their wedding on the day we announced our engagement. There were lots of press photographers there, but they were all taking photographs of us rather than the couple getting married, Annabel told me later she was furious about that! Patrick was a director at Christie's auction house and loved racing vintage cars. He'd been at Eton and Zanna and I thought it would be rather fun to ask him to write about a Fourth of June Picnic, which is such an institution at the school. It's a day which was originally to commemorate the birthday of King George III but is now just a broader celebration of the school's history. When my son Henry was there I'd call up other mothers and we would arrange to have a picnic in the grounds whilst the cricket match was going on in the background. It was rather an odd sight, especially with all the boys in their stiff winged collars.

Fourth of June Picnic
Patrick Lindsay

Agars Plough. Eton. Fourth of June 1946.
Celebrating King George III's birthday.

The Chairman and the Director of the National Gallery entertain some of their children to a picnic luncheon. Their wives sit
on the running board of the exotic V12 cylinder Lagonda Open
Tourer.

In the background the soothing snick of leather on willow
– the Eton eleven playing their annual cricket match against the
Ramblers. Peace – and peacetime at last!

It had been a poor summer. Home-grown strawberries had
not been up to scratch. Ours were flown from Israel. Cream
obtained with a struggle. My first ever *Pâté en croûte*.

Pâté en Croûte

Dough

      1½ lb (700 g) flour
      1 teaspoon salt
      4 oz (110 g) lard
      4 oz (110 g) butter
      1 egg
      ½ cup cold water

Pâté

      8 oz (225 g) veal
      8 oz (225 g) lean pork

8 oz (225 g) fat pork
2 eggs
salt and pepper
I tin truffles (optional)
2 tablespoons cognac
12 oz (350 g) lean ham
12 oz (350 g) tongue
dorure (I tablespoons milk beaten with I egg)
aspic
parsley

Mix together the dough ingredients and wrap in waxed paper. Store overnight in the refrigerator.

Line a springform loaf tin with the dough, saving some for later, and bake at gas mark 7 (425°F, 220°C) for 10 minutes. Then remove, and reduce the heat to gas mark 6 (400°F, 200°C). Mince together the veal, lean pork and fat pork. Add 2 eggs, mix well, and pound to a smooth paste. Add salt and pepper. Ignite 2 tablespoons of warmed cognac and stir in. Press the forcemeat through a sieve or purée it in a blender. Cut the ham and tongue into sticks or batons about 1 inch (2.5 cm) thick and as long as possible. Cut the contents of a can of truffles into smaller sticks.

Cover the bottom of the loaf tin with a layer of forcemeat. Arrange parallel rows of truffle and ham a tongue sticks down the length of the tin. Cover these with a layer of forcemeat and proceed in this fashion until full, arranging pink and black batons to make a cross–section pattern when the pâté is sliced. Cover with a thin layer of larding pork and with the remaining dough. Decorate the crust and make a small hole in the centre of the covering to allow steam to escape.

Bake the pâté for about 1½ hours, brushing it once or twice

with *dorure* (mix 1 tablespoon milk with beaten egg) and covering it with heavy buttered paper if it browns too quickly. Cool in the tin. Pour cool but liquid aspic through the hole in the crust to fill spaces created by shrinking during cooking. Chill the pâté well. Garnish with aspic cut-outs and ribbons of finely minced parsley and aspic, stirred to fragments with a fork.

Min Hogg

Colin was utterly thrilled when Min Hogg, who was founding editor of *World of Interiors*, came to the White House, which we had built in Tite Street in 1968, and wrote a very complimentary article about it for the magazine. We had lots of interest in the house which at the time was described as the most stylish in London. There were all sorts of funny stories about Min Hogg – rumours that she had had an affair with the film director John Huston, that she'd refused to sleep with Lucien Freud and that she had held up a very drunk Mick Jagger as they tried to dance together. I have no idea whether any of these were actually true but I do remember her as being very good fun at dinner parties, full of interesting anecdotes and stories. After my worry about choosing mushrooms in Italy I particularly love the first line of her picnic.

Autumn Mushroom Picnic
Min Hogg

If you cannot tell the difference between edible types of wild mushroom and their dangerously poisonous counterparts, this picnic plan could be the most effective way of pruning your circle of friends since dinner at the Borgias. All the same, if you cannot distinguish between them you are missing one of the most delicious of gastronomic treats. I urge you from the bottom of my heart to rectify the situation. Just check on the cost of wild mushrooms in the shops, should you be lucky enough to know of a greengrocer with the enterprise to sell them. It will be enough to convince the profoundest sceptic that they must not only be a delicacy worth trying, but also be worth the price of a guidebook on mushrooms and fungi in order to learn how to obtain the treat for free. There are masses of guides to wild mushrooms in bookshops, and one I find particularly easy to use is called *British and European Mushrooms and Fungi*, published by Chatto and Windus. It is cheap, pocket-size, and every photograph is in colour. The mixture of stern warnings and bubbling enthusiasm in its text seems like a good balance, and it certainly gave me the confidence right from the start to identify and eat what I had picked.

One pale blue morning in mid-October I gathered a basket of mixed mushrooms. They came from a Hampshire woodland spot I know, within sight and sound of the M3. You would be amazed how many rich clusters of fungi are to be found in woods close beside motorways.

Since so many lethal-looking toadstools are, in fact, edible, it is vital to educate yourself about those that have the best taste. There are lots that are either insipid or repulsively slimy, and I have never generated much enthusiasm amongst my guests for anything blue – these are the sort to leave gracing the paths and glades in which they grow. Beginners in toadstool eating should really confine themselves to the Cep and Boletus families; they are delicious and abundant and have the distinguishing feature of something looking like fine sponge rubber on their undersides in place of the gills found in ordinary shop-bought mushrooms. Incidentally, I advise scraping off this benign but slippery sponge stuff before cooking, rather in the way you remove the hairy bit attached to artichoke hearts. Apart from the guidebook, essential at all times, pickers should arm themselves with a knife to slice off the mushroom caps; wrenching the whole stem out of the ground stops other mushrooms from coming up in the same place.

While I was foraging for this picnic my guests were working like Trojans, collecting wood and building a really good fire at our chosen site beside a lake. We balanced over the fire a metal trivet large enough to take two pans: one pan for water – which I had brought as hot as possible in giant thermoses – and the other for the mushrooms. Since the fungi taste extremely rich I decided to cook them as they often do in Italy, sliced and sautéed with parsley and garlic to flavour a simple pasta. As we waited for the spaghetti water to boil I sliced the mushrooms, mixed them with the chopped parsley and crushed garlic, and fried them gently in a little butter. The best spaghetti for picnics is vermicelli. I like its thin gauge which has the inestimable advantage of cooking quickly – even on an open fire.

The minute the pasta was *al dente* and drained, I tipped the mushrooms together with the pan juices on top of it, mixed them all together, and dished them up as quickly as possible.

Nicholas Coleridge

I met Nicholas a few times, although he was mainly a friend of Zanna's. He was always highly entertaining and, of course, became the absolute king of the magazine world, and we all devoured magazines.

Picnic at the Grange
Nicholas Coleridge

I don't know of a more perfect setting for a picnic than the ruins of Grange Park. This is the astonishing Greek Revival house near Micheldever in Hampshire that C.R. Cockerell built for the Baring family, and around which there was so much controversy a few years ago when plans were made to knock it down. Now the shell of the house stands, like the ruins of Priene, at the head of a valley surrounded by cornfields with distant views of a lake beyond.

It is such a dramatic setting that any picnic staged there is a colossal leap upmarket. Even half-a-dozen bread rolls and a slice of veal and ham pie looks rather good eaten underneath the portico of the ballroom, which is the best place to set up a picnic table. All around the ruin are clumps of nettles and dock leaves which conceal quite large fragments of frieze and, if you are very lucky, pieces of broken sculpture. It is rather like scavenging over the plains of Troy except that no little boys rush up with faked antiquities for sale. Until recently you could have vandalised the Neo-Classical mantelpieces too, some of which were suspended in mid-air between floor-less rooms. We talked about it a lot, but you would have needed a crane. Last time I went, however, they had all disappeared and there were deep gaping holes in the plaster. We presumed that a Fulham antique dealer had made a hit-and-run assault with a van at dead of night.

The only disadvantage of Grange Park is that it is impossible to find. I have picnicked there several times and on each occasion driven for hours in convoy, up and down hill, endlessly three-point-turning, pulling into lay-bys at every summit and agreeing that we *must* be able to see it from here. The lanes around Micheldever all look exactly the same and only every half hour or so, when you pass the railway station for the third time, do you realise that you've been driving in a circle.

The entrance to the house is guarded by a lodge and this you must drive past at great speed. Once past, however, there is little chance of being nabbed for trespassing. Grange Park is now run by the Department of the Environment, who have surrounded it with barbed wire and 'Clear off' type signs but haven't, so far, installed a watchman.

My first Grange Park outing was with friends then at the Courtauld Institute of Art, plus Napier Miles who claims to know that part of Hampshire inside out and was map reading, but really only knows it back to front. Our intended lunch had turned into picnic tea by the time we found the house and suddenly it had become very cold. All I can remember is everybody huddled in tartan car rugs sitting on the roof. Possibly we were singing old pop songs to keep warm (I do hope that we weren't). Then someone suggested having a discotheque, with music from the cassette player in the car. This was driven across the bumpy ground to the front of the ballroom portico, and looked like a Ford Fiesta in a colour magazine advertisement. We bopped ludicrously away to David Bowie and Dolly Parton, the music blaring through the open car door. Only when it was time to go home, however, did we realise the snag. The car battery had gone flat and we had to push.

My other notable picnic there was on the hottest Bank Holiday Monday of 1980. We had only taken an hour to find the gate this time, and two even more idiosyncratic carloads were in convoy.

In the sun Grange Park looks like the Acropolis, despite the scaffolding that the Department of the Environment have put around the ballroom to make it resemble the Pompidou Centre in Paris. We were better prepared this time, with a wind-up gramophone and a far superior picnic. Also more to drink.

Could the drink have been the spur for the preposterous photocall after lunch? This was a quite unforeseen craze for recreating old master paintings for the camera. Draped in the tablecloth and lengths of barbed wire, we cut a swathe through the Renaissance to the Pre-Raphaelites in half a dozen well-chosen frames: Guido Reni's *Ecce Homo*; Poussin's *Christ Expelling the Money-lenders from the Temple*; the *Laocoon*; Burne-Jones's *Virgil and Dante Meeting at the River Styx*.

That is the secret ingredient in a Grange Park picnic – the culture factor. If you know anything at all, however banal, about art or architecture you can depend on an opportunity to show off. Certainly it is the only occasion ever that I can consciously recall utilising my end-of-bin Cambridge History of Art degree.

Larissa Haskell

Larissa was a friend of Zanna's and an eminent Russian art historian of Venetian art who had been a curator of Venetian drawings at the Hermitage Museum in St Petersburg in Russia. She married the art historian Francis Haskell and they lived in Oxford. I remember visiting the Hermitage with Colin years ago when the twins were small and he threw the most dreadful tantrum when the babushkas who guard the galleries prevented him from entering a room he was particularly keen to see. An English-speaking curator was summoned to see what the fuss was about but at that point he'd calmed down and somehow managed to charm his way into the room. I sometimes wonder whether that English-speaking curator may have been Larissa.

Russian Picnic
Larissa Haskell

Russian literature is full of poetical descriptions of food. The jolly noise of pots and pans from the kitchen follows like a musical accompaniment to the idyllic childhood of Ilya Ilyich Oblomov in Goncharov's famous novel. Succulent meals of the rich Volga merchants make a reading of Melinikov-Pechersky's novels unbearable on an empty stomach. The joys of good food are celebrated on many pages of Anton Chekhov's stories, but nowhere as vividly as in *Siren*, where a clerk's lusty dream of a festive dinner drives everyone in the office crazy.

What about picnics? A reader who is looking for a menu is likely to be disappointed here – a furtive kiss in the woods would be easier to find. But the essence of a picnic – the special pleasure of eating on grass among the trees – is nowhere expressed better than in Tolstoy's *Childhood, Boyhood, Youth*.

When we reached woods, we found the carriage already there, and, beyond all our expectations, a cart, in the midst of which sat the butler. In the shade we beheld a samovar, a cask with a form of ice cream, and some other attractive parcels and baskets. It was impossible to make any mistake: there was to be tea, ice cream and fruits in the open air. At the sight of the cart we manifested an uproarious joy; for it was considered a great treat to drink tea in the woods on the grass, and especially in a place where nobody had ever drunk tea before.

Chapter VII, translated by Isabel F. Hapgood

But if a picnic, seen through the eyes of a child, did not leave other memories than ice cream and fruit, the meal eaten by Natasha Rostov after the hunt in *War and Peace* is surprising both in its length and in its colourful description.

Liquors made from herbs, pickles, mushrooms, hot rye cakes, honey in the comb, foaming honey mead, apples, nuts both fresh and roasted and nuts in honey... Preserves made with honey and others made with sugar, ham and freshly roasted chicken...

Translated by Constance Garnett

A meal which would give many an idea to lovers of health food.

Picnics of course become especially popular with the growth of urban life, which adds a value to nature unpolluted by the presence of human beings, and so picnics have become a necessary part of recreation in present–day Russia both for the family and the courting couple seeking privacy. The favourite food is a shish kebab (called *shashlik*), cooked on charcoal in a hole dug into the earth, washed down by great quantities of vodka. I give here a few recipes which, while they are still popular today, could easily have been found in the picnic baskets of Tolstoy or Chekhov.

Pirojki with Spring Onions and Egg

Dough
> ¼ oz (7 g) fresh yeast
> I glass warm milk
> I lb (450 g) plain flour
> I tablespoon melted butter

Filling
> I lb (450 g) spring onions
> butter
> 2 hard-boiled eggs, chopped

To make the dough, dissolve the yeast in the milk. Mix this liquid with the flour and melted butter and leave in a warm place to double in size (no kneading is required) for about an hour. Preheat the oven to gas mark 6 (400°F, 200°C). When ready, cut the dough into eight portions. Mix all the filling ingredients together. Fill each portion of dough with the mixture, seal and bake for one hour. Pirojki should serve as an accompaniment to the main course, for which I propose the following.

Kurinie Kotleti – Chicken Meatballs

(Serves four)

2 boned chicken breasts
1 slice white bread
milk
1 egg
oil for frying

Mince the chicken breasts. Soak the bread in milk and beaten egg and then mix with the chicken. Roll into little balls and fry in a frying pan in hot oil for 20 minutes. The essential thing is not to let the liquid escape.

Valeria Coke

When we were children Carey and I adored swimming in the fountain at Holkham, it was freezing cold but of course when the water came out of the mouths of the dolphins it was all great fun. Valeria was married to my cousin Eddie who inherited Holkham, and she suggested basing her picnic at the fountain. We all joined in, and sat in the sun with Holkham in the background and the park and the deer and the sound of the fountain, it was just glorious.

A Picnic by the Fountain of Perseus and Andromeda, Holkham, Norfolk
Valeria Coke

We usually take our picnics to the beach, a mile away, but on one hot sunny day that I remember we moved only as far as the fountain. When it plays, the fountain is spectacular; but we turn it on only when the house is open to the public as it works on a very complicated system. A vast amount of water is pumped up seven hundred feet from a well – said to be the deepest in Norfolk – to a reservoir a mile up the hill. The pressure of water from this reservoir is so great that, when the taps are turned on, it provides a magnificent display.

On the occasion that I am recalling it was a perfect summer afternoon, and before lunch the braver children clambered down the steps into the pool to swim and play hide-and-seek behind the spouting dolphins. Our picnic consisted of sorrel soup, local Cromer crab pâté, a simple quiche decorated with samphire from the marsh, and an equally simple but delicious pudding.

Sorrel Soup

    8 oz (225 g) mixed sorrel and lettuce
    2 oz (50 g) butter
    1 pint (500 ml) chicken stock
    salt
    2 egg yolks
    ½ pint (250 ml) cream
    black pepper
    grated nutmeg

Wash and dry the leaves, removing the stalks. Heat the butter in a heavy pan, add the sorrel and lettuce and cook gently for 3 minutes. Heat the stock and pour on. Bring to simmering point, add a little salt and cover the pan. Simmer for 5 minutes. Put in a liquidiser or through a mouli and return to pan. Beat the egg yolks with the cream, stir in one ladleful of hot soup and add to the pan. Add the black pepper and nutmeg to taste. Reheat but do not boil. Serve hot or cold.

Crab Pâté

    1 clove garlic, crushed
    1 dessertspoon curry powder
    cayenne
    2–3 tablespoons mayonnaise
    1 lb (450 g) crab meat
    melted butter

Add the garlic, curry powder and cayenne to the mayonnaise, and mix with the crab meat to a firm consistency. Press down in an earthenware pot or soufflé dish. Pour on melted butter to seal. Serve with toast or fresh bread and salad.

Raspberries and White Currants in Soured Cream

Mix raspberries and topped and tailed white currants together, dredge with caster sugar, and lightly fold in soured cream.

Sylvia Combe

Aunt Sylvia was always entertaining people, if you turned up at her house the table would be laid for tea in the drawing room, for lunch in the dining room, for supper in the kitchen and for breakfast in the summer house – everything would be ready for whatever might happen. I remember her telling a story about the end of one Christmas after her children had left and she had thought it was the end of the celebrations, so she took the remains of the turkey and tied it up in a tree outside for the birds, she was very keen on birds. Later that morning she heard a car coming up the drive and suddenly remembered she'd invited the Haineses to lunch so she rushed outside, took down the turkey, gave it a quick wash and that's what they had to eat, none the wiser!

She wasn't brought up at Holkham but when the blitz started she was living in London and she wrote to her grandfather to ask if it would be possible for her to bring the children up to Norfolk because London was becoming quite dangerous. He wrote back and said he was afraid it just wouldn't be possible because the nursery footman had been called up and so wasn't available. In reality she could have taken the whole of one wing and no one would have known but the lack of a nursery footman rendered the whole thing impossible, that's just how things were then. She married Simon Combe of Watney, Combe and Reid brewers and Simon's sister married Lord Londonderry. Their daughter was Jane van Tempest Stuart who was my age and also one of the other maids of honour at the Coronation.

We were all sent up to Scotland during the war to stay with my aunt who was the Countess of Airlie. Aunt Sylvia, having not been able to stay at Holkham, also came up to Scotland where we were living in lodges on the estate. She was trained up as a VAD nurse because the main house, Cortachy Castle, had been requisitioned as part of the war effort as a rehabilitation centre for Polish soldiers. The soldiers all seemed so glamorous in their uniforms and high boots and on their days off, the VADs changed into pretty cotton dresses and they used to go on picnics together, like the one described by Aunt Sylvia in her piece.

Picnic with the Poles, 1941
Sylvia Combe

In the hot summer of 1941 many Polish soldiers found themselves in Angus, Scotland, after the fall of France. Members of the Tenth Mounted Rifle Regiment, they were very brave and gallant, good company and excellent dancers. They had a great success with the local females, though perhaps were not so popular with the males! There was Bridget's Pole, Sophie's Pole, Peggy's Pole, etc., etc. Communication was carried on in indifferent but voluble French, and a good time was had by all.

Some of the officers used to come for evening picnics held on the edge of Lintrathan Loch, a lovely lake surrounded by pine woods with distant views of the Grampian Hills. Food was scarce in those days of rationing, and quite often the picnic was delayed until the hens had laid enough eggs. Luckily the Poles were well laden with booze, which they drank in incredible mixtures – whisky, gin and sherry all together – but they had very strong heads and were never the worse for wear. After one merry evening by the loch one of the most attractive of the officers, called Richard, plunged in for a refreshing swim. He had not realised that he was swimming in the Dundee water supply reservoir, and was chased by two irate Water Board officials in a boat – and that, sadly, was the last of the Polish picnics by the lake.

Baked Omelette

eggs, beaten
seasoning
chopped herbs
finely chopped onion
finely chopped bacon or chicken

Preheat the oven to gas mark 7 (425°F, 220°C). Mix all the ingredients together. Bake in buttered shallow containers (I use small enamel plates) as many very thin, individual omelettes as required. Fold in half when cold. Freshly potted shrimps or asparagus tips may be added before folding.

Elizabeth Leicester

My sisters Carey, Sarah and I all adored our mother. When we were young she used to plan the most wonderfully exciting things to do in the holidays and would do them all with us, whether it was camping or climbing trees; my school friends all thought she was marvellous. I think perhaps because she was only nineteen years older than me she was a bit like a lovely big sister. When I was seven she went with my father to Egypt where he had been posted with the Scots Guards in the war. I remember her telling me I had to look after Carey when she was gone, which I did in a rather bossy way, poor Carey. But they were away for three years, which is really quite a long time at that age and I remember when they came back we hid behind our beloved governess Billy Williams' skirts because we were shy and only really remembered our parents from photographs. It didn't take long for our mother to win back our affections. I think she had had a pretty wild time in Egypt, she was only twenty-five or -six and very pretty and there were lots of glamorous parties and gymkhanas and picnics in the desert. She wouldn't have had any choice about going. In those days wives just went with their husbands, the children took a back seat. She was resourceful though. She started the pottery at Holkham, inspired by a prisoner of war from the camp set up on the estate who had built his own pottery wheel and kiln. I showed absolutely no aptitude for the artistic side of making the mugs and butter dishes, but I was really keen to sell and was aware of the need to try and make money for the estate. She allowed me to go on sales trips around the coast to all the fancy gift shops, selling Holkham pottery, sometimes staying with friends but often just in the hotels frequented by travelling salesmen. It seems quite a brave thing to do now, but I never had any trouble and in fact the other salesmen were often friendly and helpful to me. She was also very funny and I love the picnic she wrote about: the shooting party dinner which ends with the poor man sitting next to her going home 'as hungry at the end of the meal as he had been at the beginning!'

Holkham Shooting Lunches
Elizabeth Leicester

Holkham shooting lunches in the 1920s were spartan, to say the least. The Lord Leicester of the day was so keen on the sport that eating was considered a great waste of time. I remember in the early 1930s, one Christmas in deep snow, going out to find the trestle table in a wood. On it were a loaf of bread, a rather hollow Stilton and the famous box of small, raw Spanish onions – a Holkham tradition even today. Their strength cannot be exaggerated; there was not a dry eye round the table and a great deal of nose-blowing went on. The eagerly awaited moment produced a small glass of port, which brought some life back into frozen hands and feet.

In later years there were great improvements – lunch indoors with soup, Irish stew and treacle tart kept hot round a blazing fire, with a welcoming drink for each guest.

But the most unusual Holkham dish is velvet. There is a herd of deer in Holkham Park. In the autumn the stags shed a thick skin from their antlers which is collected, fried and served on toast. This delicacy is known as velvet, and was much prized by Lord Leicester who ate it as a savoury. Once at a dinner party we ladies proceeded to the great North Dining-room in full evening dress and wearing long kid gloves, each on the arm of a gentleman in white tie and tails. My partner was very old, nearly blind and deaf. The first course was cockles. Being under-cooked, their shells hadn't opened, so had to be speared with a fork until one gave up with badly bleeding fingers. Suckling pig, then on to the velvet, while a loud and spirited explanation of its origin went on as it congealed on the plate. My neighbour was as hungry at the end of the meal as he had been at the beginning!

Vegetable Pie

(for four approximately)

This superb dish I have never seen in any recipe book or eaten outside our family circle, so, if you get it right, you are in for a treat! We have never used weights and measures for this pie, so I hope the directions below will prove a success the first time.

6 medium-sized potatoes, cooked
2–3 medium onions, sliced and lightly fried
2–3 hard-boiled eggs, sliced

3 tomatoes, sliced
4 cupfuls cooked spaghetti broken into 3-inch lengths
I pint béchamel sauce
salt
pepper
butter

In a deep pie dish arrange a layer of sliced potatoes, sprinkle on some of the fried onion, slices of egg, tomatoes, and spaghetti. Pour a generous quantity of béchamel over and season with salt and pepper. Continue this layering, ending with potatoes. Dot with butter and put in medium oven for 15–20 minutes. Finish off under the grill until potatoes are brown.

It is important to have plenty of sauce. This can have different flavourings. One that is excellent is 1 cup of tomato sauce, ½ teaspoon mixed spice and half a dried chilli stirred into the béchamel.

Anne Glenconner

It was quite difficult for me to write about a picnic as family, Colin and friends had written about Holkham, Glen and Mustique, so I thought I would draw on the memories of a former kitchen maid for the preparation of a picnic shooting lunch. Holkham is now open to the public and I often hear the visitors' comments when they come into the Old Kitchen and see the gleaming brass containers for the picnic. They always wonder what they are for!

Preparations for a Shooting Picnic at Holkham
Anne Glenconner

On Thursday, 21 June 1979, Mrs Taylor, who had been a kitchen maid at Holkham from 1918 to 1920, returned to the house on a visit. Born Gladys Barlow in 1900, during her time as a house-maid she was never allowed in the state rooms, although on one occasion, when the family was away, a housemaid smuggled her along the ground-floor passages to peep into the Marble Hall for a few seconds. This was considered a very daring act which would have been punished if seen by any of the senior staff. Seven full-time footmen worked in the house and, when in their best livery, the powdered footmen wore black suits, yellow and black check waistcoats and white gloves. On occasions additional footmen were sent over on loan from Lord Lothian of Blickling Hall. Other staff included four kitchen maids, two kitchen porters, nine housemaids, two still-room maids and five laundry maids.

A whole carcass of lamb, calf or deer would be cooked for the household, the best cuts for the dining room or shooting picnic, next for the nursery, then senior and junior staff. One man would spend his day preparing vegetables, including a hundred weight (50 kg) of potatoes a day.

In the old kitchen Mrs Taylor pointed out three steamers in the recess to the right of the spit and said they were not used every day for cooking, but only for shooting lunches. The steam would be generated in the boiler below (now an incinerator) and the steamer would be used to cook fish and meat, with the four small containers for vegetables.

Shortly before midday the game cart would arrive at the porter's door and footmen would disconnect the unions of the steamers, which were then carried to the game cart and transported to wherever lunch was being taken. Church Paddock and Scarborough Clump were favourite places.

The rules of the kitchen were such that no unauthorised person was allowed in, and for this reason the serving hatches on either side of the kitchen door were regularly in use – one for hot food and the other for cold. The main door was not used.

Another interesting memory features the boiled egg for the children's breakfast. At about eight o'clock each morning two footmen would arrive in the kitchen with a trolley. On the trolley was a large copper container into which boiling water would be poured. An inner liner was then placed inside and this in turn would receive a number of fresh eggs. More boiling water was poured in until the eggs were completely covered. The whole was then covered with a lid and the trolley pushed from the kitchen to the nursery in the Chapel wing. The timing was such that on arrival the eggs were freshly boiled and ready for the children's breakfast.

I had great difficulty in choosing two recipes from my grand-mother's own recipe book. There were so many good ones. Finally I decided on Holkham Pudding, which I have never had anywhere else, and a delicious venison dish which travels well and has been much appreciated when I have produced it on picnics in Scotland.

Holkham Pudding

    6 oz (175 g) sifted self-raising flour
    8 oz (225 g) shredded suet
    2 eggs
    6 oz (175 g) sultanas
    5 oz (150 g) soft brown sugar
    1 small cup of milk
    a little caster sugar

Mix all the ingredients, except the caster sugar, and beat on the lowest setting of the electric whisk for 2 minutes. Leave for 1 hour. Place in a buttered pudding basin and steam for 2 hours, then turn out on an ovenproof serving dish and sprinkle with caster sugar. Bake in a hot oven for thirty minutes. Serve with hot melted butter and chilled. This pudding tastes good cut into slices and fried in hot butter or eaten cold like a cake.

Venison Chops with Chestnut Purée

6 venison chops
1 teaspoon salt
½ teaspoon pepper
1 tablespoon butter

Purée

1 lb (450 g) chestnuts
½ pint (275 ml) stock
milk to blend until right consistency is reached
1 oz (25 g) butter

Sauce

3 tablespoons redcurrant jelly
juice of 4 oranges

Neatly trim and flatten the chops, season all over with salt and pepper. Thoroughly heat butter in a pan and add the chops. Cook for 6 minutes on each side.

Split the chestnut skins at the pointed ends and put the chestnuts into a saucepan. Cover them with water and bring to the boil. Take them out of the water and skin them. Put them back in the pan with just enough stock to cover and simmer for an hour. Purée them by mashing with hot milk and butter. Place the purée in the middle of a dish and arrange the chops round them.

Remove fat from the first pan, add redcurrant jelly and mix

thoroughly until melted. Pour in orange juice, mix well, and boil for 2 minutes. Pour the sauce over the chops.

When the dish is taken on a picnic, the chestnut purée and sauce should be carried in separate containers.

Carey Basset

Carey like my mother was very artistic, she did art at City & Guilds and helped my mother to design the wonderful patterns for Holkham pottery. She had three sons, sadly one of whom died, but the youngest son, James, lives near me in Norfolk and he and my son Christopher, who are close in age, went to the same prep school and are great friends. Carey adored coming out to Mustique and Colin used to find fantastic costumes for her to wear to his fancy dress parties. We had a very happy holiday together travelling around the islands of the Caribbean. You can tell from her picnic what fun she was. I love the thought of her pretending thunderflies in the mayonnaise was actually an accident with black pepper – that was typical of her sense of humour.

Carey's Cold Collation
Carey Basset

No doubt you will think that this is an appallingly badly planned menu, and you would be right; however, try it for easiness's sake and a saving on the electricity bill. And try to arrange the picnic near somebody else's fruit orchard or garden, so that guests who are sober enough to walk can pick their own pudding.

The day of my trial picnic coincided with a plague of a million tiny thunderflies; however, I pretended I had had an accident with the black pepper while making the mayonnaise, so nobody was any the wiser.

The menu is enough for four people. With the quantities given in the recipe you will get 28 small profiteroles, 4 savoury and 3 sweet for each person. The profiteroles go soft the day after they are made, so crisp them up in a very hot oven for 4 or 5 minutes. They are best eaten fresh. Taking paper plates and cups saves washing up; knives and forks aren't needed, but paper napkins are essential as one's fingers smell awful after peeling prawns.

PS. Don't forget to take water for the dogs.

Picnic Puffs

> 7½ fl. oz (220 ml) water
> 3 oz (75 g) butter
> 3½ oz (85 g) plain flour
> 3 eggs
> baking sheets

Preheat the oven to gas mark 7 (425°F, 220°C). Put the water and butter into a fairly large saucepan. Sift the flour. Bring the pan to the boil and when bubbling draw aside. Allow the bubbles to subside, then pour in all the flour at once. Stir vigorously with a wooden spoon until the mixture comes cleanly away from the sides of the pan – this happens very quickly. Allow to cool for 5 minutes and then transfer the mixture to a Magimix bowl with the double-bladed steel knife already in position. Switch on the machine and add the eggs one by one, processing after each addition until the mixture is smooth. If you don't own a Magimix you will have to beat by hand, but I must admit I've never tried it the hard way. Grease the baking sheet or sheets and hold under the cold tap; shake off surplus water. Place teaspoons of the mixture on the sheets, leaving room for expansion, and bake for about 20 minutes. If you have an Aga, as I do, place the sheets first in the baking oven, and finish in the roasting oven for the same times as given above. When baked, put on a wire rack to cool and pierce the sides with a skewer to let the steam escape, otherwise the profiteroles will be soggy inside.

Some Savoury Fillings

> Scrambled egg with smoked salmon or anchovy pieces
> Prawns or shrimps in mayonnaise
> Lobster or crab in mayonnaise
> Minced beef or other minced meats, and onion
> Diced raw vegetables in mayonnaise
> Cream cheese on lettuce leaves
> Ham, mustard and parsley
> Diced bacon and tomatoes
> Caviar and sour cream

It's best to let people assemble their own fillings and not risk soggy profiteroles. However, the chocolate ones travel well.

Chocolate Puffs

> 4 oz (110 g) bar plain chocolate
> whipped cream

Melt the chocolate with a little water or liquid coffee in a double boiler or a basin placed over hot (not boiling) water. Split the profiteroles and fill with whipped cream. Spoon the chocolate over the tops.

Christopher Tennant

As anyone who has read *Lady in Waiting* will know my son Christopher had a terrible accident when he was nineteen, as a result of which he is disabled. He hasn't been able to work, although he's done quite a bit for the charity Headway. His lovely wife Johanna mentioned that he would like to write about what it's like for a disabled person to try and picnic, which I thought was a really good idea. He also wanted to write about Boopa who was the elephant Colin had on St Lucia, so I'm delighted we can include his picnic in this edition of the book.

A Picnic with Boopa
Christopher Tennant

Picnics have always been a big part of my life and from an early age I have memories of simple picnics by the dark, still waters of the Loch at Glen Estate as well as more opulent picnics on the white sand beaches of Mustique.

They were always fun but none more so that in 1980 when

we went with my father Colin to visit his newly purchased land in St Lucia, the Jalousie Estate. Acres of undeveloped forests and open grassy glades leading down to the crystal clear, turquoise sea.

Mum, Amy, May and I piled into Dad's old Range Rover, which had certainly seen better days, and he drove us up along a rough track by the edge of the sea, over a concrete bridge, then turned the vehicle down a steep hill and headed up an old, almost impassable, rutted, riverbed. The gears crunched, the engine revved but eventually we reached the top where there was the most incredible view looking out over the whole estate. Not a comfortable ride but well worth it!

We drove on a bit further until we reached a flat plateau of green grass where the old, now derelict, Estate House sat proudly – surrounded by old stone walls – facing out to the sea.

Mum, May, Amy and I disembarked and ran down towards the sea for a swim when suddenly, we heard a rustling in the bushes and to our amazement and excitement, a tiny baby elephant poked its head out. 'Meet Boopa,' Colin said. We were lost for words!

We swam whilst Boopa looked on from the shore, then walked back to the old house where our picnic of bread rolls, cheese, salad and fried flying fish had been laid out on the grass by Mr T. Boy and his wife, Mona. Boopa came close to the wall and stuck her trunk over, sniffing around looking for food, much to our amusement and delight. When the Banana Cream was served for pudding, she must have caught a whiff of the bananas as she stretched her trunk out as far as it could possibly reach, in an effort to sample its delights.

It was a truly magical day and one that I will never forget. Dad was a master of surprises!

★

When I met my wife Johanna, she asked me how I had coped following my accident to which I replied, 'There are not many advantages to being disabled, but the few advantages there are, I take full advantage of.'

Picnics these days are not so glamorous but, nevertheless, still great fun and a situation where I can take full advantage! Since my accident it can be challenging, to say the least, to traverse fields or any uneven ground to get to the site of a picnic. Sitting on the grass is impossible because it takes ages to get up again and requires a lot of pulling and pushing from the other guests, so the alternative is to sit in those dreadful canvas folding picnic chairs, which are far too small to fit my frame into and they always sink into the ground or fold up around me! So someone always drives me as close as they can get to where the picnic is being held. I can drink my rum straight from the bottle on the basis it is easier than trying to manage a glass, no one bats an eyelid when I eat with my hands instead of using a knife and fork, and when in need of a quick 'leak' I can just head off towards the nearest bush without anyone raising an eyebrow – though I rarely make it there on time!

Fried Flying Fish

> 8 flying fish fillets
> 1½ teaspoon salt
> juice of 1 large lime
> 1 clove of garlic crushed
> 1 teaspoon chopped chives
> 1 small onion – grated
> ½ teaspoon marjoram
> 1 dash of hot pepper sauce

60 g flour
¼ teaspoon cayenne pepper
salt and a large pinch of black pepper
1 egg, lightly beaten
60 g of breadcrumbs or cornflakes crumbed
butter for frying
2 limes for garnish

Place the fish fillets in a shallow bowl and season with salt and lime juice and set aside for 30 mins.

Drain and pat the fish dry on paper towel. In a small mixing bowl mix garlic, chives, onion, marjoram and hot pepper sauce together and rub the mixture on the fillets.

Mix the flour, cayenne pepper, salt and pepper in a shallow dish. Dip the fillets in the egg and then the flour and bread- or cornflake crumbs.

Heat the butter in a frying pan and cook the fillets for 3 minutes on each side until lightly browned.

Garnish with lime wedges and serve.

Kelvin O'Mard

Kelvin was a close friend of my son Henry. He is an actor who has worked for the Royal Shakespeare Company, the Bristol Old Vic and the Royal Court Theatre, among others. He was in a film called *Water* starring Michael Caine, which was shot in St Lucia in 1984, and not long after that he met Henry. They became really good friends, bonding in the first instance over their love of St Lucia. They were both Buddhists and when Henry was dying of AIDS, Kelvin was right there with him, looking after him together with Henry's then estranged wife Tessa. Henry adored them both. Kelvin became a firm friend of the family; he always comes to our celebrations and is a very special person. I asked him to contribute a picnic in which he could write about his first impressions of Henry and all of us and I think he's written something rather moving.

A Caribbean Picnic on Bequia
Kelvin O'Mard

Friendship has always been a very important aspect of my life, ever since I was a small boy growing up in the East End of London during the 1960s. Whether it was climbing trees to pick apples in a neighbour's garden, playing hopscotch or galavanting on the local Hackney marshes, I was always with that special person, a 'best friend' with whom I felt I shared an important bond. This was most certainly the case when I met the tall and dashing Henry Tennant with whom I shared the most special of friendships. I met Henry during the 1980s, through our mutual love of the Caribbean and a coincidental meeting that to this day I believe was written in the stars.

I had just returned from the island of St Lucia where I had just finished making the 1984 film *Water* that starred the legendary actor Sir Michael Caine. I played the rather accident prone Nado, houseboy to Sir Michael Caine's 'Governor Thwaite'. It is a role I cherish to this day and during my first ever conversation with Henry, I discovered that most of the film was shot on land on the Island of St Lucia just below the Pitons, an area that was owned by Henry's father Lord Glenconner. Henry and I would talk for hours about the Caribbean and although coming from different ends of the social spectrum, we found common ground that rested on a love of the Caribbean islands that sit close to the equator, and are surrounded by turquoise seas and bathed in glorious sunlight. It was not a surprise to learn that Henry's father, Colin Tennant, had bought the island of Mustique in the Grenadines, where history now tells the story of lavish parties and where the rich and famous established holiday homes. Most notably Princess Margaret who was gifted a stretch of land on

Mustique as a wedding present. Henry loved Mustique for its golden beaches and its remoteness and it was a place where he seemed to find himself and where he was most relaxed.

I first visited Mustique in 1986 for Colin's sixtieth birthday party. It was the party of all parties, where the celebrations lasted for four or five days. The Windstar, a sixty-berth yacht with computerised sails, ferried Colin's guests around in the most luxurious comfort. The celebrations included a treasure hunt on the island of Bequia, the largest of the islands that make up the Grenadines archipelago. The treasure hunt took Colin's guests on a wonderful mystery tour of the island, where we had to solve a clue before we could move on to the next point of the adventure. It was during this treasure hunt that Henry and I came across, and fell in love with, the village Paget Farm, which seemed stuck in time and one could describe as almost biblical. The people who live there were very friendly. After Colin's party, Henry and I decided to stay on in the Caribbean and we rented a house in Paget Farm, overlooking the sea and from which we could see Mustique in the distance. We made friends with the local fishermen who were only too happy to take us on excursions in their coloured fishing boats to neighbouring islands, all of which were uninhabited. They took us to Bird Island, which derives its name from the multitude of beautiful birds that have made the island their home, among them the tropical mockingbird, hummingbirds with their blue and green iridescent plumage and the forked-tailed, prehistoric looking frigatebirds. Surrounded by sandy beaches on one side of the island and fierce looking rocks on the other, this was to be the setting for our Caribbean picnic.

Henry and I were ferried to Bird Island in a brightly coloured motor boat, skippered by two local fishermen, Nick and Danis, who had taken it upon themselves to be our tour guides and who also provided the picnic that was concealed in a cold box and would be cooked once we had landed. On the menu was a light fish stew made with fish caught that day and spicy jerk chicken that we roasted over a barbecue.

Once we had landed on the beach, our fishermen friends immediately set about building the barbecue and lighting it, placing a small pot with water at one end. Leaving Henry and myself on the beach to tend to the fire, Nick and Danis went back to the boat, which they took a few metres out to sea and from which they dived into the water. When each appeared they gleefully held up a handful of small fish which were quickly cleaned and added to the now boiling water. A little salt was added, black pepper and pimento seeds. They also added a few small diced potatoes, a carrot and some roughly fashioned dumplings, affectionately known in the Caribbean as 'droppers'. I was keen to see what else our fishermen friends were going to pull out of their cold box. And was pleased to see they had also brought along a few beers.

The jerk chicken had been prepared the night before and was sitting in a plastic Tupperware. The pieces of chicken were placed on the barbecue, hissing and sending a waft of spicy loveliness into the air. Each piece of chicken would be carefully turned so they would be evenly cooked and not burned, and basted with a barbecue sauce which had also magically appeared from the generous cold box.

The fish stew was delicious. It was fresh and light almost like a French bouillabaisse, however with dumplings. It was the perfect starter while we waited for the jerk chicken to be properly cooked. When it was ready, the chicken was served with a simple side salad of lettuce, cucumber and coleslaw and Caribbean hard dough bread. The pieces of chicken we ate with our fingers, ensuring to pluck every morsel of the spicy flesh from the bone.

It was, as we were told by Nick and Danis, the only way to eat jerk chicken. Everything was washed down by the beers we had brought and had kept cool in the shallows.

Henry and I were to have many picnics while living on Bequia, a place where our friendship was to be sealed by such beautiful memories.

Mary Ann Sieghart

One of my closest friends is called Tim Leese. He's a garden designer and now lives with his partner in the old head gardener's house at Holkham, so I see him often. When I was writing *Lady in Waiting* he'd come and cook for me – every evening there was a delicious supper waiting, he was so kind. When his mother was on her deathbed, she told Tim that the person he had always thought was his father was not his father but in fact was Paul Sieghart. So suddenly Tim had a whole new family and Mary Ann is his half-sister, which is how I know her. We had a lovely time together at the Chalk Valley Literary Festival, which has one of the nicest green rooms of anywhere I've been, a wonderful tent all done up with comfy sofas and flowers and buffet food. She's such a brilliant journalist and talented writer that I was very keen she write a piece and I love her Poachers Picnic.

The Poacher's Pocket Picnic
Mary Ann Sieghart

I love going to the theatre, but detest the timing of it. With curtain up at 7.30 p.m., how on earth are we supposed to eat? As we normally have supper at about 8 p.m. or 8.30 p.m., I can't summon an appetite for a pre-theatre dinner at the infants' eating hour of 6 p.m. And with plays getting longer and longer, nor can I wait until we return home at about 10.30 p.m. I'd either faint with hunger during the show or annoy my neighbours with the rumbling of my stomach.

So what's the solution? The Poacher's Pocket Picnic. You assemble a small picnic that – together with an appropriate bottle – fits into the inside poacher's pocket of your husband's coat. He can then walk nonchalantly into the theatre, past the security guards checking bags, with the interval food and drink nicely stashed and undetected.

The Poacher's Pocket Picnic also solves the other theatre problem: the prohibitive cost of food and drink. Who wants to pay upwards of £15 a glass for nasty champagne or £10 a glass for even nastier wine, when you can bring a much nicer entire bottle of your own? Moreover, it saves on queues at the bar. While your fellow audience members are spending half the interval waiting to be served and the other half waiting to pee, you can be happily tucking into your PPP.

The only question is, where to eat it. At the National Theatre, there's no problem. Nobody seems to mind punters bringing in their own Tupperware. If the weather's nice, you can eat and drink on one of the balconies overlooking the Thames.

At less democratic theatres, however, you have to be rather more discreet to evade the food-and-drink police. We usually try to grab a table in the furthest corner of the bar area, pour our own drinks and hide the bottle away. We then hope they won't object to our eating our own sandwiches.

Once, though, we tried something rather more ambitious. We had seats in the gods with a rather poor view of the stage. We had a very good view, though, of an empty box, which seemed to be going to waste. So, in the interval, we found our way to the box and tried the door, which was miraculously unlocked. What a great place to eat our sandwiches and drink our champagne undisturbed!

Once ensconced, we wondered whether we dared watch the second half from these much better seats. No one was a loser, we calculated: the box would otherwise be empty, and it made no difference to the theatre whether we sat there or not. Indeed, the actors would feel less demoralised with fewer empty seats in their view. So we decided to hold our nerve and stay.

We counted down the minutes to the end of the interval, praying that we would remain unnoticed. And then, just before the lights came down, there was a knock at the door. Aghast, my husband quickly hid the champagne bottle as a uniformed member of staff came in. We had been bubbled! We were certain to be reprimanded and marched out of the theatre in disgrace. I held my breath and smiled sweetly at the theatre attendant, who merely smiled sweetly back and asked me to take my glass off the red velvet shelf in front of me, in case it fell on to an audience member below. And that was that! We enjoyed the second half all the more for the illicit satisfaction of having got away with it.

And what are the ingredients of a PPP? A bottle of chilled white Burgundy or fizz, a couple of smoked salmon and cream cheese sandwiches and a bar of seventy per cent dark chocolate. Easy to stash, easy to eat and easy to hide away. Curtains up!

Rupert Everett

I have known Rupert since he was born as I was a great friend of his mother and was one of her bridesmaids when she got married. I have huge admiration for Rupert as an actor and writer. His performance in *The Judas Kiss* as Oscar Wilde I thought was wonderful and his memoirs were both so amusing and brilliantly written. He is also one of the kindest and funniest people I know.

Bird Island Picnic
Rupert Everett

As a child, my second home was my grandparents' house at Burnham Deepdale on the north coast of Norfolk.

I had been born there and the cornerstone of my character – such as it is – was formed in the freezing north-easterly wind that blew in over the marsh. It was my favourite place in the world.

As soon as spring came my grandparents ate their meals outside and in the summer months, depending on the tide and the barometer, we might set off for a picnic to Bird Island, reachable at low tide on foot, leaving the house in a long line, through the gate at the bottom of the poplar wood and up on to the bank that held the marsh and the sea at bay from the fields and woods of Holkham. The view had not changed since Nelson looked at it. The men peeled off towards my grandfather's boat, moored in the creek, laden down with big blue bags filled with sails, rollocks and batons, while the women walked in single file along the bank, my mother, my aunts, my grandmother, my great-grandmother and their best friend, a lady called Audrey Earle, in a huge Mexican hat. They carried the picnic. I danced ahead with my shrimping net or lagged behind picking samphire from the evil smelling marsh.

Once on Bird Island the tide quickly turned and it was cut off from the mainland, which was thrilling for us children. We sat on tartan rugs in the dunes (out of the wind) and ate cold sausages, samphire and hard-boiled eggs. The grown-ups drank wine while we sipped hot Bovril from a thermos. After the meal we had to wait for an hour before going into the ice-cold sea, swimming and shrimping, in snorkels and armbands, followed by more Bovril, as we sat shivering in stripey towels. Then the whole picnic was carefully packed up again and we got into Grandpa's boat and sailed home, tacking through the creeks while he shouted 'Ready about... Leo' and we all ducked as the boom swung.

Graham Norton

One of the lovely things about *Lady in Waiting* was being asked to go on all these television shows, but it really started with Graham. Graham's been wonderful. I met him first when I was on his Radio 2 programme. I've noticed how quite often the presenter hasn't read the book, but Graham obviously had read *Lady in Waiting*, and we got on very well. At the end of the interview I rather boldly mentioned that I'd love to be on his red sofa. Fortunately, Season Three of *The Crown* had just come out and both Helena Bonham Carter and Nancy Carroll, who played me, had come to see me to talk about it. Helena told me she was going to be on *The Graham Norton Show* and very luckily they felt they wanted me on as well. I had to wait until half time to appear and I was frightfully nervous waiting backstage, looking at them all on the television in the Green Room. I was quite anxious about climbing up the ladder to get on to the stage but Graham came to help me, which was nice. Rupert Everett had said to me, 'Graham loves a bit of sexual innuendo. You should just go straight in with your honeymoon story.' So that's what I did pretty much as soon as I sat down, I just launched into it. I think Graham was slightly surprised, but the audience seemed to love it. It was all great fun, and afterwards Chadwick Boseman, who has now sadly died, came up to me and just said, 'Gee whizz, Lady,' which I though was hilarious! The programme helped me to reach a wider audience which was so nice. I've kept in touch with Graham and he has very kindly contributed a 'non' picnic which I love.

A Patch of Blue Sky
Graham Norton

Growing up in Ireland during the sixties and seventies I reacted to British picnics with a mixture of awe and bewilderment. My parents had a caravan on the coast of West Cork and that was where we would spend our summers. Walking along the road to the beach we would occasionally see a car with a UK sticker parked by a grassy patch above the cliffs and we would stare at the tourists eating their meal. Small tables were erected and to the side wicker hampers, like Mary Poppins' handbag, would disgorge plates, cutlery and glassware. The British picnickers, dexterous as magicians, would produce piles of Tupperware boxes more intricate than any Russian dolls. Whole meals would be carefully assembled and washed down with actual wine! These were picnics for Instagram before that particular portal to hell existed. Picture perfect but, in reality, far from ideal. Napkins and loose leaves of lettuce would be carried over the cliffs by the stiff sea breeze, uncomfortable fold-out chairs wobbled precariously on the uneven ground, and the whole meal was consumed while being laid siege by an assortment of seagulls, wasps and pigeons. We shook our heads. If that was how you wanted to eat, surely you should be doing it indoors?

As far as I recall, every summer, we ate all our meals sitting at the flimsy Formica-covered table inside our caravan. We may have opened the windows but that was as al fresco as we got. The most that was consumed outdoors might have been an ice cream or an unripe blackberry found in a hedgerow. What we thought of as picnics were reserved for long drives and had more to do with economy than culinary pleasure. These *picnics* tended to be enjoyed in the car with the doors open. Salad sandwiches with salad cream seeping through the bread would be followed by something sweet, perhaps a slice of fruit loaf and then, if God was good, a packet of Tayto potato crisps. This was usually washed down by some pre-diluted *MiWadi* served in a bottle that bore the label of something we would have much preferred, such as orange lemonade.

If we did venture outside to eat it was always spontaneous. Coats thrown on the ground, a hastily purchased sausage roll, actual fizzy drinks reassuringly made in a factory. Now this might sound dismal, but the beauty of such picnics was that our expectations were low. If it started to rain, or we noticed platoons of ants marching up the sleeve of our makeshift picnic blanket, nothing was lost. We might not have had as nice a time as we had hoped but we could just walk away with no regrets. The tourists by the cliff were struggling to find the right lid for the Tupperware. The table leg wouldn't fold down, their elaborate cream cake was now just sludge on a plate. It seems to me, even now after living in the UK for nearly forty years, that planning a picnic is deciding to be disappointed.

For me, the only recipe anyone needs for a successful picnic is to see a patch of blue in the sky that is, as my father used to say, 'big enough for a pair of sailor's trousers' and then pop into the nearest garage shop and stock up on some items packed with fat and salt. Consume these snacks somewhere you can at least see a tree and count yourself one of the luckiest people alive.

Lorraine Kelly

I was sitting in my dressing room at the TV Studios in London before going on Lorraine's programme to promote *Lady in Waiting*. I was having my hair and make-up done. I love all that, the false eyelashes and everything. Lorraine came in and I liked her straight away. She said she was really looking forward to talking to me and told me roughly what she was going to ask, and it was all a very nice experience. Since then I've been on her show four times. I've only met Lorraine in the studio but she's always been so incredibly nice, and was very kind to write a picnic piece for the book, which is a lovely evocation of her childhood.

A Seaside Picnic
Lorraine Kelly

When I think back to my childhood summer days, they are always illuminated in a sort of golden sunny haze of playing outdoors, and going to the seaside for picnics.

We lived in a tenement in the East End of Glasgow and it was a massive treat to take a weekend day trip to the seaside at Ayr, Troon or Seamill.

My mum would make big fat generous sandwiches out of a 'Vienna loaf', which she'd hollow out and stuff full of chicken, lettuce and mayonnaise (hugely posh and sophisticated back in the sixties) and there would be home-made chocolate cornflake cakes and potato scones lathered in butter.

When we had put up the stripy windbreaker near 'our' rock at the beach, we'd spread the tartan blanket, run into the sea for a paddle and then gorge on the goodies from my mum's old picnic basket.

Everything tasted so much better when eating out in the open, even in a gale with the threat of horizontal rain. The paper plates flew away and the hard-boiled eggs were gritty with sand, but we didn't care.

I had to keep an eye on my little brother Graham who, although he was six years younger than me, ate like a tiny piglet and always managed to snaffle all the 'Blue Riband' biscuits.

There were always other families to play with, either building sandcastles, searching for crabs in the rock pools or playing endless games of football where we made up the rules as we went along.

Our picnic feast was made even more special with pokey hats (ice-cream cones with a chocolate flake and red sweet sauce) and sticks of rock that ruined our teeth.

I'm sure it must have rained and we would have been freezing after being in the cold salty sea, and I bet my brother and I fought like scratchy cats in a basket. My poor mum must have been exhausted getting up early to prepare the food, keeping us amused and then clearing up afterwards, as well as trying to stop us beating each other up, but I remember those picnics with huge affection.

My mum gave us brilliant memories, and a love of eating al fresco that I enjoy to this day when we are off camping in the wilds of Zimbabwe or Botswana, and the sandwiches and cakes still taste better outdoors.

Gyles Brandreth

Gyles is a great admirer of royalty and friend of the Queen's. I first met him when he interviewed me onstage at Alexandra Palace. He turned up in this fabulous jumper which had crowns all over it. It was really quite a long talk with an interval in the middle, but he got the audience involved and we all laughed a lot. Afterwards I said how lovely that there were so many people there and how smart all the ladies looked in their hats, and he said, 'They aren't ladies.' It turned out they were all men in drag who came and chatted afterwards and wanted photographs taken with me. They said they imagined it's how I would have dressed as Lady-in-Waiting and I suppose they were right! One of the other joys of having written my book is that I've got quite a following among the gay community because of Henry and my work with HIV and AIDS charities. I've done several other events since then with Gyles, who very kindly agreed to write a picnic piece and sent a lovely photograph of his grandson with the Queen at the Mad Hatter's Tea Party.

Let Them Eat Cake
Gyles Brandreth

What have I brought to put in Lady Glenconner's picnic hamper? A cake. A royal cake, no less. Oh yes. When it comes to picnics, I like things to be done properly.

The first picnic, I suppose, was the one they had in the Garden of Eden. I can picture them, Adam and Eve, on a tartan rug, a few well-placed vine leaves protecting their modesty, enjoying an al fresco apple.

The first picnic I remember hearing about also featured in the Bible, but in the New Testament. I think the story of Jesus turning five loaves and two fishes into a feast for five thousand is not only the first miracle of his that is recorded, but is also the only one that features in each of the four Gospels. As a little boy in church, I do remember wondering how the miracle was achieved and being hugely impressed by the self-discipline of the five thousand because, famously, after the picnic there were several baskets of leftover food remaining. (In retrospect, I am glad not to have attended that particular picnic: crowds are not my thing. I have always avoided the Glastonbury Festival because of what can best be described as 'comfort break' anxieties.)

The first picnic that really set my imagination going was the one that took place on 4 July 1862. I wasn't there, but I have always wished that I had been. The Fourth of July 1862 was the day on which the Reverend Charles Lutwidge Dodgson, a mathematics don at Christ Church College, Oxford, better known to the world as the writer Lewis Carroll, with his friend, the Reverend Robinson Duckworth, set off on a rowing trip from Oxford to Godstow, with the three daughters of Henry Liddell, the Dean of Christ Church. The children were Lorina (known as Ina), Edith and Alice and it was on this expedition, at the picnic that the five of them enjoyed that afternoon on the river-bank, that Charles Dodgson extemporised the outline of the story that would become one of the most famous children's stories ever written.

Dodgson invented the tale for Alice Liddell and her sisters and, eventually, at Alice's insistence, wrote it down. In November 1864, when he was thirty-two and Alice was twelve, he presented her with a handwritten, illustrated manuscript entitled, *Alice's Adventures Underground.*

In 1863 he took the unfinished manuscript to a publisher who liked it immediately. After alternative titles were rejected – *Alice's Adventures Among the Fairies, Alice's Golden Hour* – the book was published in 1865, with illustrations by John Tenniel as *Alice's Adventures in Wonderland.* The rest is history, and I can claim a tiny part of it because, in the summer of 2023, I was honoured to unveil a small plaque on the Isis riverbank, marking the anniversary of the rowing trip and picnic that proved a landmark in the story of children's literature.

One of the most memorable scenes in the story, of course, is the Mad Hatter's Tea Party which, I reckon, is the best and certainly most fantastic outdoor picnic in all literature. A particular admirer of Alice, and the Mad Hatter, the March Hare and the Dormouse, was Queen Victoria who, according to legend, was so taken with Lewis Carroll's story that she commanded the author to dedicate his next book to her – and was accordingly presented with a scholarly mathematical volume entitled, *An Elementary Treatise on Determinants.*

Queen Victoria gave her name to the Victoria Sponge and, by several accounts, was partial to a slice of cake when out on a picnic herself. In Scotland, on picnics, she was also partial to the occasional cigarette – apparently to keep the midges at bay.

I know that Victoria's great-great-great-grandson Charles III also enjoys a picnic, as does his wife, Queen Camilla. I know this because Queen Camilla supports a number of projects to encourage reading, literacy, and the love of language – among them one that I instigated called Poetry Together, at which we bring older people and young people together for a poetry slam and a bit of a picnic. In fact, I have had the honour of attending a Poetry Together Mad Hatter's Tea Party with Her Majesty – at which my grandson, Rory, played the part of the Mad Hatter and the Queen brought her own cake.

> The old and the young went to tea
> With a beautiful home-made cake.
> It was Camilla's version of Victoria sponge,
> Delicious and easy to bake.
> The old and young learnt a poem by heart
> And performed it with their tea.
> 'Let's get together,' they said,
> 'Whatever the weather.'
> 'Let's get together,' they said,
> 'For poetry, cake and tea!'

That's what Poetry Together is all about – school-age children meeting up with elderly people at school or in care homes, performing a poem together that they have all learnt by heart – and having tea and cake. If you want to find out more about the project, take a look here: www.poetrytogether.com

If you fancy baking your own version of Queen Camilla's cake, Her Majesty has kindly supplied the recipe. Here it is:

Ingredients

     4 oz self-raising flour (110 g), sifted
     1 teaspoon baking powder
     4 oz (110 g) soft margarine or butter at room
       temperature
     4 oz (110 g) caster sugar
     2 large eggs
     2–3 drops of pure vanilla essence

To finish

     Lemon curd or jam (with fresh cream, optional) or
       Nutella or your filling of choice,
    and sifted icing sugar

Pre-heat the oven to gas mark 3 (325°F, 170°C).

Lightly grease two 7-inch (18 cm) sponge tins, no less than 1 inch (2.5 cm) deep and line with greaseproof paper (also greased) or silicone paper.

Take a large roomy mixing bowl and sift flour and baking powder into it, holding the sieve high to give the flour a good airing. Then simply add all the other ingredients to the bowl and whisk them – preferably with an electric hand whisk – till thoroughly combined. If the mixture doesn't drop off a wooden spoon easily when tapped on the side of the bowl, then add 1 or 2 teaspoons of tap-warm water, and whisk again.

Now divide the mixture between the two prepared tins, level off and bake on the centre shelf of the oven for about 30 minutes. When cooked leave them in the tins for only about 30 seconds, then loosen the edges by sliding a palette knife all round and turn them onto a wire cooling rack. Peel off the base papers carefully and, when cool, sandwich the cakes together with lemon curd or jam (or jam and fresh cream) or Nutella or your filling of choice, and dust with icing sugar.

(Queen Camilla loves poetry. And picnics. And chocolate, too. You can make a chocolate version of her cake if you prefer: simply omit the vanilla essence and add 1 tablespoon of cocoa powder to the basic ingredients.)

Cliff Parisi

My daughter-in-law Johanna used to work for Cliff many years ago when they both lived in north London and they have been friends ever since. Cliff played the character Minty Peterson in *Eastenders* for years and I was an avid fan, watching the show regularly. I decided to try and give up *Eastenders* but I do still watch *Call the Midwife* where he has played Fred Buckle, the caretaker, since 2012. When I celebrated my 80th birthday party at Holkham my children said they weren't going to let me drive myself, they were going to organise a driver to fetch me. I got ready and the car arrived – I suppose I wasn't really concentrating on the driver, probably worrying about not creasing my dress, although I did notice he was very smart and wearing a peaked cap. Eventually he said something to me and I looked up and he turned round and it was Cliff dressed up as a chauffeur! I couldn't quite believe it. He came in and joined the party and was absolutely mobbed by all my friends who are huge *Eastenders* fans. It was a fantastic surprise for everybody.

My Gi Tar Pic Nik
Cliff Parisi

I was bought up in north London and have absolutely no recollection of ever being taken on family picnics anywhere, not even to the local park. As a family, it was just not something we did.

I attended the local secondary school in the late seventies at a time when dyslexia was not recognised, so instead of receiving the help you needed, you were regarded as just being troublesome, disruptive and stupid. I was put in a class X where aside from suffering from dyslexia, many of the kids had extreme behavioural problems, so the classes were chaotic and I learned absolutely nothing! We were not allowed out of the classroom unless to go to the kitchen or the workshop as we were not trusted to move around the school on our own. Several years ago whilst clearing out some old boxes, I came across one of my old school reports. In all subjects there were comments from the teachers such as, 'If I knew what Cliff looked like, I might be able to write something'; 'Cliff is rarely present and does nothing when he is'; 'I am unable to report on Cliff's progress as he is rarely in class'!

So, it is no wonder, that by the age of twelve, instead of going into school, I would head to the bus stop outside the locals' favourite pub on Hornsey Rise, hop on the No.14 bus and travel down to Shaftesbury Avenue and London's Tin Pan Alley to the guitar shops.

I would spend all day looking at Fenders and Gibsons and from time to time a big car or van would pull up outside one of the shops and the musicians from a famous band like The Faces or T-Rex would pile out, head into the shop and buy a load of new equipment, often plugging in and jamming in the store. It was so much fun and better than being in school.

On the rare occasions I had any spare money, I would treat myself to a Bakewell Tart from a bakery or coffee shop and to this day, it is still my favourite cake and my idea of a perfect Pic Nik!

William Hanson

I thought it might be fun for someone to write about the 'correct' way to hold a picnic, if there is such a thing. William is an expert on and teacher of etiquette. I've always admired him when I've seen him on television and he's written several books. He sent me a proof of his latest book and on reading it I spotted one or two small mistakes so I told him and he was very grateful. I let him into a rule of thumb that Princess Margaret told me, which was never to use a French word when you can use an English one, it's such a brilliant piece of advice and immediately knocks out words like pardon and serviette. He thought that was rather good!

The Top Drawer Picnic
William Hanson

Long hot days, balmy evenings, dappled sunshine and lush meadows, soft plaid rugs, and leather-strapped wicker baskets: the perfect picnic may be the aspiration of summer outdoor entertaining, but the frisson of eating al fresco can quickly fizzle out if things don't run smoothly. Top-drawer picnic etiquette doesn't just happen; it culminates with copious consideration and plenty of practical planning.

First and foremost, comfort is king. While some rare souls are happy to eat lying down and digest horizontally, most of us left that with the Romans and prefer to sit on something upright. Picnic chairs are, therefore, a must, not only to avoid numb bums and aching limbs, but their built-in drink holders prevent unwanted spillages and nervy glass balancing. A chair also protects you from potentially hazardous surfaces, keeping food clean and eliminating the risk of sand or grass invading your plate. No one wants a sandy sausage or grassy bun.

A small picnic table should also be part of the inventory. There is no need to provide a full dining table but something just big enough to provide a solid surface for the serving dishes. A rug can also be laid down as a makeshift ground sheet, territory marker, and somewhere for those under eighteen to sit.

Call me a snob but plastic plates and cups are the sole reserve of children's birthday parties, and are never used by the enlightened in the way of decent picnic etiquette. (They are also horrid for the environment.) There are standards to be kept, so china plates and proper cutlery are essential hardware and much more eco-friendly. (Paper plates, also horrid, are, however, fine if you really can't be bothered with the washing-up.) Serving dishes should also be china and of smart buffet calibre; even if food is transported in Tupperware, there should be a quick, discreet and fuss-free transfer into something more stylish.

Food for a picnic par excellence is simple yet highly skilled. Present a spread of 1980s-inspired pork-heavy picnic fayre and your guests will be utterly underwhelmed and necking the antacids before bed. Instead, savvy hosts go for moreish, savoury munchettes that require little or no cutting – encouraging people to linger and graze – topped off with a pudding that is a touch indulgent or deliciously seasonal. After all, picnics are a time for slowing down and enjoying little luxuries and (seemingly) effortless deliciousness.

After getting this far, don't let the side down with inferior drinks and glassware. Hosts should bring a well-stocked selection (alcoholic and non-alcoholic) and a plentiful supply. It's surprising how thirsty everyone becomes when eating outdoors. If you are in pursuit of superior standards, then there would be ice to hand and bottles kept cool in wine coolers to save diving into the cool bag every time someone needs a top-up. Whether it's champagne, Chablis, cider or cola, no one wants it presented to them warm in a plastic glass. Leave the best crystal at home, but at the very least, serve drinks in decent glass glasses.

When the picnic is in full swing, hosts can sit back and admire their handy work (all the while keeping an eye on their guests' needs). After all, good etiquette and manners are all about consideration for others and bringing along a general sense of ease. Picnic planning is no different, really – perfect practicalities, fantastic food and delicious drinks, all in the hope that the weather behaves.

Rhubarb Shortbread

Shortbread ingredients
- 125 g butter, soft
- 125 g plain flour
- 25 g cornflour
- 2 level tablespoons of icing sugar

Topping ingredients

    250 g chopped rhubarb

    2 large eggs, beaten

    25 g plain flour

    200 g demerara sugar

    a few drops of vanilla essence

1 x 20 cm square tin, lined with foil and lightly greased

1. Preheat oven to 180°fan (200°C).
2. Mix butter, flours and icing sugar.
3. Press mixture into tin and prick with a fork.
4. Cook for 15–20 minutes.
5. Combine all the topping ingredients.
6. Pour onto base and return to oven for 40 minutes.
7. Allow to cool before removing from tin by foil. Cut into squares.

Picture Acknowledgements

Photographs produced courtesy of:

Pg 1: Top – Anne Glenconner
Bottom L and R – Anne Glenconner

Pg 2 – Top – Anne Glenconner
Middle – Violet Vyner
Bottom – Anne Glenconner

Pg 3 – Top – Anne Glenconner
Middle – Anne Glenconner
Bottom – Alban Donohoe

Pg 4 – Top – Christabel Holland
Middle – Anne Glenconner
Bottom – Mitch Crites

Pg 5 – Top – Rachel Johnson
Middle – Rachel Johnson
Bottom L and R – Anne Glenconner

Pg 6 – Top L – Charles Harding
Top R – Cliff Parisi
Middle – Milton Gendel
Bottom R – Julian Sainsbury

SafeLives

For too many people, home isn't a safe place and the people who are meant to love them, hurt them instead. Whether it's physical or psychological, abuse can happen to anyone, no matter where they live, how old they are, or what sort of lifestyle they have.

Thousands of survivors from all over the country have bravely shared their stories with SafeLives. Their experience tells us everything about the warning signs and the consequences of inaction. And their insight shows what works to keep victims and their families safe.

Together with survivors, SafeLives is transforming the response to domestic abuse and abusive relationships, so that those being harmed are made safer, sooner, and those doing the harming are held accountable.

If this has happened to you, or to a friend or family member, please know that you are not alone. There is help and support for you.

Domestic Abuse Helplines
- England 0808 2000 247
- Wales 080 80 10 800
- Scotland 0800 027 1234
- Northern Ireland 0808 802 1414

If you'd like to support SafeLives, please find more information at https://safelives.org.uk/support-us/

About the Author

Lady Glenconner was born Lady Anne Coke in 1932, the eldest daughter of the 5th Earl of Leicester, and grew up in their ancestral estate at Holkham Hall in Norfolk. A Maid of Honour at the Queen's Coronation, she married Lord Glenconner in 1956. They had 5 children together of whom 3 survive. In 1958 she and her husband began to transform the island of Mustique into a paradise for the rich and famous. They granted a plot of land to Princess Margaret who built her favourite home there. She was appointed Lady in Waiting to Princess Margaret in 1971 and kept this role – accompanying her on many state occasions and foreign tours – until her death in 2002. Lord Glenconner died in 2010, leaving everything in his will to his former employee. Her bestselling memoir *Lady in Waiting* was published in 2019, and she has written bestselling fiction. She now lives in a farmhouse near Kings Lynn in Norfolk.

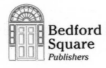

Bedford Square Publishers

Bedford Square Publishers is an independent publisher of fiction and non-fiction, founded in 2022 in the historic streets of Bedford Square London and the sea mist shrouded green of Bedford Square Brighton.

Our goal is to discover irresistible stories and voices that illuminate our world.

We are passionate about connecting our authors to readers across the globe and our independence allows us to do this in original and nimble ways.

The team at Bedford Square Publishers has years of experience and we aim to use that knowledge and creative insight, alongside evolving technology, to reach the right readers for our books. From the ones who read a lot, to the ones who don't consider themselves readers, we aim to find those who will love our books and talk about them as much as we do.

We are hunting for vital new voices from all backgrounds – with books that take the reader to new places and transform perceptions of the world we live in.

Follow us on social media for the latest Bedford Square Publishers news.

🐦 @bedsqpublishers
🅕 facebook.com/bedfordsq.publishers/
🅞 @bedfordsq.publishers

https://bedfordsquarepublishers.co.uk/